Assessment of
AUTISM
SPECTRUM
DISORDERS

Assessment of
AUTISM
SPECTRUM
DISORDERS

Edited by
Sam Goldstein
Jack A. Naglieri
Sally Ozonoff

THE GUILFORD PRESS
New York   London

© 2009 The Guilford Press
A Division of Guilford Publications, Inc.
72 Spring Street, New York, NY 10012
www.guilford.com

Printed in the United States of America

This book is printed on acid-free paper.

Last digit is print number: 9 8 7 6 5 4 3 2

Library of Congress Cataloging-in-Publication Data

Assessment of autism spectrum disorders / edited by Sam Goldstein, Jack A.
Naglieri, and Sally Ozonoff.
    p. ; cm.
  Includes bibliographical references and index.
  ISBN 978-1-59385-983-1 (hardcover : alk. paper)
  1. Autism in children—Diagnosis.   I. Goldstein, Sam, 1952–   II. Naglieri, Jack
A.   III. Ozonoff, Sally.
  [DNLM: 1. Autistic Disorder—diagnosis. 2. Child. WM 203.5 A846 2008]
  RJ506.A9A867 2009
  618.92′85882—dc22
                                                                2008026706

For Janet, Allyson, and Ryan, and for the many families who have placed their trust in me for the evaluation and care of their children

—S. G.

To my children—Andrea (and my son-in-law, Scott), Antonia, and Jack, Jr.— thank you for your love and support

—J. A. N.

To Sally Rogers and Bruce Pennington, who first taught me about assessment

—S. O.

About the Editors

Sam Goldstein, PhD, is Assistant Clinical Professor of Psychiatry at the University of Utah in Salt Lake City and an Affiliate Research Professor of Psychology at George Mason University in Fairfax, Virginia. He is also a clinical neuropsychologist and nationally certified school psychologist. Dr. Goldstein is Editor in Chief of the *Journal of Attention Disorders* and is on the editorial boards of six journals. His publications include 26 texts, numerous book chapters, and peer-reviewed research articles. With Jack A. Naglieri, he is the author of the Autism Spectrum Rating Scales.

Jack A. Naglieri, PhD, is Professor of Psychology at George Mason University and a Senior Research Scientist at the Devereux Foundation's Institute for Clinical Training and Research in Villanova, Pennsylvania. He is a Fellow of Division 16 of the American Psychological Association and recipient of its 2001 Senior Scientist Award. The author of more than 250 publications, Dr. Naglieri's recent research includes specific learning disability eligibility determination, cognitive assessment and interventions, and measurement of psychopathology and resilience. He has published a number of tests, including the Cognitive Assessment System, the Wechsler Nonverbal Scale of Ability, and the Naglieri Nonverbal Ability Tests, and books, including *Essentials of CAS Assessment*, *Essentials of Wechsler Nonverbal Assessment*, and *Helping Children Learn*.

Sally Ozonoff, PhD, is an Endowed Professor and the Vice Chair for Research in the Department of Psychiatry and Behavioral Sciences and the M.I.N.D. Institute at the University of California Davis Medical Center. Her current research focuses on onset patterns in autism, very early identification, and risk factors for autistic regression. She is also a licensed clinical psychologist whose interests are the diagnosis and assessment of autism spectrum disorders, with specializations in infant and adult diagnosis and Asperger syndrome. Dr. Ozonoff has written over 100 peer-reviewed articles and chapters and two other books, *A Parent's Guide to Asperger Syndrome and High-Functioning Autism* and *Autism Spectrum Disorders: A Research Review for Practitioners*. Her work has been showcased on the television news program *60 Minutes* as well as in many local and national newspapers. Dr. Ozonoff serves on the editorial boards of the *Journal of Autism and Developmental Disorders*, the *Journal of Child Psychology and Psychiatry*, and *Autism Research*.

Contributors

Carolyn Thorwarth Bruey, PsyD, Lancaster–Lebanon Intermediate Unit, Lititz, Pennsylvania

Vanessa Carmean, BS, Department of Psychiatry and Behavioral Sciences and M.I.N.D. Institute, University of California Davis Medical Center, Sacramento, California

Kimberly M. Chambers, BA, Department of Psychology, George Mason University, Fairfax, Virginia

Elaine Clark, PhD, Department of Educational Psychology, University of Utah, Salt Lake City, Utah

Anne Cook, PhD, Department of Educational Psychology, University of Utah, Salt Lake City, Utah

Blythe A. Corbett, PhD, Department of Psychiatry and Behavioral Sciences and M.I.N.D. Institute, University of California Davis Medical Center, Sacramento, California

Lesley Deprey, PhD, M.I.N.D. Institute, University of California Davis Medical Center, Sacramento, California

Deborah Fein, PhD, Department of Psychology, University of Connecticut, Storrs, Connecticut

Ifat Gamliel, MA, School of Education, The Hebrew University of Jerusalem, Jerusalem, Israel

Sam Goldstein, PhD, Neurology, Learning and Behavior Center, University of Utah School of Medicine, Salt Lake City, Utah

Jan S. Handleman, EdD, Douglass Developmental Disabilities Center, Rutgers, The State University of New Jersey, New Brunswick, New Jersey

Sandra L. Harris, PhD, Douglass Developmental Disabilities Center, Rutgers, The State University of New Jersey, New Brunswick, New Jersey

Kerry Hogan, PhD, Chapel Hill TEACCH Center, Department of Psychiatry, University of North Carolina School of Medicine, Chapel Hill, North Carolina

Ami Klin, PhD, Department of Child Psychology and Psychiatry, Yale University Child Study Center, New Haven, Connecticut

Laura Grofer Klinger, PhD, Department of Psychology and Autism Spectrum Disorders Research Clinic, University of Alabama, Tuscaloosa, Alabama

Lee M. Marcus, PhD, Chapel Hill TEACCH Center, Department of Psychiatry, University of North Carolina School of Medicine, Chapel Hill, North Carolina

Gary B. Mesibov, PhD, Department of Psychiatry, Carolina Institute on Developmental Disabilities, University of North Carolina at Chapel Hill, Chapel Hill, North Carolina

Joanna L. Mussey, MA, Department of Psychology, University of Alabama, Tuscaloosa, Alabama

Jack A. Naglieri, PhD, Department of Psychology, George Mason University, Fairfax, Virginia

Sarah E. O'Kelley, PhD, Autism Spectrum Disorders Research Clinic, University of Alabama, Tuscaloosa, Alabama

Sally Ozonoff, PhD, Department of Psychiatry and Behavioral Sciences and M.I.N.D. Institute, University of California Davis Medical Center, Sacramento, California

Mark J. Palmieri, PsyD, Center for Children with Special Needs, Glastonbury, Connecticut

Rhea Paul, PhD, CCC-SLP, Department of Communication Disorders, Southern Connecticut State University, New Haven, Connecticut

David Potter, MSc, The Multiple Sclerosis Society, London, United Kingdom

Victoria Shea, PhD, Department of Psychiatry, Carolina Institute on Developmental Disabilities, University of North Carolina at Chapel Hill, Chapel Hill, North Carolina

Kaitlyn P. Wilson, MS, CCC-SLP, Kennedy Krieger Institute, Kennedy Krieger High School Career and Technology Center, Baltimore, Maryland

Lorna Wing, MD, Centre for Social and Communication Disorders, Elliott House, Kent, United Kingdom

Nurit Yirmiya, PhD, Department of Psychology and School of Education, The Hebrew University of Jerusalem, Jerusalem, Israel

Preface

The prominent psychiatrist Thomas Szasz argued that mental illness is not the name of a biological condition, but rather a concept created by humankind out of a fear and rejection of diversity. Szasz asserted, as many others still do, that biological determinism clouds an appreciation of the powerful forces the environment exerts on human development, thought, and behavior. Yet autism, more than any other form of mental illness, offers an opportunity to appreciate the fallacy of Szasz's position.

As a developmental disorder beginning in early childhood and continuing throughout the lifespan, autism has been and remains a complex, often difficult concept for professionals and the public alike to appreciate. Autism was once thought to reflect the adverse outcome of cold and unaccepting parenting. Yet, as we do for so many other conditions today, we now recognize the strong biological and genetic predisposition toward autism, and acknowledge the combined biopsychosocial forces that ultimately contribute to its individual course and life outcome.

From the time of its initial descriptions—Jean Itard's reports of the wild boy of Aveyron's failure to use language or other forms of communication (Lane, 1977), Henry Maudsley's description in 1867, and Leo Kanner's first full scientific description in 1943—autism has fascinated researchers, mental health professionals, and the general public. Although even today autism occurs at a far lower incidence than the common childhood conditions of attention-deficit/hyperactivity disorder, learning disability, depression, or anxiety, the atypical nature of autistic individuals' behavior, mannerisms, habits, cognitive development, and socialization continues to challenge many of the basic theoretical models of child development and human behavior that guide our educational system and methods of raising children. Theories have come and gone, and still autism is enigmatic and perplexing; its patterns of behavior, rates of development, and at times significant improvement or worsening remain difficult to understand and explain.

As Kanner and Eisenberg (1956) eventually pointed out, autism is a reflection of an inborn dysfunction underlying affective engagement, and is now accepted as a lifelong condition. It is no longer a matter of helping autistic children through a particular developmental period, but rather directing and engineering their transition through life to prepare them to function as adults with autism.

This book arose from our interest in providing a reasoned and reasonable approach to the evaluation of autism and the spectrum of disorders associated with it. Indeed, we believe that this is the first book devoted to the evaluation of autism spectrum disorders (ASD); as such, we have attempted to set an important standard for researchers, clinicians, and caregivers. This book reflects the recent dramatic growth in the field, and it provides a strong foundation for a consistent process of assessment and a thoughtful application of diagnostic criteria. Such a process ensures proper diagnosis and, most important, avoids stigmatizing and pathologizing the typical variations in children's behavior.

One of our key goals has been to build a bridge from the available science to clinical practice. It is our intent to emphasize valid and reliable methods of assessing this complex, often perplexing group of disorders. We have also sought to cover the myriad comorbid conditions and problems that are present in many individuals with ASD. A broad assessment of such conditions is critical, given the incidence of comorbidity between ASD and many other behavioral, emotional, and developmental disorders.

The framework for this volume reflects Cohen and Volkmar's observation in 1997 that there are "enormous differences among individuals with autism in their abilities and needs; among families, in their strengths and resources; and among communities and nations, in their own viewpoints and histories" (p. xvii). We have sought to bring together many of the best-known thinkers, scientists, and clinicians from throughout the world in the field of ASD. The text begins with an overview and historical perspective, laying an important foundation and providing readers with an appreciation that autism and its kindred disorders primarily reflect social impairment. We are very pleased that autism pioneer Lorna Wing and her colleague David Potter have adapted and expanded a previous work providing a thorough review of the epidemiology of ASD; in particular, they address the issue of prevalence relative to changes in diagnostic procedures and cultural milieus.

The book continues by asking an important foundational question: Can a set of complex developmental disorders such as ASD be reliably and validly measured? We believe that we answer this question affirmatively.

The volume then proceeds with chapters providing discussions of subtypes (Ami Klin); age-related issues (Victoria Shea and Gary B. Mesibov); social behavior (Ifat Gamliel and Nurit Yirmiya); communication (Rhea Paul and Kaitlyn P. Wilson); intellectual (Laura Grofer Klinger, Sarah E. O'Kelley, and Joanna L. Mussey) and neuropsychological (Blythe A. Corbett, Vanessa Carmean, and Deborah Fein) functioning; comorbid psychiatric conditions (Lesley Deprey and Sally Ozonoff); and education (Sandra L. Harris, Carolyn Thorwarth Bruey, Mark J. Palmieri, and Jan S. Handleman). Kerry Hogan and Lee M. Marcus provide a comprehensive model for effectively utilizing assessment data to design and implement treatment. The book closes with a review of best practices and challenging issues in the assessment of ASD.

Our primary aim in preparing this volume has been to serve the needs of graduate students new to the field, as well as experienced clinicians across multiple disciplines. However, we believe that this book is also user-friendly for parents and other allied professionals interested in learning about the valid and reliable assessment of ASD. Moreover, we and our colleagues have striven to provide a scholarly addition to the field. In short, it is our hope that this volume will be widely used by all those involved in evaluating and treating ASD.

SAM GOLDSTEIN, PhD
JACK A. NAGLIERI, PhD
SALLY OZONOFF, PhD

REFERENCES

Cohen, D. J., & Volkmar, F. R. (Eds.). (1997). *Handbook of autism and pervasive developmental disorders* (2nd ed.) New York: Wiley.

Kanner, L. (1943). Autistic disturbances of affective contact. *Nervous Child, 2,* 217–250.

Kanner, L., & Eisenberg, L. (1956). Early infantile autism, 1943–1955. *American Journal of Orthopsychiatry, 26,* 55–65.

Lane, H. (1977). *The wild boy of Aveyron*. London: Allen & Unwin.

Maudsley, H. (1867). Insanity of early life. In H. Maudsley (Ed.), *The physiology and pathology of the mind* (pp. 259–386). New York: Appleton.

Contents

Contents

To the soul, there is hardly anything more healing than friendship.

—THOMAS MOORE (1779–1852)

The important thing in science is not so much to obtain new facts as to discover new ways of thinking about them.

—SIR WILLIAM BRAGG (1862–1942)

The greatest obstacle to discovery is not ignorance—it is the illusion of knowledge.

—DANIEL J. BOORSTIN (1914–)

CHAPTER ONE

Historical Perspective and Overview

Sam Goldstein
Sally Ozonoff

The assessment of disorders characterized by patterns of atypical behaviors and development, such as autism spectrum disorders (ASD), is (to say the least) complex. Though the definition and description of ASD are far less controversial than those of other childhood conditions (e.g., attention-deficit/hyperactivity disorder [ADHD]), they still involve their share of contradiction, uncertainty, and disagreement. As this book goes to press, it is still the case that the incidence of "autistic behaviors" in the general population is not fully understood; nor has the positive and negative predictive power of specific behaviors related to ASD been fully investigated. The text revision of the fourth edition of the *Diagnostic and Statistical Manual of Mental Disorders* (DSM-IV-TR; American Psychiatric Association, 2000) provides a carefully crafted description of the symptom profile, related criteria, and impairment necessary to cross diagnostic thresholds, but the application of these criteria through observation, checklists, and standardized tests presents numerous challenges. It is still the case that ASD lack a unifying theory. Are they social, learning, behavioral, developmental, or cognitive problems, or some combination of these? Despite the significant increase in research articles about ASD, and the rapid and significant advances made, the efficient assessment of these conditions and their related problems continues to present challenges—as, most importantly, does effective intervention.

The growth of a particular topic such as ASD is in part marked by the comprehensive, scientific, and clinical volumes published about it. Indeed, the field of ASD has grown to such an extent that texts related to specific issues (e.g., assessment) are now appearing. As the recognition and prevalence of these conditions increase, the risks of over- and underdiagnosis increase in parallel. The need for carefully crafted guides for assessment becomes paramount. As noted in the Preface, we have created this volume primarily to serve as a desk reference and guide for clinicians. This first chapter begins with a historical discussion of autism and other ASD. Then a short descriptive overview and the diagnostic criteria for ASD are presented, and the nature of comprehensive assessment is briefly discussed. The chapter concludes with three case studies exemplifying the complexities of assessment.

BRIEF HISTORY

Though the famous wild boy of Aveyron was thought to be a feral child living in the woods and purportedly raised by wolves in south central France at the end of the 18th century, it is more likely that he suffered from autism. The boy named Victor by the physician Jean Itard reportedly demonstrated classic signs of autism, particularly related to failure to use language or other forms of communication (Lane, 1977). In 1867, Henry Maudsley, in a text devoted to the physiology and pathology of the mind, described insanity in children. Some of his descriptions appeared consistent with today's symptoms of ASD. The qualities of stubborn, rigid, odd, and self-centered behavior have also been reported in historical figures throughout time. Interestingly, Frith (1989) hypothesized that a number of fictional characters, including Sherlock Holmes, may well have been given personalities consistent with autism.

The German word *autismus* was coined by the Swiss psychiatrist Eugen Bleuler (1911/1950). The word is derived from the Greek *autos* (self) and *ismos* (a suffix of action or of state). Bleuler, best remembered for his work in schizophrenia, first used this term to describe idiosyncratic, self-centered thinking that led to withdrawal into a private fantasy world. In 1943, Leo Kanner, in an article published in the journal *Nervous Child,* introduced the modern concept of "autism." Kanner borrowed the term from the field of schizophrenia as described by Bleuler. Kanner suggested that children with autism also live in their own world, cut off from normal social intercourse. Yet he also hypothesized that autism is distinct from schizophrenia, representing a failure of development, not a regression. Kanner also observed in the clinical histories of these children additional features reflecting problems with symbolization, abstraction, and understanding meaning. All had profound disturbances in communication.

In the 1943 article, Kanner described 11 children with "autistic distur-bances of affective contact." He suggested that they had been born lacking the usual motivation for social interaction. Kanner described these distur-bances as reflecting the absence in these children of the biological precondi-tions for psychologically metabolizing the social world and making it part of themselves. The condition was noted to lead to severe problems in social interaction and communication, as well as a need for sameness. Children with autism were described as rigid, inflexible, and reacting negatively to any change in their environment or routine.

Kanner considered autism a genetically driven condition. He also observed that the parents of some of his patients were successful in aca-demic and vocational realms. Kanner suggested that autism, though a con-genital condition, could be influenced by parenting. This led to the belief (which persisted for some time) that autism was caused by inappropriate parenting. In particular, those who espoused the psychoanalytic theory of the time came to believe that parents, particularly their child-rearing meth-ods, were the causes of autism. That the interactional problems of autism arise from the child, however, not the parents, has been well demonstrated in the research literature (Mundy, Sigman, Ungerer, & Sherman, 1986). The data today support the concept that biological and genetic factors con-vey the vulnerability to autism. Autism is also a condition that is typically observed across many generations and families. In 1956, Kanner and Eisen-berg further elaborated on this theory, providing case observations col-lected between 1943 and 1955. During this period, it appears that Kanner's concept of the condition changed only minimally.

Kanner also suggested that many children with autism are not men-tally retarded, but unmotivated to perform. A body of research now dem-onstrates that when developmentally appropriate tests are given, intel-ligence and developmental scores are in the range of mental retardation for the majority of individuals with autism (Rutter, Bailey, Bolton, & Le Couteur, 1994). Yet as the concept of autism as reflecting primarily a social learning problem has become more widely accepted, the percentage of indi-viduals on the autism spectrum who have normal intellectual abilities has increased. Though intellectual deficits were traditionally considered a key aspect of autism, current conceptualization has evolved to appreciate and recognize the differences between general intelligence on the one hand and the social learning problems characteristic of autism and other ASD on the other. These concepts are further discussed by Klinger, O'Kelley, and Mussey in Chapter 8.

The year after the publication of Kanner's original paper, Hans Asperger, a physician working in Vienna, proposed another autistic condi-tion. Although Asperger was evidently unaware of Kanner's paper or its use of the word "autism," he used a similar term in his description of the social problems these children demonstrated. In 1944, Asperger described a syndrome he referred to as "autistic psychopathy." This condition is now referred to as Asperger's disorder in DSM-IV-TR (it is also known as Asperger syndrome). His paper, published in German, was unavailable to English-speaking scientists until an account of his work was authored by Wing in 1981 and the paper was translated by Frith into English in 1991 (Asperger, 1944/1991; see also Frith, 1991).

Rutter et al. (1994) reported on Theodore Heller, a special educator in Vienna, who described an unusual condition in which children appeared normal for a number of years and then suffered a profound regression in functioning and development. This condition was originally known as "dementia infantilis" or "disintegrative psychosis." It is currently referred to as childhood disintegrative disorder in DSM-IV-TR. Another Austrian, Andreas Rett (1966), first observed females with an unusual developmental disorder characterized by a short period of normal development and a multifaceted form of intellectual and motor deterioration, with many symptoms similar to autism. In the DSM-IV-TR, this is now referred to as Rett's disorder (it is also known as Rett syndrome). Autism is also associated with many other genetic and medical conditions, occurring at a higher than expected rate in such disorders as fragile X syndrome, tuberous sclerosis, Williams syndrome, and neurofibromatosis (Gillberg, 1990).

Until the 1970s, autism was considered a form of schizophrenia. In the first and second editions of the DSM (American Psychiatric Association, 1952, 1968), only the term "childhood schizophrenia" was available to describe children with autism. It has become abundantly clear with further research that although young children with autism suffer in many other areas of their development, their behavior is very different from that seen in the psychotic disorders of later childhood or teenage years (Kolvin, 1971; for a review, see Cohen & Volkmar, 1997). The work of Cantwell, Baker, and Rutter (1980) and DeMyer, Hingtgen, and Jackson (1981) was influential in establishing the distinction between autism and schizophrenia. There is now a general consensus on the validity of autism as a separate diagnostic category, and on the majority of features central to its definition. This consensus has been contributed to by the convergence of the two major diagnostic systems that include psychiatric and developmental disorders, the DSM and the World Health Organization's *International Classification of Diseases* (ICD). Though there continue to be some differences between these two sets of diagnostic criteria, they have become more alike than different with each revision (Volkmar, 1998). In fact, autism probably has an excellent empirical basis for cross-cultural diagnostic criteria.

In this book, we focus on autism and related disorders as defined by DSM-IV-TR. Autism was first included in the DSM in its third edition (American Psychiatric Association, 1980), where it was called "infantile autism." The criteria were limited in their descriptions; specific symptoms were not outlined; and all criteria needed to be met for the diagnosis to be made (Volkmar, 1998). Major changes occurred in the revision of DSM-III, as Factor, Freeman, and Kardash (1989) noted. DSM-III-R (American Psychiatric Association, 1987) included detailed, concrete descriptions of specific behaviors and guidelines for number and patterns of symptoms that needed to be present, increasing the reliability of diagnosis. The life-long nature of the disorder was also acknowledged, in the change in name from "infantile autism" to "autistic disorder." Deficits were defined in relation to a child's mental age, and subjective words and phrases ("bizarre," "gross deficits") that may have limited applicability to an older or higher-functioning individual were removed. Both verbal and nonverbal communication difficulties, including social use of language, were highlighted, rather than simply structural language deficits. The changes were much smaller from the DSM-III-R to the DSM-IV (American Psychiatric Association, 1994), but a major one was the inclusion for the first time of Asperger's disorder. It is likely that this current diagnostic protocol (which has been retained in DSM-IV-TR) will remain active for at least another few years. However, the diagnostic criteria may change significantly if DSM-V moves toward a more dimensional versus categorical model of defining conditions such as the ASD.

DESCRIPTIVE OVERVIEW

Because of the unusual combination of behavioral weaknesses and a lack of biological models for this disorder, autism is a most perplexing condition (Schopler & Mesibov, 1987). It is best conceptualized as a biologically determined set of behaviors that occurs with varying presentation and severity, probably as the result of varying causes. Autism occurs significantly more often in boys (Smalley, Asarnow, & Spence, 1988) and presents across all socioeconomic levels (Gillberg & Schaumann, 1982). It is estimated that one out of four children with autism experiences physical problems, including epilepsy (Rutter, 1970). Up to 75% are generally found to experience intellectual deficiencies, although this proportion appears to be dropping in recent years. Lotter (1974) first suggested that level of intellectual functioning and amount of useful language by 5 years of age were the best predictors of outcome, and these findings have been consistently supported by later research (Gillberg & Steffenburg, 1987; Howlin, Goode, Hutton, & Rutter, 2004; Venter, Lord, & Schopler, 1992).

Autism as commonly defined (Kanner's autism, DSM-IV-TR autistic disorder, etc.) is actually one point on a spectrum of disorders, along which individuals can present problems ranging from those that cause almost total impairment to others that allow some but not optimal function. Children on the autism spectrum experience a wide variety of developmental difficulties, involving communication, socialization, thinking, cognitive skills, interests, activities, and motor skills. Although critics suggest that the DSM-IV-TR grouping of pervasive developmental disorders (PDD), which includes the ASD as discussed in this book, is poorly defined and inconsistent because it does not refer to all "pervasive developmental disorders" (e.g., mental retardation) and because some children experience only specific or partial impairments (Gillberg, 1990), the category of PDD and the term ASD both seem to define well the breadth of difficulties experienced by most of these children.

Rutter (1983) found that the pattern of cognitive disabilities in autistic children is distinctive, and different from that found in children with general intellectual disabilities. Language and language-related skills involving problems with semantics and pragmatics are present (Rutter, 1983). Other difficulties frequently include perceptual disorders (Ornitz & Ritvo, 1968), cognitive problems (Rutter, 1983), specific types of memory weaknesses (Boucher and Lewis, 1992), and impairment in social relations (Fein, Pennington, Markowitz, Braverman, & Waterhouse, 1986; Fein), many of which are described in detail in later chapters of this volume. Consistent with Kanner's description of autism, social impairments have been found to be the strongest predictors of receiving a diagnosis (Siegel, Vukicevic, Elliott, & Kraemer, 1989). Dimensionally measured variables such as those related to interpersonal relationships, play skills, coping, and communication are consistently impaired areas for youth with autism and other PDD. Hobson (1989) found that higher-functioning autistic children are unable to make social or emotional discriminations or read social or emotional cues well. These deficits appear to have an impact on social relations and are likely to stem from cognitive weaknesses. The inability to read social and emotional cues or to understand others' points of view leads to marked interpersonal difficulties (Baron-Cohen, 1989; MacDonald et al., 1989). Since Rutter's (1978) first description of social impairments without cognitive deficits in some higher-functioning youth with autism, diagnostic criteria for these conditions have expanded to include deficits in nonverbal behavior, peer relations, lack of shared enjoyment and pleasure, and problems with social and emotional reciprocity (American Psychiatric Association, 1994, 2000; World Health Organization, 1993). Relative to their cognitive abilities, children with these forms of ASD exhibit much lower than expected social skills, even compared to a group with mental retardation (Volkmar et al., 1987). Delays in social skills are even stronger predictors of receiving a diagnosis of autism or another PDD than are delays in communication (Volkmar, Carter, Sparrow, & Cicchetti, 1993). Clearly, impairments in social skills among those receiving diagnoses of any PDD are greater than expected relative to overall development (Loveland & Kelley, 1991).

CURRENT DIAGNOSTIC CRITERIA

The DSM-IV-TR (American Psychiatric Association, 2000) criteria for the PDD are discussed in this section. The three criteria for autistic disorder include three sets of behavioral descriptions. To qualify for the diagnosis, a child first must present at least six symptoms, with at least two from the first set of criteria and at least one from each of the second and third sets. The first set of criteria features qualitative impairment in social interaction, as manifested by (1) impairment of nonverbal behaviors, including eye contact, facial expression, body postures, and gestures of social interaction; (2) failure to develop peer relationships appropriate to the child's developmental level; (3) markedly impaired sharing of emotional states or interests with others; and/or (4) absence of social or emotional reciprocity. The second set of criteria refers to qualitative impairment in communication, as manifested by (1) a delay or complete absence of the development of spoken language, without efforts to compensate through gestures; (2) obvious impairment in the ability to initiate or sustain conversation, despite adequate speech; (3) repetitive or stereotyped use of language, or idiosyncratic language; and/or (4) lack of varied, spontaneous make-believe play or social imitative play appropriate for the child's developmental level. The third set of criteria involves repetitive and stereotypic patterns of behavior, interests, or activities, including (1) preoccupation with a certain pattern of behavior that is abnormal in focus or intensity; compulsive adherence to specific nonfunctional routines or rituals; repetitive motor mannerisms (self-stimulatory behavior); and/or persistent preoccupation with parts of objects. Once the presence of at least six symptoms from these three criteria sets has been established, a further set of criteria includes delay prior to the age of 3 in at least one of these: social interaction, language as used in social communication, and/or symbolic or imaginative play. Finally, the child's clinical description should not be better accounted for by Rett's disorder or childhood disintegrative disorder.

The DSM-IV-TR criteria describe Rett's disorder as being manifested in a child who has exhibited normal development for at least the first 5 months of life, including normal prenatal and perinatal development, apparently normal psychomotor development through the first 5 months, and normal head circumference at birth. Between 5 and 48 months, there is deceleration of head growth; loss of earlier-acquired purposeful hand movements, with the development of stereotypic hand movements (e.g., hand wringing); loss of social engagement; acquisition of poorly coordinated gait or trunk movements; and marked delay as well as impairment of expressive and receptive language, with severe psychomotor retardation.

Childhood disintegrative disorder in DSM-IV-TR is defined as involving normal development for at least the first 2 years of life, and then loss of skills in at least two of these areas: receptive or expressive language; adaptive behavior or social skills; bowel or bladder control; play; and/or motor skills. In addition, the child begins to manifest at least two of the following types of abnormal functioning: qualitative impairments in social interaction (impaired use of nonverbal behaviors, failure to develop peer relationships, absence of social or emotional reciprocity); qualitative impairments in communication (delay or total absence of spoken language, inability to sustain and initiate conversation, stereotyped or repetitive use of language, absence of varied make-believe play); and/or restrictive, repetitive, and stereotypic patterns of behavior, interests, and activities. The child's behavior should not be accounted for by another specific PDD or by schizophrenia. Thus childhood disintegrative disorder is a PDD that occurs after a longer and clearer period of normal development. Autistic disorder can also involve a regression in behavior, but it usually occurs before a child's second birthday (Kurita, Osada, & Miyake, 2004).

DSM-IV defined the criteria for a new diagnosis, Asperger's disorder, which has remained unchanged in DSM-IV-TR. Included in the diagnostic criteria are qualitative impairment in social interaction, including at least two of these symptoms: (1) obvious impairment in the use of many nonverbal behaviors, such as body posture; (2) failure to develop appropriate peer relations; (3) a lack of spontaneous seeking to share enjoyment, interests, or achievements; and/or (4) absence of social or emotional reciprocity. A second set of criteria involves restricted, repetitive, and stereotyped behaviors, interests or activities, including at least one of the following symptoms: (1) at least one restricted or stereotyped pattern of interest that is abnormal in focus or intensity; (2) inflexible adherence to specific rituals or routines; (3) repetitive motor mannerisms; and/or (4) persistent preoccupation with parts of objects. Altogether, the child's disturbance must cause clinically significant impairment in social, academic and other areas of functioning. Furthermore, for this diagnosis to be made, the child should not exhibit a significant delay in early language development, in cognitive development, or in the development of age-appropriate self-help skills and adaptive behavior. Most critically, DSM-IV-TR states that children diagnosed with Asperger's disorder cannot also meet criteria for autistic disorder. This requirement was added to make the diagnoses mutually exclusive and thus more reliable, but it has been controversial (Mayes, Calhoun, & Crites, 2001; Miller & Ozonoff, 1997), and other systems may be entertained for future DSM editions (Klin, Pauls, Schultz, & Volkmar, 2005). Other unresolved controversies regarding Asperger's disorder (Frith, 2004), such as its relation to high-functioning autism, are discussed by Klin in Chapter 4.

As with all DSM categories, a Not Otherwise Specified condition is included for the PDDs. The category Pervasive Developmental Disorder—Not Otherwise Specified (PDD-NOS; including Atypical Autism) is very briefly described in the DSM-IV-TR but does not include specific diagnostic criteria. This category is used when there is a severe and pervasive impairment in the development of reciprocal social interaction associated with impairment in either verbal or nonverbal communication skills or with the presence of stereotyped behavior, interests, and activities. However, the criteria must not be met for a specific PDD or a number of other psychiatric conditions. This category includes Atypical Autism. Such presentations may also not meet the criteria for Autistic Disorder because of late age of onset, atypical symptomatology, subthreshold symptom count, or a combination of these.

THE NATURE OF COMPREHENSIVE ASSESSMENT

As Cohen (1976) noted, the clinical provision of a diagnosis is but part of the overall diagnostic process. That is, comprehensive assessment is more than the simple application of a set of diagnostic criteria to a particular individual. It must provide an overview of the individual's history—relevant information about development (especially change over time), life course, and socialization—and, equally important, an overview of the environment in which the individual lives and functions. In short, as Cohen noted, the diagnostic process should provide a thorough overview of the individual person's assets, liabilities, and needs. A thorough history is likely to be the best assessment tool. In most clinical assessments, history is often supported by checklists and standardized instruments. It is the rule rather than the exception that most evaluations for ASD also screen broadly for comorbid developmental, emotional and behavioral problems. A comprehensive assessment for ASD thus typically evaluates a child's total functioning—intellectual, neuropsychological, communicative, behavioral, and emotional. These issues are all covered in later chapters.

CASE STUDIES

The complexities and challenges of assessing ASD are reflected in the following three brief case studies. The issues raised in these studies, as well as many others, are further addressed and elaborated throughout this volume. The majority of assessments for autism are conducted with children; these three cases reflect issues at three different age levels (4, 9, and 13 years). These three cases are taken from our clinical practice. All three youth were referred because of questions about the presence of autism.

Joey

Four-year-old Joey came from a normally functioning family without any history of ASD or other developmental delays. At 4, Joey demonstrated a number of idiosyncratic behaviors and stereotypic movements. He met many early developmental milestones within normal limits, but language was late in developing, and Joey was also fearful of sitting on the toilet. Joey would point to make his needs known, but would not point on direction. He played in parallel with other children, but preferred to play alone— often in repetitive activities, lining up toys, and becoming distressed if even a single object was moved.

The parents' responses to the Conners' Rating Scales—Revised (Conners, 1997) and the Child Behavior Checklist (Achenbach & Edelbrock, 1991)—well-known standardized childhood questionnaires—noted mild attention and thought problems, but no significant symptoms of disruptive behavior. Checklists of autistic symptoms, including the Autism Behavior Checklist (Krug, Arick, & Almond, 1980) and a research version of the Scales of Autistic Behavior (Goldstein & Naglieri, 2007), noted Joey's problems with conversational skills, avoidance of eye contact, inability to understand basic social behavior, and obsessive patterns. Nonetheless, Joey was able to smile appropriately and listen when spoken to, and he did not resist social interaction.

During a general developmental screening, Joey's overall development was deemed to be 1½ years below his chronological age. He could not complete even simple language measures, with estimated language skills at a 2- to 2½-year-old level. On Module 2 of the Autism Diagnostic Observation Schedule (ADOS; Lord, Rutter, DiLavore, & Risi, 1999), Joey's speech was noted to have a rather atypical pattern of pitch, tone, and rhythm. Joey also struggled to maintain conversation and did not point consistently, but was capable of some shared enjoyment. His performance yielded a score of 8 for Language/Communication, a score of 9 for Reciprocal Social Interactions, and a total score of 17, well above the cutoff of 12 indicative of autism.

A diagnosis of autistic disorder was provided, though it was noted that Joey possessed somewhat better-developed social engagement skills than other newly diagnosed 4-year-olds with autism. It appeared that Joey also demonstrated other developmental impairments (particularly significant language delays) that were further compounding his acquisition of developmental milestones and probably also contributing to his patterns of autistic behaviors.

John

Nine-year-old John was initially referred because of his problems with self-control and self-regulation. His parents wondered whether he might be autistic because he seemed uninterested in interacting with peers. There was no extended family history of ASD, but learning disabilities and emotional problems were present. John had been a difficult infant, irritable, and hard to comfort. He spoke his first words by 9 months of age, but then stopped speaking. After pressure equalization tubes were placed in his ears when he was 1½ years old, his language began to develop again. Toilet training was completed by 3½ years of age, although periodic daytime wetting was noted through 9 years of age. He was diagnosed at 6 years of age with ADHD, but responded adversely to stimulant medication. John was not doing well academically and did not appear particularly interested in the academic or social expectations of school. His parents noted that John "seems to not look at people as he is talking to them, and looks away talking quietly so you don't understand what he is saying."

Parent and teacher behavioral checklists noted John's problems with cognitive skills, inattention, restlessness, and social problems. He was not described as aggressive or disruptive. According to John's parents, he talked excessively about favorite topics that held limited interests for others, used certain words or phrases repetitively, interpreted conversation literally, asked irrelevant questions, struggled with conversational skills, avoided or limited eye contact with others, did not demonstrate much facial expression, did not appear to understand social behavior, and often missed social cues. John also demonstrated an extreme or obsessive interest in narrow subjects. His favorite topics of discussion were street signs and sprinkler heads. John's teacher at school noted that he was very passive but not a disruptive influence.

John's language skills were measured in the low average range, as was his overall intellectual ability. Measures of neuropsychological processes, however, noted John's very poor planning, attention, and simultaneous processing. John struggled to self-monitor, self-correct, use strategy efficiently, integrate information, and screen out detail. His motor and perceptual abilities appeared low average. His academic achievement appeared consistent with this overall neuropsychological profile. During a clinical interview, John's responses were tangential. He appeared to have difficulty sharing joint attention with the examiner and appreciating the ideas and thoughts of others.

John's problems reflected a pervasive impairment in reciprocal social interaction, communication, interests, and activities. He also appeared impaired in the use of multiple nonverbal behaviors and, despite demonstrating adequate communicative speech, demonstrated an impairment in pragmatic skills and in his ability to initiate and sustain conversation with others. Moreover, he demonstrated a pattern of interests that were mildly atypical in intensity and focus. The overall symptom profile approached but did not cross the threshold for a full-syndrome diagnosis of autistic disorder. John was provided with the diagnosis (PDD-NOS), as well as the comorbid condition ADHD, inattentive type. Although any PDD is a rule-out in most cases for making the diagnosis of ADHD, research has demonstrated that a significant percentage of children with PDD experience both conditions and suffer from elevated level of impairments because of this (Goldstein & Schwebach, 2004). Issues related to comorbidity are explored by Deprey and Ozonoff in Chapter 10.

Susan

Thirteen-year-old Susan had a history of slow overall development. As a preschooler, she had exhibited delayed language skills and had received speech–language services. She still particularly struggled with pragmatics. Susan had also been diagnosed in the past with the combined type of ADHD. During her educational career, a number of educators had raised questions as to whether Susan's problems reflected a PDD. In particular, Susan demonstrated limited social interaction, was literal in interpreting conversation, frequently asked irrelevant questions, and struggled to maintain conversation. She also appeared not to understand basic social behavior, often missing social cues. Furthermore, at times she appeared to be obsessively interested in narrow subjects. Her current favorite subjects were the characters from the children's card game Yu-Gi-Oh! Susan was an expert on each character's strengths and limitations.

At the time of assessment, Susan was in a self-contained classroom for youth with communication disorders. She was a number of grades behind her peers academically, but enjoyed reading for pleasure. She was not aggressive in the face of stress and could work for both short- and long-term rewards. There was also no extended family history of ASD or significant developmental delays. Though Susan's parents recognized and acknowledged her developmental impairments, they had never considered Susan to suffer from autism. They noted that she had enjoyed interacting with family members even as a young child. It was their impression that Susan did not demonstrate any of the symptoms they considered consistent with autism. Their responses on the Autism Diagnostic Interview—Revised (Rutter, Le Couteur, & Lord, 2003) did not strongly reflect the types of social context problems typically experienced by those with autism or other PDD. Instead, her parents attributed the majority of Susan's interpersonal difficulties to her cognitive and language impairments. Responses to parent and teacher questionnaires noted symptoms of inattention, hyperactivity, impulsivity, and cognitive difficulty. Susan's language skills were measured in the borderline to low average range. Her intelligence was measured in the mild range of mental retardation, as were her memory skills. A measure of nonverbal ability also yielded functioning in the mild range of mental retardation. Neuropsychological processes such as planning, attention, and sequencing (Das, Naglieri, & Kirby, 1994) were also measured in this very low range. Her basic academic achievement appeared well below her age level, but consistent with expectations based upon this neuropsychological profile.

Susan's interaction with the examiner was immature. Module 3 of the ADOS was administered. On this instrument, Susan showed neither echolalia nor marked speech abnormalities. She also demonstrated no excessive stereotypic behavior. However, she did not easily ask for or offer information. She did not easily report events, but could maintain a conversation in a simple way. Eye contact, though somewhat inconsistent, was not deemed to be inappropriate. Facial expression appeared generally normal, though immature. Susan could share enjoyment, but demonstrated some degree of limited insight and some difficulty sharing joint attention. Susan obtained a total score of 3 for Language/Communication (just at the autism cutoff) and 4 for Reciprocal Social Interactions (just at the cutoff for autism spectrum). Her total score of 7 was just at the cutoff reflecting autism spectrum.

Although Susan demonstrated a number of atypical symptoms consistent with a PDD, her presentation did not meet the full diagnostic criteria for autistic disorder. Moreover, differential diagnosis was clearly complicated by Susan's marked impairments in other areas of development, particularly language. Susan had also demonstrated improvement in some of her autistic symptoms, despite the fact that her development had continued to progress at a slow rate over the previous 4 years. Even with further discussion, Susan's parents found it difficult to accept that in part her problems were related to a PDD. Nonetheless, her presentation was consistent with the diagnosis of PDD-NOS. The combination of standardized historical and interactive assessment tools was helpful in understanding and appreciating Susan's symptoms and impairments (Risi et al., 2006). Clearly, Susan's comorbid problems caused by the combined type of ADHD and mild mental retardation with language impairments presented as her greatest challenges. Later chapters in this volume address the assessment of many of these related issues, particularly intelligence, socialization, language, and neuropsychological functioning. Again, Chapter 10 thoroughly covers the issue of comorbid conditions and differential diagnosis.

SUMMARY

The assessment of ASD is complex, requiring a reasoned and reasonable appreciation of diagnostic criteria, assessment tools, and comorbid problems. A brief historical review reveals that autistic qualities are not simply manifestations of 20th- and 21st-century culture, but have probably presented challenges for individuals throughout human history. The current consensus on the majority of diagnostic criteria provides a good foundation for examining and evaluating individuals with possible ASD.

REFERENCES

Achenbach, T., & Edelbrock, C. S. (1991). *Normative data for the Child Behavior Checklist: Revised.* Burlington: University of Vermont, Department of Psychiatry.

American Psychiatric Association. (1952). *Diagnostic and statistical manual of mental disorders.* Washington, DC: Author.

American Psychiatric Association (1968). *Diagnostic and statistical manual of mental disorders* (2nd ed.). Washington, DC: Author.

American Psychiatric Association. (1980). *Diagnostic and statistical manual of mental disorders* (3rd ed.). Washington, DC: Author.

American Psychiatric Association. (1987). *Diagnostic and statistical manual of mental disorders* (3rd ed., rev.). Washington, DC: Author.

American Psychiatric Association. (1994). *Diagnostic and statistical manual of mental disorders* (4th ed). Washington, DC: Author.

American Psychiatric Association. (2000). *Diagnostic and statistical manual of mental disorders* (4th ed., text rev.). Washington, DC: Author.

Asperger, H. (1991). 'Autistic psychopathy' in childhood (U. Frith, Trans.). In U. Frith (Ed.), *Autism and Asperger syndrome* (pp. 37–92). Cambridge, UK: Cambridge University Press. (Original work published 1944)

Baron-Cohen, S. (1989). Do autistic children have obsessions and compulsions? *British Journal of Clinical Psychology, 28*(3), 193–200.

Bleuler, E. (1950). *Dementia praecox or the group of schizophrenias* (J. Zinkin, trans.). New York: International Universities Press. (Original work published 1911)

Boucher, J., & Lewis, V. (1992). Unfamiliar face recognition in relatively able autistic children. *Journal of Child Psychology and Psychiatry, 33,* 843–860.

Cantwell, D. P., Baker, L., & Rutter, M. (1980). Families of autistic children and dysphasic children: Family life and direction patterns. *Advances in Family Psychiatry, 2,* 295–312.

Cohen, D. J. (1976). The diagnostic process in child psychiatry. *Psychiatric Annals, 6,* 29–56.

Cohen, D. J., & Volkmar, F. R. (1997). *Handbook of autism and pervasive developmental disorders.* New York: Wiley.

Conners, C. K. (1997). *Conners' Rating Scales—Revised.* North Tonawanda, NY: Multi-Health Systems.

Das, J. P., Naglieri, J. A., & Kirby, J. R. (1994). *Assessment of cognitive processes.* Needham Heights, MA: Allyn & Bacon.

DeMyer, M. K., Hingtgen, J. N., & Jackson, R. K. (1981). Infantile autism reviewed: A decade of research. *Schizophrenia Bulletin, 7,* 388–451.

Factor, D. C., Freeman, N. L., & Kardash, A. (1989). A comparison of DSM-III and DSM-III-R criteria for autism. *Journal of Autism and Developmental Disorders, 19,* 637–640.

Fein, D., Pennington, B., Markowitz, P., Braverman, M., & Waterhouse, L. (1986). Towards a neuropsychological model of infantile autism: Are the social deficits primary? *Journal of the American Academy of Child Psychiatry, 25,* 198–212.

Frith, U. (1989). *Autism: Explaining the enigma*. Oxford: Blackwell.

Frith, U. (1991). Asperger and his syndrome. In U. Frith (Ed.), *Autism and Asperger syndrome* (pp. 1–36). Cambridge, UK: Cambridge University Press.

Frith, U. (2004). Confusions and controversies about Asperger syndrome. *Journal of Child Psychology and Psychiatry, 45,* 672–686.

Gillberg, C. (1990). Autism and pervasive developmental disorders. *Journal of Child Psychology and Psychiatry, 31,* 99–119.

Gillberg, C., & Schaumann, H. (1982). Social class and autism: Total population aspects. *Journal of Autism and Developmental Disorders, 12,* 223–228.

Gillberg, C., & Steffenberg, S. (1987). Outcome and prognostic factors in infantile autism and similar conditions: A population-based study of 46 cases followed through puberty. *Journal of Autism and Developmental Disorders, 17,* 273–287.

Goldstein, S., & Naglieri, J. (2008). *Autistic rating scales*. Toronto: Multi-Health Systems.

Goldstein, S., & Schwebach, A. (2004). The comorbidity of pervasive developmental disorder and attention deficit hyperactivity disorder: Results of a retrospective chart review. *Journal of Autism and Developmental Disorders, 34*(3), 329–339.

Hobson, R. P. (1989). Beyond cognition: A theory of autism. In G. Dawson (Ed.), *Autism: Nature, diagnosis, and treatment* (pp. 22–48). New York: Guilford Press.

Howlin, P., Goode, S., Hutton, J., & Rutter, M. (2004). Adult outcome for children with autism. *Journal of Child Psychology and Psychiatry, 45,* 212–229.

Kanner, L. (1943). Autistic disturbances of affective contact. *Nervous Child, 2,* 217–250.

Kanner, L., & Eisenberg, L. (1956). Early infantile autism, 1943–1955. *American Journal of Orthopsychiatry, 26,* 55–65.

Klin, A., Pauls, D., Schultz, R., & Volkmar, F. (2005). Three diagnostic approaches to Asperger syndrome: Implications for research. *Journal of Autism and Developmental Disorders, 35,* 221–234.

Kolvin, I. (1971). Studies in the childhood psychoses: I. Diagnostic criteria and classification. *British Journal of Psychiatry, 118,* 381–384.

Krug, D. A., Arick, J., & Almond, P. (1980). Behavior checklist for identifying severely handicapped individuals with high levels of autistic behavior. *Journal of Child Psychology and Psychiatry 21*(3), 221–229.

Kurita, H., Osada, H., & Miyake, Y. (2004). External validity of childhood disintegrative disorder in comparison with autistic disorder. *Journal of Autism and Developmental Disorders, 34,* 355–362.

Lane, H. (1977). *The wild boy of Aveyron*. London: Allen & Unwin.

Lotter, V. (1974). Factors related to outcome in autistic children. *Journal of Autism and Child Schizophrenia, 4,* 263–277.

Lord, C., Rutter, J., & DiLavore, P. C., & Risi, S. (1999). *Autism diagnostic observation schedule (ADOS)*. Los Angeles, CA: Western Psychological Services.

Loveland, K. A., & Kelley, M. L. (1991). Development of adaptive behavior in preschoolers with autism and Down syndrome. *American Journal on Mental Retardation 96*(11), 13–20.

Macdonald, H., Rutter, M., Howlin, P., Rios, P., LeConeur, A., Evered, C., & Folstein, S. (1989). Recognition and expression of emotional cues by autistic and normal adults. *Journal of Child Psychology and Psychiatry 30*(6), 865–877.

Mayes, S. D., Calhoun, S. L., & Crites, D. L. (2001). Does DSM-IV Asperger's disorder exist? *Journal of Abnormal Child Psychology, 29*, 263–271.

Maudsley, H. (1867). Insanity of early life. In H. Maudsley (Ed.), *The physiology and pathology of the mind* (pp. 259–386). New York: Appleton.

Miller, J., & Ozonoff, S. (1997). Did Asperger's cases have Asperger disorder? *Journal of Child Psychology and Psychiatry, 38*, 247–251.

Mundy, P., Sigman, M. D., Ungerer, J., & Sherman, T. (1986). Defining the social deficits of autism: The contribution of non-verbal communication measures. *Journal of Child Psychology and Psychiatry, 27*, 657–669.

Ornitz, E. M., & Ritvo, E. R. (1968). Neurophysiological mechanisms underlying perceptual inconstancy in autistic and schizophrenic children. *Archives of General Psychiatry, 19*, 22–27.

Rett, A. (1966). Uber ein eigenartiges hirnatrophisches Syndrome bei Hyperammonie im Kindersalter. *Wien Medizinische Wochenschrift, 118*, 723–738.

Risi, S., Lord, C., Gotham, K., Crosello, C., Chrysler, C., Szatmari, P., et al. (2006). Information from multiple sources in the diagnosis of autism spectrum disorders. *Journal of the American Academy of Child and Adolescent Psychiatry, 45*, 1094–1103.

Rutter, M. (1970). Autistic children: Infancy to adulthood. *Seminars in Psychiatry, 2*, 435–450.

Rutter, M. (1978). Diagnostic validity in child psychiatry. *Advances in Biological Psychiatry, 2*, 2–22.

Rutter, M., Bailey, A., Bolton, P., & Le Couteur, A. (1994). Autism in known medical conditions: Myth and substance. *Journal of Child Psychology and Psychiatry, 35*, 311–322.

Rutter, M., Le Couteur, A., & Lord, C. (2003). *Autism Diagnostic Interview—Revised*. Los Angeles: Western Psychological Services.

Rutter, R. (1983). Cognitive deficits in the pathogenesis of autism. *Journal of Child Psychology and Psychiatry 24*(4), 513–531.

Schopler, E., & Mesibov, G. B. (Eds.). (1987). *Neurobiological issues in autism*. New York: Plenum Press.

Siegel, B., Vukicevic, J., Elliott, G. R., & Kraemer, H. C. (1989). The use of signal detection theory to assess DSM-III-R criteria for autistic disorder. *Journal of the American Academy of Child and Adolescent Psychiatry, 28*(4), 542–548.

Smalley, S., Asarnow, R., & Spence, M. (1988). Autism and genetics: A decade of research. *Archives of General Psychiatry, 45*, 953–961.

Venter, A., Lord, C., & Schopler, E. (1992). A follow-up study of high-functioning autistic children. *Journal of Child Psychology and Psychiatry, 33*, 489–507.

Volkmar, F. (1998). Categorical approaches to the diagnosis of autism: An overview of DSM-IV and ICD-10. *Autism, 2*, 45–59.

Volkmar, F., Carter, A., Sparrow, S. S., & Cicchetti, D. V. (1993). Quantifying social development in autism. *Journal of the American Academy of Child & Adolescent Psychiatry, 32*(3), 627–632.

Volkmar, F. R., Sparrow, S. S., Goudreau, D., Cicchetti, D. V., Paul, R., & Cohen, D. J. (1987). Social deficits in autism: An operational approach using the Vineland Adaptive Behavior Scales. *Journal of the American Academy of Child and Adolescent Psychiatry, 26*(2), 156–161.

Wing, L. (1981). Asperger's syndrome: A clinical account. *Psychological Medicine, 11,* 115–130.

World Health Organization. (1993). *The ICD-10 classification of mental and behavioral disorders: Diagnostic criteria for research.* Geneva: Author.

CHAPTER TWO

———

The Epidemiology
of Autism Spectrum Disorders
IS THE PREVALENCE RISING?

Lorna Wing
David Potter

For decades after Kanner's original paper on the subject was published in 1943, autism was generally considered to be a rare condition, with a prevalence of about 2–4 per 10,000 children. Then studies carried out in the 1990s and the first years of the present century reported annual rises in the incidence of autism in preschool children based on age of diagnosis and increases in the age-specific prevalence rates in children. Prevalence rates of up to 60 per 10,000 for autism and even more for the whole autism spectrum were reported. Reasons for these increases are discussed in this chapter. They include changes in diagnostic criteria, development of the concept of the wide autism spectrum, different methods used in studies, growing awareness and knowledge among parents and professional workers, and the development of specialist services, as well as the possibility of a true increase in numbers. Various environmental causes for a genuine rise in incidence have been suggested, including the triple vaccine for measles, mumps, and rubella (MMR). Not one of the possible environmental causes, including MMR, has been confirmed by independent scientific investigation, whereas there is strong evidence that complex genetic factors play a major role in etiology. The evidence suggests that most, if not all, of

18

the reported rise in incidence and prevalence is due to changes in diagnostic criteria and to increasing awareness and recognition of autism spectrum disorders (ASD). Whether there is also a genuine rise in incidence remains an open question.

This chapter is an updated version of an earlier paper of ours (Wing & Potter, 2002). The changes in findings occurring since the 2002 paper was written are noted in the relevant sections of this chapter.

The term "autism" was first used by Eugen Bleuler (1911/1950), who applied it to the social impairment of schizophrenia in adults. The concept of autism in children was introduced by Leo Kanner in his seminal paper published in 1943. He described a pattern of behavior he called "early infantile autism," characterized by severe impairment of social interaction and communication and by intense resistance to change. For decades after Kanner's publication, childhood autism was considered to be a rare condition. Then, in the late 1980s and the 1990s, this view was challenged. The most recent studies have reported progressively rising annual incidence rates, and prevalence rates considerably higher than in almost all the early studies.

DEFINITION OF INCIDENCE AND PREVALENCE

There are particular implications for the use of the terms "incidence" and "prevalence" in relation to the ASD. "Incidence" refers to the number of individuals in a specified population in whom the condition being studied *begins* within a specified time period, such as 1 year. "Prevalence" refers to the number of individuals in a specified population who have the condition being studied at a specified time, such as a particular day, regardless of when it began. The usefulness of each index varies with the nature of the condition being studied. With a condition such as measles—which has an obvious onset, lasts about 2 weeks unless there are complications, and has an obvious endpoint—the annual incidence will be larger and usually of more practical interest than the 1-day prevalence. Variations on the theme of incidence, such as changes with different seasons, may also be important. The problems with calculating incidence rates for autistic conditions are that the age of onset is difficult to define and to ascertain, and that the conditions are (in most if not all cases) lifelong. There is strong evidence, to be discussed later in this chapter, that genetic factors are of major importance in etiology. Because autistic conditions are long-lasting, prevalence for age groups at which all cases should, in theory, be diagnosed must be larger than the annual incidence; this is of particular importance for estimating the services needed. If they could be calculated accurately, incidence rates would be more sensitive indicators than prevalence of changes in etiological factors.

STUDIES OF INCIDENCE

Because of the difficulties of defining onset, there have been only a few studies of the annual incidence of ASD. They include the studies in the United Kingdom by Taylor et al. (1999), Powell et al. (2000), who also calculated prevalence, Kaye, Melero-Montes, and Jick (2001), and Smeeth et al. (2004), and in the United States by Dales, Hammer, and Smith (2001). These covered birth cohorts in the 1980s and 1990s. All showed a marked rise in incidence of ASD, but all relied on case records of children diagnosed as having ASD and used the year of diagnosis as the year of onset (see discussion later). The children in these studies were not seen by the research workers to confirm the diagnoses.

These studies used the year in which the children were *diagnosed* as the year of onset. Howlin and Asgharian (1999) found that although parents had begun to be worried much earlier, the average age when a diagnosis was confirmed by professionals was 5.5 years for autism and 11.0 years for Asperger syndrome. Volkmar, Cicchetti, and Bregman (1985) pointed out that the age of diagnosis is more appropriately called the "age of recognition" and should not be assumed to be the real age of onset. Increasing awareness and changes in diagnostic practice, leading to a continuing trend for more and earlier diagnoses, would affect the results of incidence studies that use age of diagnosis as age of onset. It would appear that incidence has been rising until a lower age of diagnosis has become the clinical norm.

STUDIES OF PREVALENCE

Most epidemiological studies of ASD have examined prevalence. Table 2.1 gives a list of 38 studies of prevalence published in or before 2002 in the English language or with detailed abstracts in English. It can be seen that there was a marked tendency over time for an increase in the rates found.

Table 2.2 lists 11 studies published since 2002. It shows that the higher rates found in the later part of the 20th century have been maintained. The last paper in the first section of Table 2.2 (Baird et al., 2006) found a prevalence for all ASD in the South Thames region of London of 116 per 10,000 children. This is close to the rate found in Karlstad, Sweden (Kadesjö, Gillberg, & Hagberg, 1999) of 120 per 10,000, the highest of any so far. Baird et al. (2006) pointed out that they did not include children in mainstream schools who were not "statemented" (i.e., not recognized as

TABLE 2.1. Prevalence Studies before and in 2002: Age-Specific Rates per 10,000 Children

Authors (Year)	Area studied	Rate of autism[a]/ other ASD[b]	Criteria used for autism/other ASD
Studies giving rates of autism (some also give rates of other ASD)			
Lotter (1966)	Middlesex, England	4.5/–	Kanner/–
Brask (1972)[c]	Aarhus, Denmark	4.3/–	Kanner/–
Treffert (1970)	Wisconsin, United States	0.7/2.4	Kanner/DSM-II
Wing & Gould (1979)[c,d]	Camberwell, England	4.6/15.7	Kanner/triad[e]
Hoshino et al. (1982)	Fukushima, Japan	5.0/–	Kanner
Bohman et al. (1983)	Vasterbotten, Sweden	3.0/2.6	Rutter/Rutter
Ishii &Takahashi (1983)[c]	Toyota, Japan	16.0/–	Rutter/–
McCarthy et al. (1984)	E. Health Bd., Ireland	4.3/–	Kanner/–
Gillberg (1984)	Gothenburg, Sweden	2.0/1.9	DSM-III/DSM-III
Gillberg et al. (1986) [c,d]	Gothenburg, Sweden	3.3/14.3	DSMIII/triad[e]
Steffenburg & Gillberg (1986)	Gothenburg, Sweden	4.7/2.8	DSM-III/DSM-III
Steinhausen et al. (1986)	W. Berlin, Germany	1.9/–	Rutter/–
Matsuishi et al. (1987) [c]	Kurume City, Japan	15.5/–	DSM-III/–
Burd et al. (1987)	North Dakota, United States	1.2/2.1	DSM-III/DSM-III
Tanoue et al. (1988)	Ibaraki, Japan	13.8/–	DSM-III
Bryson et al. (1988) [c]	Nova Scotia, Canada	10.1/–	DSM-III-R/–
Ritvo et al. (1989)	Utah, United States	4.0/–	DSM-III/–
Sugiyama & Abe (1989)[c]	Nagoya, Japan	13.0/–	DSM-III/–
Cialdella & Mamelle (1989)	Rhone, France	5.1/5.2	DSM-III/DSM-III
Gillberg et al. (1991)	Gothenburg, Sweden	8.4/3.2	DSM-III-R/DSM-III-R
Fombonne & DuMazaubrun (1992)	Four Regions, France	4.9/–	ICD-10/–
Honda et al. (1996)[c]	Yokohama, Japan	21.1/–	ICD-10/–

(continued)

TABLE 2.1. *(continued)*

Authors (Year)	Area studied	Rate of autism[a]/ other ASD[b]	Criteria used for autism/other ASD
Fombonne et al. (1997)	Three Departments, France	5.4/10.9	ICD-10/ICD-10
Arvidsson et al. (1997)[c]	Mölnlycke, Sweden	31.0/15.0	ICD-10/ICD-10
Webb et al. (1997)	S. Glamorgan, Wales	7.2/–	DSM-III-R/–
Sponheim & Skjeldae (1998)	Akershus, Norway	3.8/1.4	ICD-10/ICD-10
Tomita (1998)[c]	Tokyo, Japan	32.0/58.0	ICD-10/ICD-10
Kadesjö et al. (1999)[c]	Karlstad, Sweden	60.0/60.0	ICD-10/Gillberg[f]
Kielinen et al. (2000)	N. Finland	12.2/1.7	DSM-IV/DSM-IV
Baird et al. (2000)[c]	S.E. Thames, England	30.8/27.1	ICD-10/ICD-10
Powell et al.	W. Midlands, England	16.2/17.5	DSM-III-R or ICD-10
Mágnússon & Saemundsen	Iceland	8.6/4.6	ICD-10/ICD-10
Bertrand et al.	Brick Township, New Jersey, United States	40.0/27.0	DSM-IV/DSM-IV
Croen et al.	California, United States	11.0/–	DSM-III-R or DSM-IV
Chakrabarti & Fombonne	Staffordshire, England	16.8/45.8	DSM-IV/DSM-IV

Studies giving combined rates for autism and other ASD			
Fombonne et al.	Great Britain	26.1	DSM-IV
Scott et al.	Cambridge, England	57.0	DSM-IV

Studies giving combined rates for Asperger syndrome and high-functioning autism			
Ehlers & Gillberg	Gothenburg, Sweden	36.0 + 35[g]	Gillberg[f]

Note. Age ranges vary. [a]"Autism" includes Kanner's early infantile autism, childhood autism, and autistic disorder, as defined in the relevant sets of criteria. [b]"Other ASD" includes subgroups of the autistic spectrum other than "autism." These differ among the studies listed. [c]Population studied < 50,000. [d]All participants in these studies had IQ below 70. [e]Triad of social, communication, and imagination impairments (Wing & Gould, 1979). [f]Gillberg's criteria for Asperger syndrome (Ehlers & Gillberg, 1993). [g]The rate in italics is for children with marked social impairment, but not the full picture of Asperger syndrome.

TABLE 2.2. Prevalence Studies 2003–2006: Age-Specific Rates per 10,000 Children

Authors (Year)	Area studied	Rate of autism[a]/ other ASD[b]	Criteria used for autism/other ASD
Studies giving rates of autism (some also give rates of other ASD)			
Lauritsen et al. (2004)	Denmark	11.8/22.6	ICD-10/ICD-10
Honda et al. (2005)[c]	Yokohama, Japan	27.2/–	ICD-10/–
Chakrabarti & Fombonne (2005)[c]	Staffordshire, England	22.0/36.7	DSM-IV/ DSM-IV
Fombonne et al. (2006)	Montréal, Québec, Canada	21.6/42.9	DSM-IV/ DSM-IV
Gillberg et al. (2006)	Gothenburg, Sweden	20.5/32.9	DSM-IV/ Gillberg[d]
Baird et al. (2006)	S. Thames, London, England	38.9/77.2	ICD-10/ICD-10
Studies giving combined rates for autism and other ASD			
Yeargin-Allsopp et al. (2003)	Metropolitan Atlanta, Georgia, United States	34.0	DSM-IV
Keen & Ward (2004)	Doncaster, England	40.0	Triad[e]
Green et al. (2005)	Great Britain	90.0	ICD-10
Montes & Halterman (2006)[c]	Rochester, New York, United States	66.0	Parent report
Studies giving rates for Asperger syndrome and high-functioning autism			
Webb et al. (2003)[c]	Cardiff, Wales	20.2	ICD-10

Note. Age ranges vary. [a]"Autism" includes Kanner's early infantile autism, childhood autism, and autistic disorder, as defined in the relevant sets of criteria. [b]"Other ASD" includes subgroups of the autistic spectrum other than "autism." These differ among the studies listed. [c]Population studied < 50,000. [d]Gillberg's criteria for Asperger syndrome (Ehlers & Gillberg, 1993). [e]Triad of social, communication, and imagination impairments (Wing & Gould, 1979).

having any special educational needs). The study may therefore have missed an unknown number of more able children with ASD.

POSSIBLE REASONS FOR INCREASE IN INCIDENCE AND PREVALENCE

Changes in Diagnostic Criteria

Evolution of Terminology

There are no definitive diagnostic tests for autism or other ASD. Diagnosis is based on a detailed developmental history and observation of behavior in structured and unstructured situations. This process is fraught with difficulties of definition and standardization. Over the years since Kanner described the pattern of behavior he called "early infantile autism," research in the field has resulted in the development of the concept of a spectrum of autistic disorders (Wing & Gould, 1979), which is considerably wider than Kanner's original group. There have been numerous suggestions for diagnostic criteria, but the discussion in this section is confined to criteria used in the prevalence studies in Table 2.1.

Kanner and Eisenberg (1956) published a list of diagnostic criteria for early infantile autism. They emphasized two behavioral features as necessary and sufficient: first, aloofness and indifference to others; second, intense resistance to change in the child's own repetitive routines, which had to be *elaborate* in form. These features also had to be present by 24 months at the latest. Rutter (1978) published criteria for defining what he called "childhood autism." These were onset before 30 months, impaired social development, delayed and deviant language development, and insistence on sameness. He described each of these behavioral features in detail.

The term "autism" as a childhood condition did not appear in the international classification systems until more than 20 years after Kanner's first publication. The first mention was as a subgroup of the schizophrenias, in the eighth revision of the *International Classification of Diseases* (ICD-8; World Health Organization, 1967). A major change in the concept of childhood autism was evident in the third edition of the *Diagnostic and Statistical Manual of Mental Disorders* (DSM-III; American Psychiatric Association, 1980). DSM-III introduced the term "pervasive developmental disorders" (PDD) as a general category, thus acknowledging the shift in the concept of autism from a psychiatric to a developmental disorder. Brief diagnostic criteria were given for two subgroups: "infantile autism," with onset before 30 months, and "childhood onset PDD," with onset after 30 months but before 12 years.

Another influence in the field was the work of Asperger (1944/1991), which was not well known in English-speaking countries until the 1980s. The children he described made inappropriate social approaches. They had good grammar and vocabulary, but used this only to talk about a narrow range of special interests, unique to each child. These children were usually of average or high intelligence, but often had specific learning disorders. They were also socially and often physically clumsy and inept. Asperger believed his syndrome to be different from Kanner's autism. This is still debated, but most authors now consider it to be part of an autism spectrum (Frith, 1991). As a result of studies they carried out in the 1970s, and their interest in Asperger's work, Wing and Gould (1979) developed the concept of the spectrum of autistic disorders—the essential features of which were a triad of impairments of social interaction, social communication, and flexible social imagination (the last being replaced by a narrow, repetitive range of interests or activities). These are familiar features appearing in virtually all sets of criteria. The essential point of the spectrum concept was that each of the elements of the triad could occur in widely varying degrees of severity and in many different manifestations. For example, social impairment could be shown as passivity in social interaction or as active but inappropriate and repetitive approaches to others, not just aloofness as in Kanner's criteria.

The concept of a spectrum began to be seen in DSM-III-R (American Psychiatric Association, 1987). This kept the general category of PDD, but the subgroups were labeled "autistic disorder" and "PDD not otherwise specified" (PDD-NOS). The definitions of the subgroups differed from those in DSM-III and were given as formal diagnostic criteria covering a range of relevant features of behavior. The age-of-onset criterion was no longer included. DSM-IV (American Psychiatric Association, 1994; see also DSM-IV-TR, American Psychiatric Association, 2000) also retained the overall category of PDD, but introduced new subgroups in addition to autistic disorder. These were Rett's disorder, childhood disintegrative disorder, and (for the first time) Asperger syndrome, referred to as Asperger's disorder. The residual subgroup of PDD-NOS was retained. Detailed criteria for the subgroups that could be used in research were given; those for autistic disorder now included onset before 36 months. ICD-10 had closely similar subgroups and research criteria (World Health Organization, 1993).

Effects of Diagnostic Criteria Used in Prevalence Studies

The boundaries between ASD, other developmental disorders, and typical development are difficult to define with any precision. Children with ASD but with high ability may not be seen by their parents or teachers as requiring any form of special help. They may be identified only in studies in which every child in a complete population of children in a specified age range is examined in detail—as, for example, in the Gothenburg study (Ehlers & Gillberg, 1993). Posserud, Lundervold, and Gillberg (2006), using the Autism Spectrum Screening Questionnaire (Ehlers, Gillberg, & Wing, 1999), found a continuous distribution of scores in a population of school children, with a smooth falloff in the number of children showing no symptoms down to those with many symptoms.

Moreover, given the nature of the diagnostic criteria for different subgroups of ASD, there can be no doubt that there were variations in the ways these were interpreted by different researchers. The most careful operational definitions, and training in their use, could not completely remove these differences. Nor can the degree to which they affected the results be measured. It is very possible that the rules dividing autistic disorder, however defined, from other ASD were applied differently by different investigators, which may explain some of the variations shown in Tables 2.1 and 2.2. Particular problems arise in relation to autistic disorder and Asperger syndrome. DSM-IV/ICD-10 rules specify, for Asperger's disorder/Asperger syndrome, age-appropriate development of language, adaptive skills, and curiosity up to 3 years. If these criteria are applied strictly, they diagnose Asperger syndrome significantly less and autistic disorder significantly more often than do Gillberg's criteria (Gillberg, Gillberg, Rastam, & Wentz, 2001), which are more closely based on Asperger's own descriptions (Leekam, Libby, Wing, Gould, & Gillberg, 2000). This is relevant to Fombonne's (2001) observation that in all the studies he surveyed, the rates for Asperger syndrome were lower than those for autistic disorder. These problems add to the difficulty of interpreting data from the published epidemiological studies. Even if the studies purport to count ASD, it is not always clear what clinical pictures were included.

Table 2.3 shows the numbers of studies that purportedly used each of the different criteria sets for ASD. The ranges of the rates for each set of criteria are also given. The column labeled "autism" covers the following: early infantile autism, as defined by Kanner and Eisenberg (1956); infantile autism, as in DSM-III; autistic disorder, as in DSM-III-R or DSM-IV; and childhood autism, as defined by Rutter (1978) or as in ICD-10. (As noted above, the DSM-IV and ICD-10 criteria are virtually identical.) The column labeled "Other ASD" covers some or all of the other subgroups defined by the different sets of criteria. These differ widely in different studies; for example, some exclude Asperger or Rett syndrome. For this reason, only the mean rates for "autism" (however defined) are given.

As can be seen from Table 2.3, the mean rates for studies using Kanner and Eisenberg's (1956) criteria were the lowest of all. The combination of social aloofness and elaborate repetitive routines is comparatively rare, because aloofness is strongly associated with severe or profound

TABLE 2.3. Age-Specific Rates per 10,000 by Criteria Used: Means and Ranges

Criteria used in studies	No. of studies of autism	Mean rate for autism	Range of rates	No. of studies of other ASD	Range of rates
		Studies in or before 2002			
Kanner	6	3.9	0.7–5.0	–	–
DSM-II	–	–	–	1	2.4
Rutter	3	7.0	1.9–16.0	1	2.6
DSM-III	9	7.0	1.2–15.5	5	1.9–5.2
DSM-III-R	3	8.6	7.2–10.1	1	3.2
DSM-IV/ ICD-10	14	21.0	3.8–60.0	10	1.4–58.0
Triad[a]	–	–	–	2	14.3–15.7
Gillberg[b]	–	–	–	1	60.0
		Studies in 2003–2006			
DSM-IV/ ICD-10	6	23.7	11.8–38.9	5	22.6–77.2

Note. Includes only studies giving rates for autism separately from other ASD. [a]Triad of social, communication, and imagination impairments (Wing & Gould, 1979). The rates are for children with IQ < 70. [b]Gillberg's criteria for Asperger syndrome—first version (Ehlers & Gillberg, 1993). The rate is for children of all IQ levels.

mental retardation (IQ below 35). Elaborate rituals and routines, on the other hand, require the cognitive ability to organize aspects of the environment, such as using objects to make complex repetitive patterns or insisting on lengthy bedtime routines (Wing & Gould, 1979). Four studies—one early one in Camberwell (Wing & Gould, 1979) and three later ones in, respectively, Mölnlycke, Sweden (Arvidsson et al., 1997), Karlstad, Sweden (Kadesjö et al., 1999), and northern Finland (Kielinen, Linna, & Moilanen, 2000)—applied both Kanner's criteria and ICD-10 childhood autism criteria to the same children. In the Camberwell study, ICD-10 criteria were applied retrospectively to the original data. All children fitting Kanner's criteria also fitted the DSM-IV/ICD-10 criteria, but in each study, the numbers fitting the former set were markedly lower than those fitting the latter two sets. Specifically, the proportions meeting Kanner's criteria ranged from 33% to 45% of all those diagnosed as meeting DSM-IV/ICD-10 criteria in the four studies. The mean rates for studies using Rutter's or DSM-III criteria were just under double those for studies using Kanner's criteria. The Rutter and DSM-III systems were similar to each other, and neither insisted that the repetitive activities had to be elaborate. Both also raised the upper limit of age of onset to 30 months.

DSM-III-R was used for only three studies. The mean rate for DSM-III-R autistic disorder was just over double that for Kanner and Eisenberg's (1956) criteria. The highest rates, with a mean over five times that for Kanner and Eisenberg's criteria, were found in studies using DSM-IV/ICD-10. This was maintained in studies published from 2003 to 2006, but with only a small rise in the mean and a narrower range of rates. Both DSM-III-R and DSM-IV/ICD-10 allowed for a wide range of types of social and communication impairment and of repetitive activities, even within the subgroup of autistic disorder. Unlike Kanner's and Rutter's criteria, DSM-III-R and DSM-IV/ICD-10 did not insist on language delay or deviance as long as some other type of communication impairment was present, such as poor intonation or inappropriate use of speech in relation to the social context. Volkmar et al. (1992), in a field trial carried out before DSM-IV was published, found that DSM-III-R, in contrast to ICD-10, was significantly overinclusive when compared with clinicians' diagnoses. The authors suggested that one reason why autistic disorder in ICD-10 was more specific was that ICD-10 included a number of other subgroups in which individuals could be classified, compared with only one (PDD-NOS), in DSM-III-R. It is not likely that the lack of an upper limit for age of onset in DSM-III-R was a significant factor. Volkmar, Stier, and Cohen (1985) found that only 5 children out of 129 (4%) diagnosed as having PDD when DSM-III was used apparently had an age of onset after 30 months. In the light of these findings, it appears paradoxical that the highest prevalence rates for autism have been found in studies using DSM-IV/ICD-10. When this is taken together with the very wide range of rates associated with each set of criteria, it is evident that other factors in addition to the definitions of criteria must have been involved in order to explain the overall rise in rates.

DSM-IV and ICD-10 criteria were also associated with the highest rates found for other ASD, as shown in Table 2.3. This has continued in studies carried out in 2003–2006.

Differences in Methods Used in Studies

Differences among the studies included variations in the sizes and types of target populations, as well as in methods of identifying cases (Fombonne, Simmons, Ford, Meltzer, & Goodman, 2001).

Size of Target Populations

Honda, Shimizu, Misumi, Nimi, and Ohashi (1996) examined 18 prevalence studies in the English language or with English summaries, in print at the time they were writing (all included in Table 2.1). They found that rates for autism (plus other ASD if reported) of over 10.0 per 10,000 were reported significantly more often in studies covering target populations of fewer than 50,000. The same analysis for the larger number of studies reported here gave a similar result. Seventeen of the studies in Table 2.1 using target populations under 50,000 found age-specific rates for all ASD (however defined) above 10 per 10,000, and only one reported a rate of under 10. In contrast, only 6 out of 19 using larger populations found rates over 10 per 10,000 (χ^2 = 15.5, df = 1, p < .001). The five studies with target populations under 10,000 that used DSM-IV/ICD-10 criteria (Honda et al., 1996; Arvidsson et al., 1997; Tomita, 1998; Kadesjö et al., 1999; Bertrand et al., 2001) gave rates per 10,000 for all ASD ranging from 21 to 120. The study of Asperger syndrome and other high-functioning autistic disorders in Gothenburg, Sweden (Ehlers & Gillberg, 1993) covering a population of only 1,519 children, found a rate of 71 per 10,000 for this group. Honda et al. (1996) concluded that studies of large populations gave results with smaller confidence intervals, but made it much more difficult to be sure of finding all eligible children. They noted that accurate case finding was much easier with small target populations.

However, in studies of autism and/or all ASD published after 2002 shown in Table 2.2, six covered target populations of more than 50,000 (Lauritsen, Pedersen, & Mortensen, 2004; Gillberg et al., 2006; Baird et al., 2006; Yeargin-Allsopp et al., 2003; Keen & Ward, 2004; Green, McGinnity, Meltzer, Ford, & Goodman, 2005), and only four investigated populations below this level. All found rates for childhood autism and/or all ASD above 10 per 10,000. The mean rate for all ASD in the six larger studies was 61.3 per 10,000. For the three smaller studies that gave rates for the whole spectrum (Chakrabarti & Fombonne, 2005; Fombonne et al., 2006; Montes & Halterman, 2006), the mean was 63.1. The study in Yokohama (Honda, Shimizu, Imai, & Nitto, 2005), covering a population below 50,000, found a rate for childhood autism of 27.2, similar to the rates found in most of the other studies in Table 2.2. The study in Cardiff (Webb et al., 2003) in Table 2.2, giving a rate of 20.2 for children with high-functioning autistic disorders, was a small-scale study but was confined to children in mainstream schools.

Methods of Case Finding

The authors of almost all of the studies in Table 2.1 used medical and/ or educational agencies to find eligible children. The method of case finding that generally produced the highest rates was close involvement with routine developmental checks for preschool children. Eight of the 15 rates for autism of over 10.0 per 10,000 were based on repeated developmental checks (Matsuishi et al., 1987; Tanoue, Oda, Asano, & Kawashima, 1988; Sugiyama & Abe, 1989; Honda et al., 1996; Arvidsson et al., 1997;

Tomita, 1998; Baird et al., 2000; Chakrabarti & Fombonne, 2001), compared with none of the 20 rates below this level ($\chi^2 = 13.83$, $df = 1$, $p < .001$). Japanese researchers in particular found this approach particularly useful, because about 90% of Japanese children undergo these developmental examinations (Honda et al., 1996); five of the eight studies using this method were carried out in Japan. Assessments for ASD were integrated with the routine examinations, and repeated checks were carried out over several years. As noted above, the highest rate of all was found from detailed examination of a small target population (Kadesjö et al., 1999). The lowest rate (0.7) was found in Wisconsin (Treffert, 1970). This was one of the earliest studies, published in 1970 before diagnostic criteria for autism appeared in the ICD or DSM classification systems. The rate was based upon computer printouts of clinical and demographic details of children known to agencies throughout the state who had been given a diagnosis of childhood schizophrenia according to DSM-II criteria. Treffert used the records to rediagnose some as having autism, based on Kanner's criteria and the absence of any evidence of "organicity." None was seen by the author. All these factors combined to give a very low rate for "classic autism."

Over the years since the Treffert (1970) study was published, there have been major changes in the collection of information for educational and health records in many countries. Administrative decisions can have an effect on the level of awareness of particular conditions. In the United States, in 1991, autism was included for the first time in the Individuals with Disabilities Education Act (IDEA). This was about the time that the numbers of children diagnosed as having autism began to rise, so it seems likely that IDEA contributed to the increase. Recording of specific diagnoses of ASD by educational authorities started about a decade later in Great Britain, except for England. It did not start in England until 2004, although the rise in reported prevalence began well before this. The researchers carrying out prevalence studies since 2002 have benefited from the greatly improved systems of diagnosing and recording.

Increasing Awareness of the Existence of ASD

Until the 1960s, there was little general interest in or awareness of ASD. Then the development of voluntary associations of parents—later to include interested professionals—began in the United States and the United Kingdom in the 1960s. Their aims were to push for educational and treatment services for their children and to encourage research. These groups were followed over the ensuing years by associations in many other countries throughout the world. Together, these associations were energetic in ensuring publicity concerning these children and their needs through all the media.

Professional interest was stimulated by the development, also beginning in the United States and United Kingdom in the 1960s, of scientific investigation into the nature of autism (e.g., DeMyer, 1975; Hermelin & O'Connor, 1970; Lotter, 1966; Rutter, 1970, 1978; Schopler & Reichler, 1976). Awareness of the widening of the criteria for autistic conditions and the concept of Asperger syndrome (Wing, 1981, 2005) has also grown. There has been a profound change since the days when autism was considered a rare condition, to be diagnosed only by using Kanner's strict criteria. The appearance of various methods of eliciting the diagnostic criteria for autism and other ASD has contributed to the greater willingness of clinicians to diagnose these disorders. In the 1990s, two diagnostic interview schedules for obtaining information on developmental history and behavior patterns were designed and tested. These were the Autism Diagnostic Interview—Revised (ADI-R; Lord, Rutter, & Le Couteur, 1994) and the Diagnostic Interview for Social and Communication Disorders (DISCO; Wing, Leekam, Libby, Gould, & Larcombe, 2002). The latter had a long history since it evolved from the Handicaps, Behaviour and Skills schedule (Wing & Gould, 1978), first used in research in the Camberwell study (Wing & Gould, 1979) in the 1970s. More recently, the Developmental, Dimensional and Diagnostic Interview (3di) for ASD has been published (Skuse et al., 2004). These schedules were designed for different aspects of diagnostic assessment, and each has its advantages and disadvantages. For each of these schedules, training courses have been organized for professional workers, thus helping to spread knowledge in the field. Schedules for systematic methods of observation and psychological assessment, such as the Autism Observation Diagnostic Schedule (ADOS; Lord et al., 2000), and the training course for psychologists associated with the DISCO have also helped to increase interest and awareness among professionals.

From the end of the 1990s, public attention has been brought to bear on ASD through media publicity concerning a suggested link between autism and vaccination with MMR vaccine or with childhood vaccines containing mercury in a preservative. These possibilities have had a powerful influence in making the general public aware of the existence of autistic conditions, although current scientific evidence does not support either hypothesis (see discussion later in this chapter).

Since the paper on which this chapter is based was first published, the mass media's interest in ASD, already increasing, has escalated to a remarkable degree. Many books by parents and by people with ASD have been published. Movies, television programs, and novels with characters with autistic conditions have appeared, including at least two detective stories. In 1962, when a group of parents in the United Kingdom set up an association that was to become the British National Autistic Society, the members tried to obtain publicity through the press. The one newspaper that did publish an article headed it "Problems of Artistic Children." Now autism is so well known and of such interest that a character with autism seems to guarantee success in virtually any of the media.

Recognition That ASD Can Be Associated with Other Conditions

Mental Retardation

Kanner (1943) at first believed that children with his syndrome were of potentially normal intelligence. Scientific studies that measured intellectual ability showed that autism and mental retardation at all levels could and often did coexist (Rutter, 1970; Lotter, 1966; Wing & Gould, 1979). It took time for this fact to affect clinical practice, but awareness has increased over the years.

In the United States, Croen, Grether, Hoogstrate, and Selvin (2002) examined statistics from the Department of Developmental Services (DDS) of the California Health and Human Services Agency. These showed a marked increase in the numbers of persons with autism entering the official counting system annually over the previous 11 years. Croen et al., using DDS data, examined the rates of DSM-III-R or DSM-IV autistic disorder (depending on when the diagnosis was made) and found an overall rate for the 11 years studied of 11.0 per 10,000. The annual prevalence rates showed a more or less steady increase, from 5.78 in 1987 to 14.89 in 1994. The annual prevalence rates for the same years for mental retardation of unknown cause showed a more or less steady *decrease,* from 28.76 in 1987 to 19.52 in 1994. Blaxill, Baskin, and Spitzer (2003) criticized Croen et al.'s conclusion that at least part of the rise in reported prevalence of autism was due to substitution of this diagnosis for idiopathic mental retardation. In their response, Croen and Grether (2003) agreed that there were problems in their methodology and that more research was needed. Gurney et al. (2003) found a substantial rise in ASD rates in Minnesota, from 3 per 10,000 in 1991–1992 to 52 per 10,000 in 2001–2002. These authors did not find a corresponding drop in other special education disability categories, except for a slight decrease for mild mental retardation. They nevertheless concluded that federal and state administrative changes in policy and law favoring better identification of autism were likely to have contributed to the rise.

In the United Kingdom, studies were done that examined the relationship of autism and mental retardation clinically rather than by using administrative records. In 1980, Shah, Holmes, and Wing (1982) carried out a study of an institution for adults with mental retardation before it was finally closed. At the time of the study, the residents' years of birth ranged from 1880 to 1964. The research team assessed each of the 893 residents and found that 339 (38%) were socially impaired as in ASD; that is, they were aloof, passive, or active but odd in social interaction. Out of all those with social impairment, 134 (40%) had autism as classically defined by Kanner (Shah et al., 1982). Only a few of the youngest residents had previously been diagnosed as having autism. It is not possible to make any calculation of population prevalence rates from these results, but they do show that many adults with undiagnosed autistic conditions were to be found in mental retardation institutions in the United Kingdom. A follow-up study showed very little change in the prevalence of social impairment among those who were surviving, most of whom were living in the small residences for adults with mental retardation that replaced the institutions (Beadle-Brown et al., 2002). In Sweden, Gillberg, Steffenburg, and Schaumann (1991) observed that the increase in rates found over the three studies in Gothenburg (Gillberg, 1984; Steffenburg & Gillberg, 1986; Gillberg et al., 1991) was due partly to better detection of autism among children with severe mental retardation as well as among those with intelligence in the average or high range.

In the United Kingdom, the general tendency until the 1970s was to label as "mentally retarded" or "maladjusted" children whose learning disabilities or behavioral disturbances were too severe to be accommodated in mainstream schools. Few of these children were assessed in pediatric clinics or given any other diagnosis. For example, out of the 50 school-age children in the Camberwell study (Wing & Gould, 1979) diagnosed by the researchers as having ASD, in 1971 only 7 (14%) were known to the educational and school medical services as having autism. Six of the seven fitted Kanner and Eisenberg's (1956) diagnostic criteria. Seven other children were diagnosed by the research team with this type of autism, but they were not recorded by the services as having any type of autistic condition. This meant that just over half (57%) of the children over 5 years of age with the most classic form of autism had not been diagnosed. Only 1 of the remaining 36 school-age children with other ASD was recorded as having autism (Wing, Yeates, Brierly, & Gould, 1976). The rest of the 50 school-age children were recorded as mildly or severely mentally retarded or, in a few cases, as "maladjusted." During the 1970s, child development centers began to be set up in the United Kingdom. More and more children were referred for detailed developmental assessments, and pediatricians began to develop interest and expertise in the field of ASD. This change was accelerated in the 1980s when autistic conditions were classified in the DSM and later in the ICD as disorders of development caused by brain dysfunction, instead of being regarded as rare psychiatric conditions.

Average or High Intellectual Ability

As noted earlier, Asperger's work was hardly known in English-speaking countries until the 1980s. Most of the children he described had average or high intellectual ability, although Asperger (1944/1991) noted that he had seen the pattern of behavior he described in children with mental retardation. Spreading knowledge of Asperger's syndrome heightened awareness that autistic conditions, even Kanner's classic autism, could be found in children and adults of high ability. This shift of emphasis allowed the inclusion in the spectrum of children with the more subtle as well as those with the most obvious features of autism (Denckla, 1986). Wolff (1995) described a group of adults whom she had followed up from childhood when they had subtle signs of ASD. She referred to them as having "schizoid personality disorder of childhood," but, in her book written in 1995, she acknowledged that their pattern of skills, disabilities, and behavior fitted into the most able end of the whole autism spectrum. This work made yet another contribution to the widening of the concept of the spectrum. Wolff found that the future outlook for this group was good on the whole, with most becoming independent as adults and some being high achievers in their work. A small minority had a history of psychiatric conditions, alcohol or drug problems, or delinquency.

Other Developmental and Physical Disorders

Another of Kanner's beliefs that probably affected diagnostic practice in the early years was that autism was a unique condition, separate from all other childhood disorders. It is now recognized that ASD can occur together with any other developmental or physical disability. Epileptic fits are commonly associated with ASD (Rutter, 1970). Language disorders, especially affecting semantics and pragmatics (Brook & Bowler, 1992; Rapin & Dunn, 1997), and motor coordination problems (Smith, 2000) are important aspects of the pattern of disabilities in ASD and can cause diagnostic confusion if the underlying social impairment is not recognized (Gillberg & Billstedt, 2000). Research is now being undertaken on the association of autism or some features of autism with an ever-growing range of identifiable chromosomal abnormalities, including fragile X syndrome (Turk & Graham, 1997), Turner syndrome (Creswell & Skuse, 1999), tuberous sclerosis (Hunt & Dennis, 1987), Tourette syndrome (Kadesjö & Gillberg, 2000), and Down syndrome (Howlin, Wing, & Gould, 1995). Howlin et al. (1995) observed that because of the stereotyped view of children with Down syndrome as very sociable and outgoing, the presence of autism, which occurs in about 10% of those with the syndrome, has often not been diagnosed. The apparent sociability of children with Williams syndrome has given rise to the view that it is the opposite of autism, but cases are reported of the co-occurrence of Williams syndrome and autism (Herguner & Mukaddes, 2006). The same is true of Cohen syndrome (Howlin, Karpf, & Turk, 2005).

Psychiatric Conditions

Before and for years after Kanner's first paper on his syndrome, autistic conditions were often diagnosed as childhood schizophrenia. The studies of Kolvin and his colleagues (Kolvin, 1971) were important in clarifying the differences between these diagnoses. It is likely that in the past, while some adults with autism were diagnosed as having mental retardation and placed in the relevant institutions, others were given a lifelong label of schizophrenia and lived in institutions for the mentally ill. No studies of the prevalence of autistic conditions among residents in the latter institutions before they were closed have been published. Ryan (1992) suggested that some individuals diagnosed as having "treatment-resistant" mental illnesses such as schizophrenia, bipolar disorder, or obsessive–compulsive disorder may have had Asperger syndrome. Wing and Shah (2000) found that 17% of people referred to a specialist center and diagnosed as having an ASD at age 15 or over had marked catatonic features. Some had previously been diagnosed as having catatonic schizophrenia, because the possibility of autism had not been considered. Tantam (1988) studied 60 adults who had been referred to a psychiatrist because of lifelong social isolation and conspicuous eccentricity. They had had a variety of psychiatric diagnoses, including both neuroses and psychoses. When Tantam examined their histories in detail, he found that 46 of the 60 fitted the criteria for autistic disorder or Asperger syndrome. Nylander and Gillberg (2001) found that 16 out of 499 adults (3.2%) attending a treatment center for psychiatric disorders had an ASD; in almost all cases, it had not been previously diagnosed. The findings were similar to those of studies of special hospitals for mentally ill offenders in England (Hare, Gould, Mills, & Wing, 1999; Scragg & Shah, 1994). Bejerot, Nylander, and Lindstrom (2001) found that 20% of 64 individuals diagnosed with obsessive–compulsive disorder had marked autistic traits. Gillberg and Rastam (1992) described a subgroup of teenagers with anorexia nervosa who also had autism-like conditions. It is not possible to calculate the prevalence of psychiatric disorders among those with ASD from these findings—nor, conversely, to calculate the proportion of those with ASD among all those with psychiatric conditions. However, it is clear that in the past, some individuals with ASD have been misdiagnosed as having a psychiatric illness. In other cases, a psychiatric illness has been correctly diagnosed, but an associated ASD has been missed. Such mistakes still occur, though it is to be hoped that they are becoming less common.

Development of Specialist Services

Two different trends in service provision in the United Kingdom have affected patterns of referrals and the numbers of children and adults with ASD seen by different professionals. On the one hand, the numbers of large institutions for people with mental retardation, and special schools for children with mild mental retardation, specific learning disabilities, and/or disturbed behavior, have gradually diminished since the late 1970s. As discussed above, in the past children and adults, including some with ASD, would have been admitted to these services because of their learning or behavior problems without having any specialized diagnostic assessment. On the other hand, all kinds of specialist provisions for children and adults with ASD have been developed since the 1970s. They include diagnostic services for ASD and related conditions, family support services, special schools, special classes or individual support within mainstream schools, residential homes for adults, occupational services, specialized leisure opportunities, and social training groups for more able people with autistic conditions (Wing, 2001). There is still a long way to go before provision is anywhere near adequate for everyone involved, but progress has been made. The improvement in and increasing availability of services over time have made parents more willing to think of the possibility of an ASD if they are worried about their child's development. Parents of a preschool child are often reluctant to accept a diagnosis of an autistic condition, but tend to become more willing as their child grows older if the autistic traits become more obvious. Professionals are also more likely to be willing to make a diagnosis of an autistic condition if they know that it will lead to appropriate help for the child or adult and the family concerned.

Possible Causes of a Hypothetical Real Increase in Prevalence

Genetic Factors

There is strong evidence from twin studies that genetic factors are of major importance in the etiology of over 90% of cases of autistic disorder diagnosed according to DSM-IV (Rutter, 2000). It appears that an unknown number of different genes are likely to be involved. Studies of families of children with autistic disorder suggest that genetic factors are also important in relation to the wider autism spectrum (Bolton et al., 1994). Asperger (1944/1991) observed that traits related to his syndrome were often seen in the parents of the children concerned.

Baron-Cohen et al. (2006) have demonstrated, in a small group of parents of children with Asperger syndrome, that both mothers and fathers showed atypical brain function in the direction of hypermasculinity. In another paper, Baron-Cohen (2006) has discussed the possibility of assortative mating. He suggests that there is a tendency for men and women with this type of brain function to mate and therefore to increase the chances of having a child with an ASD. Baron-Cohen has raised the interesting question of whether modern patterns of education, work, and leisure make it more likely for such men and women to meet than was the case in the past.

Reichenberg et al. (2006) reported evidence for an association between advancing paternal age and the chances of having a child with autism. Offspring of fathers age 40 years or older were particularly at risk. It is possible that the modern tendency to have children later in life has had an effect on incidence and prevalence. The consequences of lowering mortality among very premature babies, and of the various forms of artificial conception, have yet to be studied in relation to autism.

Medical Conditions

In their review, Gillberg and Coleman (1996) found that estimates made by different researchers of the proportions of children with autistic disorders with medical conditions that could possibly have caused the autism vary from about 11% to 37%. The proportions were related to the intensity of the medical investigations. (Although epilepsy is common in people with ASD, affecting one-quarter or more of those with typical autistic disorder [Rutter, 1970], it was not included as a possible causal condition. It was considered to be an additional effect of whatever brain dysfunction had led to the autism.) The percentages with diagnosable medical conditions were higher for those with severe or profound mental retardation. The proportions for other ASD varied from 12% to 53%. However, the great majority of the medical conditions listed were also genetic (such as tuberous sclerosis), or prenatal in origin (such as maternal rubella). There are only a few reported examples of typical autistic behavior beginning some years after birth following, for example, herpes simplex encephalitis (Gillberg, 1986). These findings suggest that in most cases, the basic pathology underlying ASD is present from before birth. There is no evidence of a change in prevalence of the medical genetic conditions associated with autism, although it is possible that infants with these conditions have a better chance of survival than in the past.

Pre- or postnatal infections may have a role in causing autism (Gillberg & Coleman, 1996). The spread of rubella in an unvaccinated population, as occurred among immigrants from the Caribbean in Camberwell (Wing, 1980), could affect the numbers of cases of maternal rubella and the incidence and prevalence of autism in the area involved. There is evidence that thalidomide taken in the 20th to the 24th day of gestation (Rodier, Ingram, Tisdale, & Croog, 1997), and the anticonvulsant valproic acid taken during pregnancy (Miyazaki, Narita, & Narita, 2005; Williams et al., 2001) may be associated with autism. ASD have also been found in children with fetal alcohol syndrome (Nanson, 1993; Kielinen, Rantala, Timonen, Linna, & Moilanen, 2004).

Other Environmental Factors

Genetic factors alone are very unlikely to account for the large rise in rates that has been reported. If there is a real rise that is continuing, nongenetic factors must be involved. Monozygotic twins are mostly but not always concordant for autism. When both are in the spectrum, the manifestations in each may be different. Including the broader autistic phenotype raises the concordance from 60% to 92% in monozygotic twins and from 0% to 10% in dizygotic twins (Muhle, Trentacoste, & Rapin, 2004). This suggests that in at least some cases, nongenetic factors within or outside the uterus or before, during, or after birth have an effect. Many suggestions have been made concerning possible causes—including constituents of the diet, environmental pollutants, antibiotics, allergies, vaccines, and traces of neurotoxins (such as mercury present in preservatives used for some vaccines, though not in the MMR vaccine now used in the United Kingdom)— but none of these has as yet been scientifically validated. At the time of writing, there is continuing public concern that the combined MMR vaccine is responsible for the observed increase in autistic conditions, but there is no scientific evidence for this.

"Regressive" Autism and the MMR Vaccine

There is a delay of varying length before parents of children with ASD become aware that their children are not developing as expected. Studies of home videos taken in the first year of life of children later diagnosed as having autism showed subtle symptoms of autism that could be reliably identified by the researchers (Werner, Dawson, Osterling, & Dinno, 2000; Baranek, 1999). Baranek noted that caregivers used strategies to compensate for their children's unresponsiveness before they reported any autistic symptoms. Volkmar et al. (1985) found that only 4% of 129 children and adults diagnosed as having PDD were reported to have had an onset after 30 months, and they were indistinguishable in their behavior from the rest of the group. Some parents of the children with PDD reported that their children had begun to develop some limited speech (sometimes mainly echolalia), and then stopped speaking during their second or third year. This is not the same thing as the condition known in DSM-IV-(-TR)/ICD-10 as childhood disintegrative disorder, in which there is good evidence of completely normal development for at least 2 years and then a catastrophic loss of self-care and other skills. This has a prevalence of less than 1 per 10,000, and Fombonne and Chakrabarti (2001) found no evidence of any increase in this condition.

Wakefield et al. (1998) and Wakefield and Montgomery (2000) examined children with ASD referred to a pediatric gastroenterologist because of gastrointestinal symptoms such as chronic diarrhea or constipation. They described what they considered to be a particular form of inflammatory bowel disease. They put forward the hypothesis that this was due to MMR vaccination, which was causing a new variant of "regressive" autism— that is, loss of some previously acquired skills, together with gastrointestinal problems. They considered that the observed rise in rates of ASD was related to this new condition. Wakefield and colleagues did not examine children with ASD who did not have gastrointestinal problems; nor did they examine children with severe chronic constipation without any form of autism. Black, Kaye, and Jick (2002) carried out a nested case–control study and found that 9% of children diagnosed with autism and 9% of nonautistic controls had recorded gastrointestinal disorders.

Four of the incidence studies discussed earlier in this chapter (Taylor et al., 1999; Powell et al., 2000; Kaye et al., 2001; Dales et al., 2001) were designed to examine whether the introduction of MMR affected the annual incidence of autistic disorder and other ASD. As noted previously, all found a steady rise year by year, but the slopes of the graphs were unaffected by the introduction of MMR vaccination. This was considered to be strong evidence that the triple vaccine was not causing the observed rise in the incidence of autistic conditions. The studies did not reveal the reasons for the annual rises, but the authors suggested that increasing awareness of ASD among parents and professionals was an important factor. Chen and De Stefano (1998) pointed out the lack of evidence from large databases of any significant link between MMR and chronic bowel or behavior problems. Fombonne and Chakrabarti (2001) examined epidemiological data concerning children with ASD, some diagnosed before MMR vaccination and some after. They found no evidence to support a distinct syndrome of MMR-induced autism or of "autistic enterocolitis."

Richler et al. (2006) found in a multisite study that 72% of 163 children, who were reported by parents to have lost some skills they had previously acquired, had had atypical development prior to the loss. The children who "regressed" had slightly poorer outcomes in Verbal IQ and social reciprocity, and more gastrointestinal symptoms, than children with autism who did not "regress." However, the authors found no relationship between some loss of skills in young children with ASD and MMR vaccination. Lingam et al. (2003) examined the effects on parents of publicity concerning the MMR vaccine and "autistic regression." They found that after the publicity in 1997, parents were more likely to report regression after MMR vaccination, even though their children's records showed concerns about development before they were vaccinated.

It remains a possibility that MMR vaccination precipitates autism or other ASD in a small number of children who are vulnerable, perhaps because of genetic loading that would otherwise be insufficient to produce overt ASD. The number would be too small to be evident in the large-scale studies that have shown no effects from MMR. All types of immunization carry a very small risk of adverse effects, but this has to be balanced against the very much higher risk of death or severe disability from the illnesses against which the vaccines provide protection. Some parents are demanding that their children be given each of the MMR vaccines separately, but this policy could allow infections to occur during the interval between each vaccination. In any case, there is no published evidence for or against the safety of this procedure as compared with giving the combined MMR vaccine. Despite the lack of objective scientific evidence to show that MMR vaccination can be associated with ASD, the controversy still rages.

Migration and Ethnicity

A significantly higher prevalence rate for autism was reported among children of first-generation immigrant parents in the studies in Camberwell (Wing & Gould, 1979), Gothenburg (Gillberg et al., 1991; see also Gillberg, Steffenburg, Borjesson, & Andersson, 1987), and Mölnlycke (Arvidsson et al., 1997). Akinsola and Fryers (1986) reported a higher rate of "social impairments" among children of immigrants in Manchester, England. Goodman and Richards (1995) found a higher proportion of autistic disorders in children born to Afro-Caribbean immigrants than in children born to parents who were both born in Britain. The study in Ibaraki (Tanoue et al., 1988) showed a higher prevalence of autism among children with parents who had moved to the area from other parts of Japan. Six other studies in Table 2.1 (Ritvo et al., 1989; Webb, Lobo, Hervas, Scourfield, & Fraser, 1997; Powell et al., 2000; Mágnússon & Saemundsen, 2001; Bertrand et al., 2001; Croen et al., 2002) and one in Table 2.2 (Keen & Ward, 2004) found no evidence to support the hypothesis of a raised prevalence in children with immigrant parents. The question remains whether *first*-generation immigrants face environmental hazards against which they are unprotected compared with the resident population, which would include those whose ancestors were immigrants more than one generation ago. The effect of maternal rubella among children of first-generation immigrants from the Caribbean noted in the Camberwell study (Wing & Gould, 1979) is one example. Another possibility is that parents who are likely for genetic reasons to have children with ASD tend to migrate more often than others, but no scientific evidence on this is available. In contrast to other findings, one study in Israel (Kamer, Zohar, & Youngman, 2004) found a significantly higher rate of PDD among native Israeli children than among all immigrant children.

The possible effect of ethnic origin is a different question from that of migration. All the studies listed in Tables 2.1 and 2.2 were carried out in Europe, North America, or Japan. The published studies do not provide evidence for or against the possibility that particular regions, countries, or areas within countries, or particular ethnic groups, differ significantly in their prevalence rates. As noted below, the marked tendency shown in Table 2.1 for studies in Japan to find higher rates was probably due to the method of case finding. Table 2.2 shows that rates in other countries have now caught up with Japanese rates. Fombonne (2005a) examined in detail the problems of evaluating findings in prevalence studies of autistic disorders, including the effect of immigrant status, and concluded that the hypothesis of higher prevalence among immigrants or particular ethnic groups has not been supported by proper statistical analysis of results so far. The same author (Fombonne, 2005b) suggests that in the future, more sophisticated studies of this and other issues might provide clearer answers. Dyches, Wilder, Sudweeks, Obiakor, and Algozzine (2004) have noted how little is known about the relationship of migration, ethnicity, and autism— either concerning prevalence or concerning how families from different ethnic backgrounds cope with the stresses. They emphasize the importance of research on this subject.

HAS THERE BEEN A TRUE INCREASE IN NUMBERS?

Even if MMR vaccination is not responsible for the increase in numbers, it is still possible that there is a real and continuing rise. From the evidence presented, some or all the factors discussed above have contributed to the observed rise in rates of ASD, but there is no certainty as to how much of the rise they explain.

Evidence against a True Increase

In the section above on possible causes of a hypothetical real increase, some of the causes discussed might have caused a rise in incidence and therefore prevalence, but it is unlikely that any of them would have had more than a very small effect.

Three small but intensive studies, one in Camberwell and two in Gothenburg, are of particular interest when we consider the possibility of a rise in rates from whatever cause. In the Camberwell study (Wing & Gould, 1979), because of the methodology used, only 3 children among those identified as having ASD had an overall IQ of 70 or above. The rest, a total of 71 children under age 15 years, had an IQ under 70. The age-specific prevalence for all ASD based on these 71 children was 20 per 10,000 children under age 15 years. A study in Gothenburg (Gillberg, Persson, Grufman, & Themner, 1986), also counting all ASD in those with IQ under 70 using comparable diagnostic criteria, found 18 per 10,000—very close to the Camberwell finding. A later study in Gothenburg (Ehlers & Gillberg, 1993) examined children ages 13–17 with IQ of 70 and above, in order to identify all with high-functioning ASD. The age-specific rates found were 36 per 10,000 for Asperger syndrome diagnosed according to Gillberg's criteria, and 35 per 10,000 for children with social impairment but not the full criteria for Asperger syndrome. Adding all the findings from the two Gothenburg studies gave a rate of 89 per 10,000 for all IQ levels and all ASD.

The important point about these studies is that the Camberwell children were born in the years 1956–1970, the Gothenburg children with IQ under 70 were born in 1966–1970, and the Gothenburg children with IQ of 70 and above were born in 1975–1983. In other words, all these children were born well before the time when rising numbers began to be reported, but the rate found for the whole IQ range and the whole spectrum was higher than in all but two of the other studies in Table 2.1—one in Tokyo (Tomita, 1998) giving almost the same rate (90 per 10,000), and the other a very small-scale study in Karlstad, Sweden (Kadesjö et al., 1999) reporting a rate of 120 per 10,000. Among studies carried out after 2002, one for the whole of Great Britain (Green et al., 2005) gave the closely similar prevalence of 90 per 10,000, and one in the South Thames region of London (Baird et al., 2006) gave a prevalence of 116 per 10,000.

Taken at face value, these findings suggest that if the case finding had been as thorough and the same criteria for the whole autism spectrum had been applied in all the early epidemiological studies, the rates found would have been higher even than most of those found recently. Furthermore, the annual rise in incidence found in the studies quoted above would have been likely to continue until all children with ASD were diagnosed in their preschool years.

However, the findings have to be viewed with caution. The Camberwell and Gothenburg studies of children with IQ under 70 had total populations of children in the age range studied of approximately 35,000 and 24,000, respectively, whereas the Gothenburg study of the more able children had a total population in the age range of only 1,519 children. Nevertheless, it should be noted that the studies were particularly intensive, and that all the children who were suspected of having an ASD were examined in detail by the researchers.

Prevalence among Adults

If the numbers of children with ASD have always been so large, it is legitimate to ask where all the adults are with these conditions. Many are still living with their parents. Some are in residential homes, either specifically for individuals with ASD or for persons with a variety of disabilities. Torben, Mouridsen, and Rich (1999) followed up 341 children with ASD for an average of 24 years, until they were 14–48 years old, and found a crude mortality rate of 3.5%—almost double the expected rate for the general population of the same age.

The findings reported above concerning adults diagnosed with mental retardation or mental illness suggest that there is an unknown but possibly large number of adults with undiagnosed ASD among these groups. The social impairment can lead such individuals into conflict with the law, and some may be found in special hospitals (Hare et al., 1999; Scragg & Shah, 1994). Although clinical experience has shown that there are some people with ASD in prisons and others who are homeless and living on the streets, no relevant epidemiological studies have yet been published. Follow-up studies show a wide variation in outcome, from total dependence to full independence in adult life (Gillberg, 1991; Howlin, 2000; Larsen & Mouridsen, 1997; Rutter, 1970), but no studies of the overall prevalence of ASD in adults of any age have been done. One of the many difficulties of such a study would be the identification of adults with ASD who are of high ability and who are well adjusted in their work and personal lives. This brings up the problem of deciding whether to include or exclude those who are not in need of any services. Some may have had difficulties as children that would have made them eligible for an ASD in their childhood, but overcame these to become independent as adults. There are no easy answers to such questions.

SUGGESTIONS FOR FUTURE RESEARCH

A number of authors have discussed possible reasons for the rise in the reported prevalence of ASD (including Charman, 2002; Prior, 2003; Tidmarsh & Volkmar, 2003; Gernsbacher, Dawson, & Goldsmith, 2005; Fombonne, 2005a, b; Rutter, 2005; Williams, Higgins, & Brayne, 2006). All agree that much, if not all, of the reported rise in incidence and prevalence is due to considerable widening of diagnostic criteria and to greater awareness among both parents and professionals. They also agree that it remains an open question whether there has also been a genuine rise in the numbers of children with ASD—and, if so, what the reasons are, how large it is, and whether it is still continuing. The findings of this chapter are in line with these conclusions.

It is not possible to return to the past in order to apply current diagnostic criteria to all the early studies. The question of whether there are really more children with ASD now than in the past cannot be answered definitively. Some studies can be done to examine aspects of the problems of incidence and prevalence. For example, Kanner's very strict criteria as used in Lotter's (1966) study could be applied to any new prevalence study, in addition to the much wider criteria for ASD now in use. This might indicate whether the rate for this particular subgroup has changed.

Research on MMR vaccination is important, because parental concern has led to a drop in the numbers of children being vaccinated—with the consequent danger of epidemics of measles, mumps, or rubella, all of which can cause long-term disability or death in a small but significant number of children. A study in which children were assessed regularly for any features of ASD from birth until 5 years of age, when the diagnosis should be clear for most participants, would be of interest. It would not be ethical to demand that some be given MMR vaccine in one dose, that some receive it in separate injections, and that some not be vaccinated at all, but the parents' own decisions are likely to vary. It would be appropriate to ensure the inclusion of some siblings of children with ASD, because they are known to have a higher risk of developing such conditions. At least one large population cohort of children exists who were screened for communication impairment at 18 months (Baird et al., 2000). They have been followed up, and those with autism, those with developmental disorders without autism, and those with typical development have been identified. A cohort of this kind would provide the basis for a detailed study of a potential causal role for MMR vaccination and abnormalities of the immune system. Examination of the hypotheses concerning MMR vaccine, ASD, and abnormalities in the bowel would be helpful, but performing ileocolonoscopy in children for research purposes presents major ethical problems.

Establishing the age of onset for each child with an ASD is crucial for studies of incidence and for examining the significance of any environmental factors operating before or after birth. It is also important for investigation of the so-called "regressive" autism. In order to develop infant assessment methods, more work is needed on the behavior and abilities of babies who are later found to have an ASD. Again, the siblings of children with ASD would be appropriate participants, but children who possibly have other types of developmental disorders and those likely to have typical development should also be included for comparison.

The problem underlying all research into the causes of ASD is that the human and financial resources required to carry out any studies that can answer the questions considered in this chapter would be immense. The numbers of participating infants and children required in order to be sure of finding enough with ASD to give statistically meaningful results are daunting. This will continue to be the case unless and until reliable physical or psychological methods of identifying these conditions are found. The effort and cost of large-scale studies would be worthwhile if clear-cut results were obtained. However, regardless of the reasons, the prevalence of ASD is much higher than the first epidemiological studies suggested, and this has major implications for all the individuals, their families, and the helping agencies involved.

ACKNOWLEDGMENT

This chapter is adapted from Wing and Potter (2002). Copyright 2002 by John Wiley & Sons, Inc. Adapted by permission.

REFERENCES

Akinsola, H., & Fryers, T. (1986). A comparison of patterns of disability in severely mentally handicapped children of different ethnic origins. *Psychological Medicine, 16,* 127–133.

American Psychiatric Association. (1980). *Diagnostic and statistical manual of mental disorders* (3rd ed.). Washington, DC: Author.

American Psychiatric Association. (1987). *Diagnostic and statistical manual of mental disorders* (3rd ed., rev.). Washington, DC: Author.

American Psychiatric Association. (1994). *Diagnostic and statistical manual of mental disorders* (4th ed.). Washington, DC: Author.

American Psychiatric Association. (2000). *Diagnostic and statistical manual of mental disorders* (4th ed., text rev.). Washington, DC: Author.

Arvidsson, T., Danielsson, B., Forsberg, P., Gillberg, C., Johansson, M., & Kjellgren, G. (1997). Autism in 3–6 year-old children in a suburb of Goteborg, Sweden. *Autism 1,* 163–171.

Asperger, H. (1991). 'Autistic psychopathy' in childhood (U. Frith, Trans.). In U. Frith (Ed.), *Autism and Asperger syndrome* (pp. 37–92). Cambridge, UK: Cambridge University Press. (Original work published 1944)

Baird, G., Charman, T., Baron-Cohen, S., Cox, A., Swettenham, J., Wheelwright, S., et al. (2000). A screening instrument for autism at 18 months of age: A 6 year follow-up study. *Journal of the American Academy of Child and Adolescent Psychiatry, 39,* 694–702.

Baird, G., Simonoff, E., Pickles, A., Chandler, S., Loucas, T., Meldrum, D., et al. (2006). Prevalence of disorders of the autistic spectrum in a population cohort of children in South Thames: The Special Needs and Autism Project (SNAP). *Lancet, 368,* 210–215.

Baranek, G. T. (1999). Autism during infancy: A retrospective video analysis of sensory–motor and social behaviors at 9–12 months of age. *Journal of Autism and Developmental Disorders, 29,* 213–224.

Baron-Cohen, S. (2006). Two new theories of autism: Hyper-systematising and assortative mating. *Archives of Disease in Childhood, 91,* 2–5.

Baron-Cohen, S., Ring, H., Chitnis, X., Wheelwright, S., Gregory, L., Williams, S., et al. (2006). fMRI of parents of children with Asperger syndrome: A pilot study. *Brain and Cognition, 61,* 122–130.

Beadle-Brown, J., Murphy, G., Wing, L., Gould, J., Shah, A., & Holmes, N. (2002). Changes in social impairment for people with intellectual disabilities: A follow-up of the Camberwell cohort. *Journal of Autism and Developmental Disorders, 32,* 195–206.

Bejerot, S., Nylander, L., & Lindstrom, E. (2001). Autistic traits in obsessive–compulsive disorder. *Nordic Journal of Psychiatry, 55,* 169–176.

Bertrand, J., Mars, A., Boyle, C., Bove, F., Yeargin-Allsop, M., & Decoufle, P. (2001). Prevalence of autism in a United States population: The Brick Township, New Jersey, investigation. *Pediatrics, 108,* 1155–1161.

Black, C., Kaye, J. A., & Jick, H. (2002). Relation of childhood gastrointestinal disorders to autism: Nested case–control study using data from the UK General Practice Research Database. *British Medical Journal, 325,* 419–421.

Blaxill, M. F., Baskin, D. S., & Spitzer, W. A. (2003). Commentary: Blaxill, Baskin and Spitzer on Croen et al. (2002). "The changing prevalence of autism in California." *Journal of Autism and Developmental Disorders, 33,* 223–226.

Bleuler E. (1950). *Dementia praecox or the group of schizophrenias* (J. Zinkin, Trans.) New York: International Universities Press. (Original work published 1911)

Bohman, M., Bohman, I., Bjorck, P., & Sjoholm, E. (1983). Childhood psychosis in a northern Swedish county: Some preliminary findings from an epidemiological survey. In M. Schmidt & H. Remschmidt (Eds.), *Epidemiological approaches in child psychiatry: II* (pp. 164–173). New York: Thieme-Stratton.

Bolton, P., Macdonald, H., Pickles, A., Bios, P., Goode, S., Crowson, M., et al. (1994). A case–control family history study of autism. *Journal of Child Psychology and Psychiatry, 35,* 877–900.

Brask, B. H. (1972). A prevalence investigation of childhood psychoses. In *Nordic Symposium on the Comprehensive Care of Psychotic Children* (pp. 145–153). Oslo: Barnepsykiatrist Forening.

Brook, S. L., & Bowler, D. M. (1992). Autism by another name?: Semantic and pragmatic impairments in children. *Journal of Autism and Developmental Disorders, 22,* 61–81.

Bryson, S. E., Clark, B. S., & Smith, I. M. (1988). First report of a Canadian epidemiological study of autistic syndromes. *Journal of Child Psychology and Psychiatry, 29,* 433–446.

Burd, L., Fisher, W., & Kerbeshian, J. (1987). A prevalence study of pervasive developmental disorders in North Dakota. *Journal of the American Academy of Child and Adolescent Psychiatry, 26,* 704–710.

Chakrabarti, S., & Fombonne, E. (2001). Pervasive developmental disorder in preschool children. *Journal of the American Medical Association, 285,* 3093–3099.

Chakrabarti, S., & Fombonne, E. (2005). Pervasive developmental disorder in preschool children: Confirmation of high prevalence. *American Journal of Psychiatry, 162,* 1133–1141.

Charman, T. (2002). The prevalence of autism spectrum disorders: Recent evidence and future challenges. *European Child and Adolescent Psychiatry, 11,* 249–256.

Chen, R. T., & De Stefano, F. (1998). Vaccine adverse effects: Causal or coincidental? *Lancet, 351,* 611–612.

Cialdella, P., & Mamelle, N. (1989). An epidemiological study of infantile autism in a French department (Rhone): A research note. *Journal of Child Psychology and Psychiatry, 30,* 165–176.

Creswell, C. S., & Skuse, D. H. (1999). Autism in association with Turner syndrome: Genetic implications for male vulnerability to pervasive developmental disorders. *NeuroCase, 5,* 511–518.

Croen, L., & Grether, K. G. (2003). Response: A response to Blaxill, Baskin and Spitzer on Croen et al. (2002). "The changing prevalence of autism in California." *Journal of Autism and Developmental Disorders, 33,* 227–230.

Croen, L., Grether, J., Hoogstrate, J. & Selvin, S. (2002). The changing prevalence of autism in California. *Journal of Autism and Developmental Disorders, 32,* 207–215.

Dales, L., Hammer, S. J., & Smith, N. J. (2001). Time trends in autism and in MMR immunization coverage in California. *Journal of the American Medical Association, 285*(1), 183–1185.

DeMyer, M. (1975). Research in infantile autism: A strategy and its results. *Biological Psychiatry, 10,* 433–452.

Denckla, M. B. (1986). Editorial: New diagnostic criteria for autism and related behavior disorders: Guidelines for research protocols. *Journal of the American Academy of Child and Adolescent Psychiatry, 25,* 221–224.

Dyches, T. T., Wilder, L. K., Sudweeks, R. R., Obiakor, F. E.. & Algozzine, B. (2004). Multicultural issues in autism. *Journal of Autism and Developmental Disorders, 34,* 211–222.

Ehlers, S., & Gillberg, C. (1993). The epidemiology of Asperger syndrome. A total population study. *Journal of Child Psychology and Psychiatry, 34,* 1327–1350.

Ehlers, S., Gillberg, C., & Wing, L. (1999). A screening questionnaire for Asperger syndrome and other high functioning autistic spectrum disorders in school-age children. *Journal of Autism and Developmental Disorders, 29,* 129–141.

Fombonne, E. (2001). What is the prevalence of Asperger disorder? *Journal of Autism and Developmental Disorders, 31,* 363–364.

Fombonne, E. (2005a). Epidemiological studies of pervasive developmental disorders. In F. Volkmar, R. Paul, A. Klin, D. & Cohen (Eds.) *Handbook of autism and pervasive developmental disorders* (3rd ed., Vol 1, pp. 42–69). Hoboken, NJ: Wiley.

Fombonne, E. (2005b). The changing epidemiology of autism. *Journal of Applied Research in Intellectual Disabilities, 18,* 281–290.

Fombonne, E., & Chakrabarti, S. (2001). No evidence for a new variant of measles–mumps–rubella-induced autism. *Pediatrics, 108,* E58.

Fombonne, E., & Du Mazaubrun, C. (1992). Prevalence of infantile autism in four French regions. *Social Psychiatry and Psychiatric Epidemiology, 27,* 203–210.

Fombonne, E., Du Mazaubrun, C., Cans, C. & Grandjean, H. (1997). Autism and associated medical disorders in a French epidemiological survey. *Journal of the American Academy of Child and Adolescent Psychiatry, 36,* 1561–1569.

Fombonne, E., Simmons, H., Ford, T. Meltzer, H., & Goodman, R. (2001). Prevalence of pervasive developmental disorder in the British Nationwide Survey of Child Mental Health. *Journal of the American Academy of Child and Adolescent Psychiatry, 40,* 820–827.

Fombonne, E., Zakarian, R., Bennett, A. Meng, L., & McLean-Heywood, D. (2006). Pervasive developmental disorders in Montréal, Québec, Canada: Prevalence and links with immunisations. *Paediatrics, 118,* e139–e150.

Frith, U. (1991). Asperger and his syndrome. In U. Frith (Ed.), *Autism and Asperger syndrome* (pp. 1–36). Cambridge, UK: Cambridge University Press.

Gernsbacher, M., Dawson, M., & Goldsmith, H. (2005). Three reasons not to believe in an autism epidemic. *Current Directions in Psychological Science, 14,* 55–58.

Gillberg, C. (1984). Infantile autism and other childhood psychoses in a Swedish urban region: Epidemiological aspects. *Journal of Child Psychology and Psychiatry, 25,* 35–43.

Gillberg, C. (1986). Onset at age 14 of a typical autistic syndrome: A case report of a girl with herpes simplex encephalitis. *Journal of Autism and Developmental Disorders, 16,* 369–375.

Gillberg, C. (1991). Outcome in autism and autistic-like conditions. *Journal of the American Academy of Child and Adolescent Psychiatry, 30,* 375–382.

Gillberg, C., & Billstedt, E. (2000). Autism and Asperger syndrome: Coexistence with other clinical disorders. *Acta Psychiatrica Scandinavica, 102,* 321–330.

Gillberg, C., & Coleman, M. (1996). Autism and medical disorders: a review of the literature. *Developmental Medicine and Child Neurology, 38,* 191–202.

Gillberg, C., Cederlund, M., Lamberg, K., & Zeijion, L. (2006). Brief report: "The autism epidemic." The registered prevalence of autism in a Swedish urban area. *Journal of Autism and Developmental Disorders, 36,* 429–435.

Gillberg, C., Gillberg, C., Rastam, M., & Wentz, E. (2001). Asperger Syndrome (and high functioning autism) Diagnostic Interview (ASDI): A preliminary study of a new structured clinical interview. *Autism, 5,* 57–66.

Gillberg, C., Persson, E., Grufman, M., & Themner, U. (1986). Psychiatric disorders in mildly and severely mentally retarded urban children and adolescents: Epidemiological aspects. *British Journal of Psychiatry, 149,* 68–74.

Gillberg, C., & Rastam, M. (1992). Do some cases of anorexia nervosa reflect underlying autistic-like conditions? *Behavioural Neurology, 5,* 27–32.

Gillberg, C., Steffenburg, S., Borjesson, B., & Andersson, L. (1987). Infantile autism in children of immigrant parents: A population-based study from Göteborg, Sweden. *British Journal of Psychiatry, 150,* 856–857.

Gillberg, C., Steffenburg, S., & Schaumann, H. (1991). Is autism more common now than ten years ago? *British Journal of Psychiatry, 158,* 403–409.

Goodman, R., & Richards, H. (1995). Child and adolescent psychiatric presentations of second-generation Afro-Caribbeans in Britain. *British Journal of Psychiatry, 167,* 362–369.

Green, H., McGinnity, A., Meltzer, H., Ford, T., & Goodman, R. (2005). *Mental health of children and young people in Great Britain 2004.* Basingstoke, UK: Palgrave Macmillan.

Gurney, J. G., Fritz, M. S., Ness, K. K. Sievers, P., Newschaffer, C. J., & Shapiro, E. G. (2003). Analysis of the prevalence trends of autism spectrum disorder in Minnesota. *Archives of Pediatrics and Adolescent Medicine, 157,* 622–627.

Hare, D., Gould, J., Mills, R., & Wing, L. (1999). *A preliminary study of individuals with autistic spectrum disorders in three special hospitals in England.* London: National Autistic Society.

Herguner, S., & Mukaddes, N. M., (2006). Autism and Williams syndrome: A case report. *World Journal of Biological Psychiatry, 7,* 186–188.

Hermelin, B., & O'Connor, N. (1970). *Psychological experiments with autistic children.* Oxford: Pergamon Press.

Honda, H., Shimizu, Y., Imai, M., & Nitto, Y (2005). Cumulative incidence of childhood autism: A total population study of better accuracy and precision. *Developmental Medicine and Child Neurology, 47,* 10–18.

Honda, H., Shimizu, Y., Misumi, K., Nimi, M., & Ohashi, Y. (1996). Cumulative incidence and prevalence of childhood autism in children in Japan. *British Journal of Psychiatry, 169,* 228–235.

Hoshino, Y., Kumashiro, H., Yashima, Y., Tachibana, R., & Watanabe, M. (1982). The epidemiological study of autism in Fukushima-ken. *Folio Psychiatrica et Neurologica Japonica, 36,* 115–124.

Howlin, P. (2000). Outcome in adult life for more able individuals with autism and Asperger syndrome. *Autism, 4,* 63–83.

Howlin, P., & Asgharian, A. (1999). The diagnosis of autism and Asperger syndrome: Findings from a survey of 770 families. *Developmental Medicine and Child Neurology, 41,* 834–839.

Howlin, P., Karpf, J., & Turk, J. (2005). Behavioural characteristics and autistic features in individuals with Cohen syndrome. *European Journal of Child and Adolescent Psychiatry, 40,* 57–64.

Howlin, P., Wing, L., & Gould, J. (1995). The recognition of autism in children with Down syndrome: Implications for intervention and some speculations about pathology. *Developmental Medicine and Child Neurology, 37,* 398–414.

Hunt, A., & Dennis, J. (1987). Psychiatric disorder among children with tuberous sclerosis. *Developmental Medicine and Child Neurology, 29,* 190–198.

Ishii, T., & Takahashi, O. (1983). The epidemiology of autistic children in Toyota, Japan: Prevalence. *Japanese Journal of Child and Adolescent Psychiatry, 24,* 311–321.

Kadesjö, B., & Gillberg, C. (2000). Tourette's disorder: Epidemiology and comorbidity in primary school children. *Journal of the American Academy of Child and Adolescent Psychiatry, 39,* 548–555.

Kadesjö, B., Gillberg, C., & Hagberg, B. (1999). Brief report: Autism and Asperger syndrome in seven-year-old children. *Journal of Autism and Developmental Disorders, 29,* 327–332.

Kamer, A., Zohar, A., & Youngman, R. (2004). A prevalence estimate of pervasive developmental disorder among immigrants to Israel and Israeli natives: A file review study. *Social Psychiatry and Psychiatric Epidemiology, 39,* 141–145.

Kanner, L. (1943). Autistic disturbances of affective contact. *Nervous Child, 2,* 217–250.

Kanner, L., & Eisenberg, L. (1956). Early infantile autism, 1943–1955. *American Journal of Orthopsychiatry, 26,* 55–65.

Kaye, J. A., Melero-Montes, M., & Jick, H. (2001). Mumps measles and rubella vaccine and the incidence of autism recorded by general practitioners: A time trend analysis. *British Medical Journal, 322,* 460–463.

Keen, D., & Ward, S. (2004). Autistic spectrum disorder: A child population profile. *Autism, 8,* 39–48.

Kielinen, M., Linna, S.-L., & Moilanen, I. (2000). Autism in northern Finland. *European Child and Adolescent Psychiatry, 9,* 162–167.

Kielinen, M., Rantala, M., Timonen, E. Linna, S.-L., & Moilanen, I. (2004). Associated medical disorders and disabilities in children with autistic disorder: A population-based study.*Autism, 8,* 49–60.

Kolvin, I. (1971). Studies in the childhood psychoses: I. Diagnostic criteria and classification. *British Journal of Psychiatry, 118,* 381–384.

Larsen, F. W., & Mouridsen, S. E. (1997). The outcome in children with childhood autism and Asperger syndrome originally diagnosed as psychotic: A 30-year follow-up study of subjects hospitalised as children. *European Child and Adolescent Psychiatry, 6,* 181–190.

Lauritsen, M., Pedersen, C., & Mortensen, P. (2004). The incidence and prevalence of pervasive developmental disorders: A Danish population-based study. *Psychological Medicine, 34,* 1339–1346.

Leekam, S., Libby, S., Wing, L., Gould, J., & Gillberg, C. (2000). Comparison of ICD-10 and Gillberg's criteria for Asperger syndrome. *Autism, 4,* 11–28.

Lingam, R., Simmons, A., Andrews, N., Miller, E., Stowe, J., & Taylor, B. (2003). Prevalence of autism and parentally reported triggers in a north east London population. *Archives of Disease in Childhood, 88,* 666–670.

Lord, C., Risi, S., Lambrecht, L., Cook, E. H., Leventhal, B. L., DiLavore, P. C., et al., (2000). The Autism Diagnostic Observation Schedule—Generic: A standard measure of social and communication deficits associated with the spectrum of autism. *Journal of Autism and Developmental Disorders, 30,* 205–223.

Lord, C., Rutter, M., & Le Couteur, A. (1994). Autism Diagnostic Interview—Revised: a revised version of a diagnostic interview for caregivers of individuals with possible pervasive developmental disorders. *Journal of Autism and Developmental Disorders, 24,* 659–686.

Lotter, V. (1966). Epidemiology of autistic conditions in young children: I. Prevalence. *Social Psychiatry, 1,* 124–137.

Mágnússon, P., & Sæmundsen, E. (2001). Prevalence of autism in Iceland. *Journal of Autism and Developmental Disorders, 31,* 153–163.

Matsuishi, T., Shiotsuki, Y., Yoshimura, K., Shoji, H., Imuta, F., & Yamashita, F. (1987). High prevalence of infantile autism in Kurume City. *Japanese Journal of Child Neurology, 2,* 268–271.

McCarthy, P., Fitzgerald, M., & Smith, M. (1984). Prevalence of childhood autism in Ireland. *Irish Medical Journal, 77,* 129–130.

Miyazaki, K., Narita, N., & Narita, M. (2005). Maternal administration of thalidomide or valproic acid causes abnormal serotonergic neurons in the offspring: Implications for pathogenesis of autism. *Journal of Developmental Neuroscience, 23,* 287–297.

Montes, G., & Halterman, J. (2006). Characteristics of school-age children with autism. *Journal of Developmental and Behavioral Pediatrics, 27,* 379–385.

Muhle, R., Trentacoste, S. V., & Rapin, I. (2004). The genetics of autism. *Pediatrics, 113,* 72–86.

Nanson, J. (1993). Autism in the foetal alcohol syndrome: A report of six cases. *Alcoholism: Clinical and Experimental Research, 17,* 926–928.

Nylander, L., & Gillberg, C. (2001). Screening for autism spectrum disorders in adult psychiatric out-patients: A preliminary report. *Acta Psychiatrica Scandinavica, 103,* 428–434.

Posserud, M., Lundervold, A., & Gillberg, C. (2006). Autistic features in a total population of 7–9-year-old children assessed by the ASSQ (Autism Spectrum Screening Questionnaire). *Journal of Child Psychology and Psychiatry, 47,* 167–175.

Powell, J. E., Edwards, A., Edwards, M., Pandit, B. S., Sungum-Paliwal, S. R., & Whitehouse, W. (2000). Changes in the incidence of childhood autism and other autistic spectrum disorders in preschool children from two areas of the West Midlands, UK. *Developmental Medicine and Child Neurology, 42,* 624–628.

Prior, M. (2003). Is there an increase in the prevalence of autism spectrum disorders? *Journal of Paediatrics and Child Health, 39,* 81–82.

Rapin, I., & Dunn, M. (1997). Language disorders in children with autism. *Seminars in Pediatric Neurology, 4,* 86–89.

Reichenberg, A., Gross, R., Weiser, M., Bresnahan, M., Silverman, J., Harlap, S., et al. (2006). Advancing paternal age and autism. *Archives of General Psychiatry, 63,* 1026–1032.

Richler, J., Luyster, R., Risi, S., Hsu, W.-L., Dawson, G., Bernier, R., et al. (2006). Is there a 'regressive phenotype' of autism spectrum disorder associated with the measles–mumps–rubella vaccine?: A CPEA study. *Journal of Autism and Developmental Disorders, 36,* 299–360.

Ritvo, E. R., Freeman, B. J., Pingree, C., Mason-Brothers, A., Jorde, L., Jenson, W. R., et al. (1989). The UCLA–University of Utah epidemiological study of autism: Prevalence. *American Journal of Psychiatry, 146,* 194–245.

Rodier, P., Ingram, H., Tisdale, B., & Croog, V. (1997). Linking aetiologies in humans and animal models: Studies of autism. *Reproductive Toxicology, 11,* 417–422.

Rutter, M. (1970). Autistic children: Infancy to adulthood. *Seminars in Psychiatry, 2,* 435–450.

Rutter, M. (1978). Diagnosis and definition. In M. Rutter & E. Schopler (Eds.).

Autism: A reappraisal of concepts and treatment (pp. 1–25). New York: Plenum Press.

Rutter, M. (2000). Genetic studies of autism: From the 1970s into the millennium. *Journal of Abnormal Child Psychology, 28,* 3–14.

Rutter, M. (2005). Incidence of autism spectrum disorders: Changes over time and their meaning. *Acta Paediatrica, 94,* 2–15.

Ryan, R. M. (1992). Treatment resistant chronic mental illness: Is it Asperger's syndrome? *Hospital and Community Psychiatry, 48,* 807–811.

Schopler, E., & Reichler, R. J. (Eds.). (1976). *Psychopathology and child development: Research and treatment.* New York: Plenum Press.

Scott, F., Baron-Cohen, S., Bolton, P., & Brayne, C. (2002). Brief report: Prevalence of autism spectrum conditions in children aged 5 to 11 years in Cambridgeshire. *Autism, 6,* 231–238.

Scragg, P., & Shah, A. (1994). Prevalence of Asperger's syndrome in a secure hospital. *British Journal of Psychiatry, 165,* 679–682.

Shah, A., Holmes, N., & Wing, L. (1982). Prevalence of autism and related conditions in adults in a mental handicap hospital. *Applied Research in Mental Retardation, 3,* 303–317.

Skuse, D., Warrington, R., Bishop, D. Chowdhury, U., Lau, J., Mandy, W., et al. (2004). The Developmental, Dimensional and Diagnostic Interview (3di): A novel computerized assessment for autism spectrum disorders. *Journal of the American Academy of Child and Adolescent Psychiatry, 43,* 548–558.

Smeeth, L., Cook, C., Fombonne, E., Heavey, L., Rodriguez, L. C., Smith, P. G., et al. (2004). Rate of first recorded diagnosis of autism and other pervasive developmental disorders in United Kingdom general practice 1988 to 2001. Retrieved from www.biomedcentral.com/1741-7015/2/39.

Smith, I. (2000). Motor functioning in Asperger syndrome. In A. Klin, F. R. Volkmar, & S. S. Sparrow (Eds.), *Asperger syndrome* (pp. 97–124). New York: Guilford Press.

Sponheim, E., & Skjeldal, O. (1998). Autism and related disorders in a Norwegian study using ICD-10 diagnostic criteria. *Journal of Autism and Developmental Disorders, 28,* 217–227.

Steffenburg, S., & Gillberg, C. (1986). Autism and autistic-like conditions in Swedish rural and urban areas: A population study. *British Journal of Psychiatry, 149,* 81–87.

Steinhausen, H., Gobel, D., Breinlinger, M., & Wohlleben, B. (1986). A community survey of infantile autism. *Journal of the American Academy of Child Psychiatry, 25,* 186–189.

Sugiyama, T., & Abe, T. (1989). The prevalence of autism in Nagoya, Japan: A total population study. *Journal of Autism and Developmental Disorders, 19,* 87–96.

Tanoue, Y., Oda, S., Asano, F., & Kawashima, K. (1988). Epidemiology of infantile autism in the Southern Ibaraki, Japan. *Journal of Autism and Developmental Disorders, 18,* 155–167.

Tantam, D. (1988). Lifelong eccentricity and social isolation: I. Psychiatric, social and forensic aspects. *British Journal of Psychiatry, 153,* 777–782.

Taylor, B., Miller, E., Farrington, C. P., Petropoulos, M. C., Favot-Mayaud,

I., Li, J., et al. (1999). Autism and measles, mumps and rubella vaccine: No epidemiological evidence for a causal association. *Lancet, 353,* 2026–2029.

Tidmarsh, L., & Volkmar, F. (2003). Diagnosis and epidemiology of autism spectrum disorders. *Canadian Journal of Psychiatry, 48,* 517–525.

Torben, I., Mouridsen, S., & Rich, B. (1999). Mortality and causes of death in pervasive developmental disorders. *Autism, 3,* 7–16.

Tomita, M. (1998). *Prevalence, subgroups, developmental level and polarization of preschool autistic spectrum children assessed in Japanese community.* Paper presented at the 39th Annual Conference of the Japanese Association of Child and Adolescent Psychiatry, Tokyo.

Treffert, D. A. (1970). Epidemiology of infantile autism. *Archives of General Psychiatry, 22,* 431–438.

Turk, J., & Graham, P. (1997). Fragile X syndrome, autism and autistic features. *Autism, 1,* 175–197.

Volkmar, F. R., Cicchetti, D. V., & Bregman, J. (1992). Three diagnostic systems for autism: DSM-III, DSM-III-R and ICD-10. *Journal of Autism and Developmental Disorders, 22,* 483–492.

Volkmar, F. R., Stier, D. M., & Cohen, D. J. (1985). Age of recognition of pervasive developmental disorder. *American Journal of Psychiatry, 142,* 1450–1452.

Wakefield, A. J., & Montgomery, S. (2000). Measles mumps rubella vaccine: through a glass darkly. *Adverse Drug Reactions and Toxicological Reviews, 19,* 265–283.

Wakefield, A, J., Murch, S. H., Anthony, A., Linnell, J., Casson, D. M., Malik, M., et al. (1998). Ileal–lymphoid–nodular hyperplasia, non-specific colitis and pervasive developmental disorder in children. *Lancet, 351,* 637–641.

Webb, E. V., Lobo, S., Hervas, A., Scourfield, J., & Fraser, W. I. (1997). The changing prevalence of autistic disorder in a Welsh health district. *Developmental Medicine and Child Neurology, 39,* 150–152.

Webb, E., Morey, J., Thompson, W., Butler, C., Barber, M., & Fraser, W. I. (2003). Prevalence of autistic spectrum disorder in mainstream schools in a Welsh education authority. *Developmental Medicine and Child Neurology, 45,* 377–384.

Werner, E., Dawson, G., Osterling, J., & Dinno, N. (2000). Brief report: Recognition of autism spectrum disorder before one year of age: A retrospective study based on home videotapes. *Journal of Autism and Developmental Disorders, 30,* 157–162.

Williams, G., King, J., Cunningham, M., Stephan, M., Kerr, B., & Hersh, J. H. (2001). Fetal valproate syndrome and autism: Additional evidence of an association. *Developmental Medicine and Child Neurology, 43,* 202–206.

Williams, J., Higgins, J., & Brayne, C. (2006). Systematic review of prevalence studies of autism spectrum disorders. *Archives of Disease in Childhood, 91,* 8–15.

Wing, L. (1980). Childhood autism and social class: A question of selection? *British Journal of Psychiatry, 137,* 410–417.

Wing, L. (1981). Asperger's syndrome: A clinical account. *Psychological Medicine, 11,* 115–130.

Wing, L. (2001). *The autistic spectrum: A parent's guide to understanding and helping your child.* Berkeley, CA: Ulysses Press.

Wing, L. (2005). Reflections on opening Pandora's box. *Journal of Autism and Developmental Disorders, 35,* 197–203.

Wing, L., & Gould, J. (1978). Systematic recording of behaviours and skills of retarded and psychotic children. *Journal of Autism and Childhood Schizophrenia, 8,* 79–97.

Wing, L., & Gould, J. (1979). Severe impairments of social interaction and associated abnormalities in children: Epidemiology and classification. *Journal of Autism and Developmental Disorders, 9,* 11–29.

Wing, L., Leekam, S., Libby, S., Gould, J., & Larcombe, M. (2002). The Diagnostic Interview for Social and Communication Disorders: Background, interrater reliability and clinical use. *Journal of Child Psychology and Psychiatry, 43,* 307–325.

Wing, L., & Potter, D. (2002). The epidemiology of autistic spectrum disorders: Is the prevalence rising? *Mental Retardation and Developmental Disabilities Research Reviews, 8,* 151–161.

Wing, L., & Shah, A. (2000). Catatonia in autistic spectrum disorders. *British Journal of Psychiatry, 176,* 357–362.

Wing, L., Yeates, S., Brierley, L., & Gould, J. (1976). The prevalence of early childhood autism: A comparison of administrative and epidemiological studies. *Psychological Medicine, 6,* 89–100.

Wolff, S. (1995). *Loners: The life path of unusual children.* London: Routledge.

World Health Organization. (1967). *Manual of the international statistical classification of diseases, injuries and causes of death* (8th rev., Vol. 1). Geneva: Author.

World Health Organization. (1993). *The ICD-10 classification of mental and behavioral disorders: Diagnostic criteria for research.* Geneva: Author.

Yeargin-Allsopp, M., Rice, C., Karapurkar, T., Doernberg, N., Boyle, C., & Murphy, C. (2003). Prevalence of autism in a US metropolitan area. *Journal of the American Medical Association, 289,* 49–55.

CHAPTER THREE

Psychometric Issues and Current Scales
for Assessing Autism Spectrum Disorders

Jack A. Naglieri

Kimberly M. Chambers

The study of any psychological disorder is dependent upon the tools that are used, as these tools directly influence what is learned about the subject in research as well as clinical practice. As in all areas of science, what we discover depends upon the quality of the instruments we use and the information they provide. Better-made instruments yield more accurate and reliable information. Instruments that uncover more information relevant to the subject being examined will have better validity, and ultimately will more completely inform both researchers and clinicians. The tools we use for diagnosis have a substantial impact on the reliability and validity of the information we obtain and the decisions we make. Simply put, the better the tool, the more valid and reliable the decisions, the more useful the information obtained, and the better the services that are eventually provided. In this chapter, the tools used for assessing the characteristics of children and adolescents who have autism spectrum disorders (ASD) are examined.

This chapter has two goals. First, we review the important psychometric qualities of test reliability and validity. The aim of this first section is to illustrate the relevance of reliability and validity for the decisions made by clinicians and researchers whose goal is to understand ASD better. We emphasize the practical implications these psychometric issues have for the assessment of ASD, and the implications they have for interpretation of results within and across instruments. Special attention is also paid to scale development procedures, particularly methods used to develop derived scores. The second section of this chapter focuses on the various measures used to assess ASD. The structure, reliability, and validity of each instrument are summarized. The overall aim of the chapter is to provide an examination of the relevant psychometric issues and the extent to which researchers and clinicians can have confidence in the tools they use to assess ASD.

Psychometric Issues

Reliability

The reliability of any variable, test, or scale is critical for clinical practice as well as research purposes. It is important to know the reliability of a test, so that the amount of accuracy in a score can be determined and used to calculate the amount of error in the measurement of the construct. The higher the reliability, the smaller the error, and the smaller the range of scores that are used to build the confidence interval around the estimated true score. The smaller the range, the more precision and confidence practitioners can have in their interpretation of the results.

Bracken (1987) provided levels for acceptable test reliability. He stated that individual scales from a test (e.g., a subtest or subscale) should have a reliability of .80 or greater, and that total tests should have an internal consistency of .90 or greater. The reason for testing and the importance of the decisions made could also influence the level of precision required. That is, if a score is used for screening purposes (where overidentification is preferred to underidentification), a .80 reliability standard for a total score may be acceptable. However, if decisions are made, for example, about special educational placement, then a higher reliability (e.g., .95) would be more appropriate (Nunnally & Bernstein, 1994).

Every score obtained from any test is composed of the true score plus error (Crocker & Algina, 1986). We can never obtain the true score, so we describe it on the basis of a range of values within which the person's score falls at a specific level of certainty (e.g., 90% probability). The range of scores (called the confidence interval) is computed by first obtaining the standard error of measurement (SEM) from the reliability coefficient and the standard deviation (SD) of the score in the following formula (Crocker & Algina, 1986):

$$SEM = SD \times \sqrt{1 - \text{reliability}}$$

The confidence interval should be used in practice, to better describe the range of scores that is likely to contain the true score. In practice, we say that a child earned an IQ score of 105 (± 5), and state that there is a 90% likelihood that the child's true IQ score falls within the range of 100 to 110 (105 ± 5).

The confidence interval is based on the *SEM*, which is the average *SD* of a person's scores around the true score. For this reason, we can say that there is a 68% chance (the percentage of scores contained within ±1 *SD*) that the person's true score is within that range. Recall that 68% of cases in a normal distribution fall within +1 and −1 *SD*. The *SEM* is multiplied by a *z* value of, for example, 1.64 or 1.96, to obtain a confidence interval at the 90% or 95% level, respectively. The resulting value is added to and subtracted from the obtained score to yield the confidence interval. So in the example provided above, the confidence interval for an obtained score of 100 is 95 (100 − 5) to 105 (100 + 5). Figure 3.1 provides confidence intervals (95% level of confidence) for a standard score of 100 that would be obtained for measures with reliability of .50 through .99. As would be expected, the range within which the true score is expected to fall varies considerably as a function of the reliability coefficient, and the lower the reliability, the wider the range of scores that can be expected to include the true score.

Technically, however, the confidence interval (and *SEM*) is centered on the estimated true score rather than the obtained score (Nunnally & Bernstein, 1994). In many published tests—for example, the Wechsler Intelligence Scale for Children—Fourth Edition (Wechsler, 2003) and the Cognitive Assessment System (Naglieri & Das, 1997)—the confidence intervals are provided in the test manual's table for converting sums of subtest scores

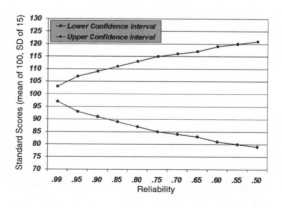

FIGURE 3.1. Relationships between reliability and confidence intervals.

to standard scores, and the range is already centered on the estimated true score. The relationships among the various scores are illustrated in Table 3.1, which provides the obtained score, estimated true score, and lower and upper ranges of the confidence intervals for standard scores (mean of 100, SD of 15) for a hypothetical test with a reliability of .90 at the 90% level of confidence.

Examination of these scores shows that the confidence interval is equally distributed around a score of 100 (92 and 108 are both 8 points from the obtained score), but the interval becomes less symmetrical as the obtained score deviates from the mean. For example, ranges for standard scores that are below the mean are *higher* than the obtained score. As shown in Table 3.1, the range for a standard score of 80 is 74 to 90 (6 points below 80 and 10 points above 80). In contrast scores for standard scores that are above the mean are *lower* than the obtained score. The range for a standard score of 120 is 110 to 126 (10 points below 120 and 6 points above 120). This difference is the result of centering the range of scores on the estimated true score rather than the obtained score. Note that the size of the confidence interval is constant (±8 points) in all instances. Regardless of how the confidence intervals are constructed, the important point is that measurement error must be known and taken into consideration when scores from any measuring system are used. Confidence intervals, especially those that are based on the estimated true score, should be provided for all test scores including rating scales.

TABLE 3.1. Relationships among Obtained Standard Scores, Estimated True Scores, and Confidence Intervals across the 40–160 Range

Obtained standard score	Estimated true score	True minus obtained score	Lower confidence interval	Upper confidence interval	Upper minus lower confidence interval
40	46	6	38	54	16
50	55	5	47	63	16
60	64	4	56	72	16
70	73	3	65	81	16
80	82	2	74	90	16
90	91	1	83	99	16
100	100	0	92	108	16
110	109	−1	101	117	16
120	118	−2	110	126	16
130	127	−3	119	135	16
140	136	−4	128	144	16
150	145	−5	137	153	16
160	154	−6	146	162	16

Note. This table assumes a reliability coefficient of .90 and a 90% confidence interval.

The importance of the *SEM* becomes most relevant when two scores are compared. The lower the reliability, the larger the *SEM*, and the more likely an individual's scores are to differ on the basis of chance. For example, when a child's score on a measure of self-regulation is compared to scores on a measure of social skills, the reliability of these measures will influence their consistency and therefore the size of the difference between them. The lower the reliability, the more likely they are to be different by chance alone. The formula for determining how different two scores need to be includes the *SEM* of each score and the *z* score associated with a specified level of significance. The difference can be computed by using the following formula:

$$Difference = Z \times \sqrt{SEM1_2 + SEM2_2}$$

The difference needed for significance when one is comparing two variables with reliability coefficients of .85 and .78, using an *SD* of 15, is easily calculated with the formula above. To illustrate, scores on measures of self-regulation (with a reliability of .85) and social skills (reliability of .78) would have to differ by 19 points (more than an entire *SD*) to be significant. Figure 3.2 provides the values that would be needed for comparing two scores with the same reliability, ranging from very good (.95) to very poor (.40) at the .05 level of significance, and a standard score that has an *SD* of 15. This figure shows that when one is comparing two scores with reliabilities of .70, differences of more than 20 points would be attributed to *measurement error alone*. Clearly, in both research and clinical settings, variables with high reliability are needed.

It is therefore important that researchers and clinicians who assess behaviors associated with ASD use measures that have a reliability coef-

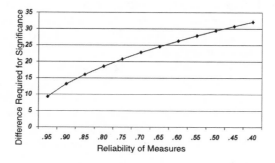

FIGURE 3.2. Relationships between reliability and the differences needed for significance when one is comparing two scores. Note that this figure assumes two variables with the same reliability and an *SD* of 15 at the 95% level of confidence.

ficient of .80 or higher and composite score reliabilities of at least .90. If a test or rating scale does not meet these requirements, then its inclusion in research should be questioned. This is particularly important in correlational research, because the extent to which two variables correlate is influenced by the reliability of each variable. Clinicians are advised not to use measures that do not meet reliability standards, because there will be too much error in the obtained scores to allow for reliable interpretation. This is especially important, because the decisions clinicians make can have significant and long-lasting impact on the lives of examinees.

Validity

Although reliability is important, reliable measurement of a construct with little validity would be of limited utility to the clinician and researcher. Validity is described as the degree to which empirical evidence supports an interpretation of scores that represent a construct of interest. For example, a measure of ASD should contain carefully crafted questions that accurately reflect the disorder. Researchers who study ASD and authors who develop tools to be used during the diagnostic process are especially burdened with the responsibility to carefully and clearly define the behaviors associated with these disorders. When the behaviors and characteristics associated with a disorder are thoroughly operationalized, then further development of the dimensions or factors that can be used for diagnosis may be clarified. This depends, of course on the extent to which the items have adequate reliability.

Given the fact that methods for evaluating ASD, as well as our understanding of the underlying aspects of these disorders, are evolving, we have a particular responsibility to provide validity evidence of the effectiveness of any method we choose (rating scales, tests, interviews, etc.). This is not as simple a task as demonstrating reliability, because validity is harder to demonstrate and the findings will be directly related to the content of the tools used to study ASD, as well as the methodology employed. For example, the items included in a rating scale define and limit the scope of the information that is obtained. This can provide a broad or truncated view of the behaviors associated with a disorder. Choosing the standard against which measures are validated is also not foolproof, because today's so-called diagnostic "gold standard" (i.e., the *Diagnostic and Statistical Manual of Mental Disorders,* fourth edition, text revision [DSM-IV-TR]; American Psychiatric Association, 2000) will undoubtedly evolve to reflect future research findings. Similarly, research methodology is also important, particularly when typical children are being compared to those who have ASD. Special attention should be made to ensure that research findings provide a sufficient number of control groups to determine how those with ASD differ from typical children, as well as from those with other types of disorders.

In summary, the very nature of our understanding of ASD is influenced by the psychometric quality of the tests and methods we use to study these disorders, as well as by the selection of variables we use in our research. Clinicians should be mindful, however, that until there is sufficient maturity in the scope and quality of the instruments used during the diagnostic process, a good understanding of the strengths and weaknesses of all the methods used is necessary. This includes a careful understanding of the manner in which any measure of ASD is constructed.

Development of Scales to Assess ASD

There is a need for a number of well-standardized measures of ASD that have demonstrated reliability and validity. At this writing, there are several behavior rating scales that have been used in both applied and research settings, as well as structured clinical interviews and direct assessments that have varying degrees of reliability and validity. This amplifies the need for practitioners and researchers to have a good understanding of the psychometric qualities and standardization samples associated with these methods. Researchers and practitioners should also be informed about the development of any scale used to aid in the diagnosis of ASD; the test's development should be carefully described by its authors. Development of any scale should follow a series of steps to ensure the highest quality and validity. The development of tools to help diagnose ASD is a task that demands well-known procedures amply described by Crocker and Algina (1986) and by Nunnally and Bernstein (1994). These are now summarized.

Initial test development should begin with a clear definition of the behaviors that represent autism and other ASD. These behaviors and other defining characteristics must be written with sufficient clarity that they can be assessed reliably over time and across raters. Behaviors should be included that represent the characteristics that define children with autism or other ASD as completely as possible, are specific to these disorders, and reflect current conceptualizations of the disorders (such as the behaviors included in DSM-IV-TR). Definitional clarity is *required* for good item writing.

The next step is to develop an initial pool of questions, followed by pilot testing of the items. Pilot tests are designed to evaluate the clarity of the instructions and items, as well as the structure of the form and other logistical issues. For instance, it is important to be cognizant of the ways items are presented on the page, size of the fonts, clarity of the directions, colors used on the form, position of the items on the paper, and so forth. Analyses of reliability and validity are typically not of interest at this point, because sample size usually precludes adequate examination of these issues. Instead, the goal of pilot testing is to answer essential questions such as these: Does the form seem to work? Do the users understand what they need to do? Are the items clear? Can the rater respond to each question?

In contrast, conducting experiments with larger samples that allow for an examination of the psychometric qualities of the items and their correspondence to the constructs of interest is the next important step. This effort is repeated until there is sufficient confidence that the items and the scales have been adequately operationalized. In each phase of the process, experimental evidence within the context of the practical demands facing clinical application should guide development, but some essential analyses such as the following should be conducted:

- Means and SDs, and p values (if dichotomous items are used), should be obtained for each item.
- Items designed to measure the same construct should correlate with a total score obtained from the sum of all those items designed to measure that same construct. If the correlations are low, their inclusion in the scale should be questioned.
- The contribution each item makes to the reliability of the scale(s) on which it is placed should be evaluated.
- An item designed to measure a particular construct should correlate more strongly with other items designed to measure that same construct than with items designed to measure different constructs. If this is not found, the item may be eliminated.
- The internal reliability of those items organized to measure each construct should be computed, as should the reliability of a composite score.
- The factor structure of the set of items may be examined to test the extent to which items or scales form groups, or factors, whose validity can be examined.

The procedures used at this phase are repeated until the scale is ready for standardization. The number of times these activities are repeated depends upon the (1) quality of the original concepts; (2) quality of the initial pool of items; (3) quality of the sampling used to study the instrument; and (4) consistency of the results that are obtained. The overall aim is to produce an experimental version of an instrument that is ready to be subjected to a larger-scale and more costly national standardization study. This would include sufficient data collection efforts to establish the reliability and validity of the final measure. Standardization requires that a sample of persons who represent the population of the country in which the scale will be used are administered the questions in a uniform manner, so that normative values can be computed. Standardization samples are ordinarily designed to be representative of the normal population, so that those that differ from normality can be identified and the extent to which they differ from the norm (50th percentile) can be calibrated as a standard score to reflect dispersion around the mean. Development of norms is an art as much as a science, and there are several ways in which this task can be accomplished (see Crocker & Algina, 1986; Nunnally & Bernstein, 1994; Thorndike, 1982). The next tasks at this stage are collection and analysis of data for establishing reliability (internal, test–retest, interrater, intrarater) and validity (e.g., construct, predictive, and content). Of these two, validity is more difficult to establish and should be examined by using a number of different methodologies, with emphasis on assessing the extent to which the scale is valid for its intended purposes.

There are many different types of validity, making it impossible for validity to be determined by a single study. According to the *Standards for Educational and Psychological Testing* volume (American Educational Research Association [AERA], American Psychological Association, & National Council on Measurement Education, 1999), evidence for validity "integrates various strands of evidence into a coherent account of the degree to which existing evidence and theory support the intended interpretation of test scores for specific uses" (p. 17). There are 24 standards relating to validity issues that should be addressed by authors and test development companies. Some of the more salient issues include the need to provide evidence that supports the following:

- Interpretations based on the scores the instrument yields.
- The appropriate relationships between the instrument's scores and one or more relevant criterion variables.
- The utility of the measure across a wide variety of demographic groups, or its limitations based on race, ethnicity, language, culture, and so forth.
- The expectation that the scores provided differentiate between groups as intended.
- The alignment of the factorial structure of the items or subtests with the scale configuration provided by the authors.

There is wide variation in the extent to which test authors document the development, standardization, reliability, and validity of their measures in test manuals. Some manuals provide sufficient descriptions that bring out the strengths of the scale; others provide limited details. Readers interested in illustrative manuals might look at those developed for the Universal Nonverbal Intelligence Test (Bracken & McCallum, 1997), the Kaufman Assessment Battery for Children—Second Edition (Kaufman & Kaufman, 2004), and the Cognitive Assessment System (Naglieri & Das, 1997). These examples illustrate how to provide detailed discussion of the various phases of development, as well as instructions about how the scores should be interpreted for the various purposes for which the measures were intended.

Documentation of development may end with the writing of the sections in the manual that describe the construction, standardization, and reliability/validity of the instrument, but authors also have the responsibility to inform users about how the scores should be interpreted (AERA et al., 1999). This includes how test scores should be compared with one another, and authors should especially provide the values needed for significance when the various scores a measure provides are compared. This information is critically important if clinicians are to interpret the scores from any instrument in a manner that is psychometrically defensible.

Researchers and clinicians have a responsibility to choose measures that have been developed according to the highest standards available, because important decisions will be made on the basis of the information these measures provide. We suggest that for a scale to be considered acceptable for clinical practice, in addition to being reliable, it must have a standardized administration and scoring format with norms based on a large sample that represents the country in which the scale is used. This includes ample documentation of methods used to develop the measure, as well as ample evidence of validity and explicit instructions for interpretation of the scores that are obtained.

Obtaining information about the psychometric characteristics of instruments that could be used as part of the diagnostic process is a time-consuming and sometimes confusing task. Manuals provide different types of information; sometimes the information is clear and concise, and at other times it is hard to ascertain enough details to fully evaluate the results being presented. Comparisons across instruments are complicated by this inconsistency and by the logistical task of collecting the information. In the next section of this chapter, we provide a systematic examination of the scales used to assess the behaviors associated with ASD. Our goal is to be informative about the specific details associated with important issues, such as reliability, validity, and standardization samples. The discussion of each test includes a general description of the scale, as well as reliability and validity information provided by the authors of these instruments in their respective test manuals. We end the chapter with a commentary on the relative advantages of these scales.

DESCRIPTIONS OF SCALES USED TO ASSESS ASD

Autism Diagnostic Observation Schedule

Description

The Autism Diagnostic Observation Schedule (ADOS; Lord, Rutter, DiLavore, & Risi, 2002) is a semistructured assessment of communication, social interaction, and play in children or adults suspected of having ASD. The present ADOS, the ADOS-Generic or ADOS-G, is a combination of the 1989 ADOS (Lord et al., 1989) and the Pre-Linguistic Autism Diagnostic Observation Schedule (PL-ADOS; DiLavore, Lord, & Rutter, 1995). A referred individual is assessed with one of the four modules contained in the ADOS. Each module can be administered in 30–45 minutes and is geared for a child or adult at a particular developmental and language level. Each module consists of a variety of standard activities and materials that allow the examiner to observe an individual engaging in behaviors typical of persons with ASD within a standardized setting in order to aid diagnosis.

Module 1 is most appropriate for children who are at the preverbal or single-word language level. It consists of 10 activities that focus on the playful use of toys. Module 2 also focuses on the playful use of toys and contains 14 separate activities geared toward individuals at the phrase speech language level. Module 3 is intended for children and adolescents who are verbally fluent and focuses on social, communicative, and language behaviors through 14 different activities. Finally, Module 4 consists of 10 mandatory activities and 5 optional activities that also examine social, communication, and language behavior through unstructured conversation, structured situations, and interview questions. This module is used in the assessment of verbally fluent adolescents and adults.

Examiners take notes during ADOS administration, and ratings are made immediately following the administration. Guidelines for ratings are provided in each module, and algorithms are used to formulate diagnosis. Separate algorithms are used for the interpretation of each module. The ADOS uses cutoff scores for two separate domains (Social Interaction and Communication), as well as a Communication–Social Interaction total cutoff score, in order to make the diagnostic distinction between autism and the broader category of ASD. Although the ADOS has many similarities to the DSM-IV-TR and *International Classification of Diseases,* 10th revision (ICD-10) models of diagnosing ASD, the ADOS algorithm included in the manual does not include a measure of restricted, repetitive, and stereotyped patterns of behavior identified by the DSM-IV-TR and ICD-10. However, these behaviors are coded in a separate domain called Stereotyped Behaviors and Restricted Interests. In addition, the ADOS does not include information about the age of onset or early history required for a DSM-IV-TR or ICD-10 diagnosis. Recently, however, new algorithms for the ADOS have been published (Gotham, Risi, Pickles, & Lord, 2007) that do include restricted/repetitive/stereotyped behaviors and no longer have separate Social Interaction and Communication domains.

Description of the Comparison Group

The validation sample of the ADOS consisted of individuals who were referred to the Developmental Disorders Clinic at the University of Chicago. These individuals were evaluated and assigned a clinical diagnosis of autism, pervasive developmental disorder not otherwise specified (PDD-NOS), or "non-spectrum" by a child psychologist and child psychiatrist through various measures and observations. In addition to the initial sample of participants, individuals were also recruited from various other locations in order to obtain three samples (autism, PDD-NOS, and non-spectrum) in each module that were of adequate size and roughly equivalent in verbal mental age or verbal IQ. Within each module, participants were chosen from the three groups to constitute samples that would be similar with regard to chronological age, gender, and ethnicity. Participants in the validity study were then selected for inclusion in one of four module samples on the basis of verbal ability. In contrast to the other modules, Module 1 included a group with low-functioning autism because of the importance of documenting autism in very young, severely delayed children.

The composition of the sample in each module was as follows:

> Module 1: lower functioning autism (n = 20), matched autism (n = 20), PDD-NOS (n = 17), and non-spectrum (n = 17)
>
> Module 2: autism (n = 21), PDD-NOS (n = 18), and non-spectrum (n = 16)
>
> Module 3: autism (n = 21), PDD-NOS (n = 20), and non-spectrum (n = 18)
>
> Module 4: autism (n = 16), PDD-NOS (n = 14), and non-spectrum (n = 15)

For each module, information within each diagnostic group of each module was further broken down by gender, chronological age, verbal mental age, and nonverbal mental age (this information is available in the test manual).

The authors further report that the ethnicities of the participants in the study were comparable across modules and groups and were as follows: European American (80%), African American (11%), Hispanic (4%), Asian American (2%), and other or mixed ethnic groups (2%). All participants in the study were native English speakers. In addition, all participants had nothing more than mild hearing or visual impairments and were all ambulatory. Finally, with the exception of one boy with Williams syndrome, there were no participants with identifiable syndromes.

Reliability

In order to evaluate the reliability of individual items on the ADOS, the test authors obtained interrater reliability information for each module. For Module 1, interrater reliability had a mean exact agreement of 91.5%, and all items had more than 80% exact agreement across raters. With the exception of items describing repetitive behaviors and sensory abnormalities, the mean weighted kappa coefficients exceeded .60 (mean = .78). Items describing repetitive behaviors and sensory abnormalities were less frequently scored as abnormal within the autistic sample and proved more difficult to score. One item, "behavior when interrupted," was eliminated due to poor reliability.

The mean agreement for Module 2 items was 89%, and all items exceeded 80% agreement. Out of the 26 items, kappa for 15 items exceeded .60 (mean = .70), and kappa for the remaining items equaled .50, with the exception of 4 items. "unusual sensory interest in play material/person,", "unusually repetitive interests or stereotyped behaviors," "facial expressions directed to others," and "shared enjoyment in interaction" had kappa values ranging from .38 to .49, with agreements from 78% to 93%. These items were either edited or eliminated due to poor reliability.

For Module 3, the mean exact agreement was 88.2%. Many items (17) had kappa values of .60 or better (mean = .65), and all but two items received 80% or more agreement. The item "stereotyped/idiosyncratic use of words or phrases" was rewritten, and "communication of own affect," "social Distance," "pedantic speech," and "emotional gestures" were either eliminated or collapsed within another item due to poor reliability.

Finally, Module 4 had a minimum of 80% exact agreement, with kappa coefficients exceeding .60 for 22 of the items (mean = .66), and the remaining items having kappa values of .50 or higher. "Excessive interest in or references to unusual or highly specific topics or objects or repetitive behavior" had a kappa value of .41, and "responsibility" had a kappa value of .48. The items were kept because the agreement for both equaled 85%. "Attention to irrelevant details" and "social disinhibition" were eliminated due to poor reliability.

Interclass correlations were computed for algorithm subtotals and totals for each module and the combined modules. For the separate modules, interclass correlations ranged from .88 to.97 for the Social Interaction domain, .74 to .90 for the Communication domain, .84 to .98 for the Communication–Social Interaction total, and .75 to .90 for Stereotyped Behaviors and Restricted Interests.

Interrater agreement for diagnostic classification for autism versus non-spectrum was examined. For Modules 1 and 3, agreement was 100%; for Module 2, agreement was 91%; and for Module 4, agreement was 90%. However, when participants with PDD-NOS were included, agreement dropped: It was 93% for Module 1, 87% for Module 2, 81% for Module 3, and 84% for Module 4. The authors reported that when Fisher's exact test was used to compare the diagnostic groups, results were significant at $p < .01$, and that disagreements were mostly between PDD-NOS and autism.

When data were collapsed across all modules, interrater correlations for domain and total scores ranged from .82 to .93. In addition, interclass correlations of ratings during the testing session with ratings immediately after testing ranged from .80 to .92. These ratings were made by observing videotapes of the same administration. The interclass correlations ranged from .72 to .92. Finally, test–retest interclass correlations ranged from .59 to .82. Test–retest periods averaged approximately 9 months. The mean differences in domain scores for time 1 and time 2 were 1.19 (SD = 1.6) for Communication, 1.26 (SD = 1.39) for Stereotyped Behaviors and Restricted Interests, 1.78 (SD = 1.93) for Social Interaction, and 2.67 (SD = 1.93) for Communication–Social Interaction total. Group means changed less than 0.50 for each domain, with the exception of the Communication–Social Interaction total (M = −0.94, SD = 2.63). Scores for 6 children in the test–retest sample changed ADOS classification.

Validity

The authors of the ADOS have provided results from factor-analytic studies of their scale. They reported that items from the Social Interaction and Communication domains loaded highly on the first factor, and a second factor consisted of items dealing with speech and gesturing. Few details are provided in the manual.

Comparisons of children with autism, those with PDD-NOS, and those not on the spectrum are provided in the manual for each ADOS module. Typically, children with autism earned significantly higher scores on those items included in the modules than those with PDD-NOS, and the lowest scores were obtained by those not on the spectrum. The sample sizes by module and by group ranged from a low of 14 to a high of 21. These findings were augmented by analyses of classification rates. The sample sizes for these analyses by module for the groups based on clinical diagnosis (lower-functioning autism, autism, PDD-NOS, non-spectrum) ranged from 0 to 21. The results of these analyses, which are provided for various combinations and cutoff scores for the domains measured by the ADOS, generally suggest that the instrument had specificity values in the upper 80% to low 90% range, and sensitivity in the upper 90% range.

Autism Diagnostic Interview—Revised

Description

The Autism Diagnostic Interview—Revised (ADI-R; Rutter, Le Couteur, & Lord, 2003b) is an extended interview that produces information needed to diagnose autism and assist in assessing other ASD. The ADI-R consists of

93 questions focusing primarily on three domains: Language/Communication; Reciprocal Social Interactions; and Restricted, Repetitive, and Stereotyped Behaviors and Interests. This interview should be administered by an experienced clinician to an informant familiar with the assessed individual's behavior and development. The assessed individual must have a mental age of at least 2 years. The interview takes approximately 1½–2½ hours to complete.

The interviewer records and codes detailed responses to the 93 questions, using the Interview Protocol. The interviewer then scores the interview, using one or more of the five algorithm forms. Algorithms are used to code up to 42 of the interview items in order to produce formal and interpretable results. The algorithms consist of both Diagnostic and Current Behavior Algorithms. Diagnostic Algorithms are used for diagnosis and focuses on the individual's developmental history at ages 4–5 years, whereas Current Behavior Algorithms reflect symptoms at the time of testing and can be used for treatment and/or educational planning.

Summary scores are calculated for each of four domains (Qualitative Abnormalities in Reciprocal Social Interaction; Qualitative Abnormalities in Communication; Restrictive, Repetitive, and Stereotypic Patterns of Behavior, and whether the manifestations of behavior were evident [i.e., before 36 months of age]) for the Diagnostic Algorithms. Cutoff scores are then used to determine the presence of ASD. There is only one cutoff for ASD, rather than separate cutoffs for autism and ASD as on the ADOS.

Description of the Comparison Group

The ADI-R comparison group was developed by administering the ADI-R to several hundred caregivers of individuals both with and without autism; the individuals' ages ranged from preschool to early adulthood. Interviews were conducted as initial clinical assessments and research evaluations. No further information is provided on this sample of several hundred.

Reliability

The ADI-R manual presents interrater and test–retest reliability coefficients. Weighted kappa values are provided for the behavioral items of the four diagnostic algorithm domains. These coefficients are broken down by age and come from one of two studies. In a sample of 19 children 36–59 months of age, the weighted kappa coefficients ranged from .63 to .89. In a sample of 22 individuals ages 5–29 years, weighted kappa coefficients ranged from .37 to .95. Test–retest reliability coefficients are also presented from a study of 94 preschool children with a test–retest period of 2–5 months. Coefficients were provided for the behavioral items, including Reciprocal Social

Interaction, Abnormalities in Communication, and Restricted, Repetitive, and Stereotyped Patterns of Behavior of the Diagnostic Algorithm domains (excluding Age of First Manifestation). Intraclass correlation coefficients ranged from .93 to .97.

Validity

The associations between the ADI-R and the Social Communication Questionnaire (SCQ; Rutter, Bailey, & Lord, 2003a; see the description of that instrument later in this chapter), which is essentially a short form of the ADI-R were examined for a sample of children with developmental language disorders to assess concurrent validity (Bishop & Norbury, 2002). The ADI-R was scored to distinguish those students meeting the full DSM-IV/ICD-10 criteria for autism (this applied to 8 out of a total sample of 21 children and 8 out of the 14 with ASD), as well as those qualifying for a broad designation of ASD (children meeting criteria for two out of the three domains). Of the 8 children meeting the full criteria on the ADI-R, 6 children scored 15 or more on the SCQ. Intercorrelations between the ADI-R and SCQ for the three ADI-R domains were examined. The Reciprocal Social Interaction domain had a Pearson correlation of .92; the Language/Communication domain correlation was .73; and the Restricted, Repetitive, and Stereotyped Behaviors and Interests domain correlation was .89. Within the ADI-R and SCQ, the cross-correlations between the Reciprocal Social Interaction and Language/Communication domains were .77 for the SCQ and .70 for the ADI-R. The Restricted, Repetitive, and Stereotyped Behaviors and Interests correlations with the other two domains were .48 and .53 for the SCQ, and .41 and .54 for the ADI-R.

Item-by-item agreement between the ADI-R and SCQ was provided. The ADI-R items were classified as present if a score of 1, 2, or 3 was obtained, whereas a score of 1 indicated agreement on the SCQ. Agreement between the items on the two tests ranged from 45% to 85%, with an average of 70.8%.

Autism Spectrum Rating Scale

Description

The Autism Spectrum Rating Scale (ASRS; Goldstein & Naglieri, 2009) is an observer-completed rating scale designed to aid in the diagnosis of individuals who may have ASD. The ASRS is completed by parents (or similar caregivers) or teachers (or similar professionals) who rate behaviors characteristic of children ages 2–6 years (Early Childhood version) and older children ages 7–18 years (School Age form). All forms ask the rater to consider behaviors during the past month. The items measure behaviors characteristic of ASD and are organized to yield both empirically and rationally defined scales. There are three empirically derived scales (Self-Regulation, Social/Communication, and Stereotypical Behaviors) and an ASRS Total Scale. In addition to the factorially derived scales, there are several scales developed on the basis of locally organized item groups: Adult Socialization, Attention, Behavioral Rigidity, Emotionality, Peer Socialization, Language, Sensory Sensitivity, and Unusual Interests. The score for each of these scales is a *T* score with a normative mean of 50 and *SD* of 10. In addition, a short Screening version of the ASRS is provided, consisting of 15 items.

The authors state that the ASRS was developed to measure ASD and autism-related problems, in order to allow clinicians to compare an individual to norm-based expectations in an objective and reliable manner. Because the ASRS items are linked to DSM-IV-TR symptoms of autistic disorder, Asperger's disorder, and PDD-NOS, the information provided can also facilitate the process of differential diagnosis. Used in combination with other assessment information, results from the ASRS provide valuable information to guide diagnostic decisions. The results can also be used to help form individualized intervention plans and suggest behaviors to target in treatment, as well as to evaluate an individual's response to treatment. Finally, the 15-item ASRS Screening scale is intended to be used in large-scale prevention programs.

Description of the Comparison Group

The ASRS was standardized on a large sample of children and adolescents who were selected to be representative of the United States, with a proportional sample from Canada. Two samples of data were collected, one for the Early Childhood version and one for the School Age version, to create norms for parent and teacher raters. Equal numbers of males and females, who ranged in age from 2 years, 0 months through 18 years, 11 months, were included.

Reliability

The internal reliability coefficients for the empirically based scales for the Early Childhood ASRS are as follows: Stereotypical Behaviors (25 items; reliability of .79 for parents and .77 for teachers), Social/Communication (21 items; reliability of .83 and .85 for parents and teachers, respectively), and Self-Regulation (11 items; reliability of .75 for parents and .80 for teachers). The internal reliability coefficients for the empirically based scales for the School Age ASRS are as follows: Stereotypical Behaviors (19 items; reliability of .81 for parents and .83 for teachers), Social/Communication (21 items; reliability of .86 and .88 for parents and teachers, respectively), and Self-Regulation (14 items; reliability of .79 for parents and .82 for teachers). The 15-item ASRS Screening scale's reliability coefficients are .87 and .90, for parents and teachers, respectively, on the Early Childhood version, and .89 and .90 for parents and teachers, respectively, on the School Age form.

Validity

At the time of this writing the ASRS is in final stages of development, and the validity studies have yet to be completed. Readers interested in seeing the results of the item factor analysis, comparison of the scores obtained on the ASRS with other measures of ASD, rates of accurate differentiation of children with and without ASD using the ASRS, and other validity studies should see the manual.

Childhood Autism Rating Scale

Description

The Childhood Autism Rating Scale (CARS; Schopler, Reichler, & Renner, 1988) is a 15-item behavior rating scale developed to help identify children with autism and to evaluate varying degrees of the disorder. The CARS was also developed to differentiate autistic children from those with other developmental disorders, particularly those with moderate to severe mental retardation. CARS ratings are based on a clinician's observations or on parent report. Behaviors are rated on a scale of 1 (within normal limits), 2 (mildly abnormal), 3 (moderately abnormal), and 4 (severely abnormal for that age), based on a one- or two-sentence description of the behavior being evaluated. Item scores are summed and categorized as follows: 15–29.5 is considered the nonautistic range, 30–36.5 is considered the range of mild to moderate autism, and 37–60 is considered the severely autistic range. The 15 items included in the CARS are based on the diagnostic criteria from Kanner (1943), the nine dimensions by Creek (1961), Rutter's (1978) definition, and the criteria proposed by the National Society for Autistic Children (1978).

Description of the Comparison Group

The CARS scores are based on a comparison to the ratings of over 1,500 children who were referred to the North Carolina program for the Treatment and Education of Autistic and related Communication-handicapped

Children (TEACCH). This comparison group comprised a referred sample of children suspected of having autism who had CARS scores below 30 (46%). The remaining 54% were identified as having autism. About half of the sample with autism had CARS scores that fell in the mild to moderate range, and half met the criteria for severe autism. This sample consisted of 24.3% females and 75.7% males, whose racial background was European American (66.9%), African American (30.2%), or other (2.9%). The authors describe the sample as predominantly from low socioeconomic levels, based on the Hollingshead–Redlich two-factor index. Over one-fourth (26.3%) of the sample fell in the lowest socioeconomic category (V) identified by the index. The rest of the sample was distributed as follows: IV (33%), III (22.4%), II (9.3%), and I (9.1%). The sample was further described on the basis of IQ as follows: 70.6% < 70, 16.5% = 70–84, and 12.8% = 85 and above. Finally, the children varied in age as follows: < 6 years = 56.4%, 6–10 years = 32.0%, and 11 and above = 11.4%. No data on the minimum or maximum ages of the children included in the sample, or other characteristics (e.g., parental education) were provided. The degree to which this sample represents a population of children with autism in the state of North Carolina or the country was not provided. Importantly, these data were collected from the late 1960s through the late 1980s, according to the CARS manual.

Reliability

The CARS manual presents internal, test–retest, and interrater reliability coefficients. Internal reliability is reported, but the manual does not specify for what sample the coefficient (alpha = .94) was calculated. Test–retest reliability was computed for 91 individuals assessed over a period of about 1 year, but details of the exact test–retest interval and characteristics of the sample are not provided. There were no significant differences between the mean raw score earned at each rating, and the reliability coefficient (kappa) was .64. The average interrater reliability was .71 for a sample of 280 individuals (no further information on the sample is provided in the test manual). Interrater reliabilities for each of the 15 items ranged from .62 to .93.

Validity

The authors assessed criterion-related validity for the CARS by comparing total scores to clinical ratings obtained during the same diagnostic session (r = .85, $p < .001$). Total scores were also correlated with independent clinical assessments made by a child psychologist and a child psychiatrist. This was based on information obtained from referral records, parent interviews, and nonstructured clinical interviews ($r = .80$, $p < .001$).

The validity of CARS ratings made under alternate conditions was also examined. Because the CARS was originally developed to be used during the administration of the Psychoeducational Profile (PEP), different groups of children were rated on the basis of information gathered both during a PEP session and in a parent interview, a classroom observation, or a chart history. Children ($N = 41$) were rated by a therapist after a meeting with each child's parents. CARS scores that were based on the parent interview were compared to CARS scores during the PEP session. There was no significant difference between the two scores (PEP mean = 32.7; interview mean = 33.7; $t = -1.26$, $p > .10$). Correlation between the scores indicated good agreement ($r = .82$, $p < .01$). CARS screening diagnosis from the parent interview and PEP administration agreed in 90% of the cases (kappa coefficient was .75).

Raters visited classrooms for 1- to 2-hour observations of 20 children who would also receive the PEP in the clinic. Mean ratings based on observations in the classroom did not differ significantly from mean ratings based on observations made during PEP administration (PEP $\overline{X} = 32.48$, classroom $\overline{X} = 34.18$; $t = -1.55$, $p > .10$). The correlation of the ratings was .73 ($p < .01$). The classroom observations and PEP administration agreed in 86% of the cases (kappa coefficient was .86).

Raters also provided CARS ratings using the behavioral information contained in the case history charts of 61 children and by PEP administration. The mean ratings did not differ significantly (PEP $\overline{X} = 32.34$, chart review $\overline{X} = 32.47$; $t = 0.20$, $p > .10$). The correlation of these ratings was .82 ($p < .01$). CARS screening diagnosis using the two methods agreed in 82% of the cases (kappa coefficient was .63).

The validity of CARS ratings made by professionals in other disciplines was also examined. Professionals in related fields were given brief introductions to the CARS and asked to make ratings based on their observations of behavior during PEP administration. One hour prior to observations, professionals read the CARS manual and observed a training video. Ratings made by visiting professionals were compared with the criterion ratings made by clinical directors observing the same session. The 18 visiting professionals consisted of medical students, pediatric residents and interns, special educators, school psychologists, speech pathologists, and audiologists. The mean CARS ratings scores were not significantly different from the mean of the clinical directors (visitor $\overline{X} = 32.46$, clinical director $\overline{X} = 33.15$; $t = 0.92$, $p > .10$). The scores were also correlated with each other ($r = .83$, $p < .01$). Diagnostic screening categorizations resulting from CARS ratings of the two groups showed 92% agreement (kappa coefficient was .81).

Psychoeducational Profile—Third Edition

Description

The Psychoeducational Profile—Third Edition (PEP-3; Schopler, Lansing, Reichler, & Marcus, 2005) is an instrument designed to evaluate cognitive skills and behaviors typical of individuals characterized as having ASD and other developmental disabilities. This instrument is appropriate for children between the ages of 6 months and 7 years, for the purposes of planning educational programming and in the diagnosis of autism and other ASD. The test manual outlines four specific purposes of the PEP-3: to identify an individual's strengths and weaknesses, to aid in diagnosis, to establish developmental and adaptive level, and to serve as a research tool.

The PEP-3 has two major components: the Performance Part and the Caregiver Report. The Performance Part is administered through direct observation and testing, and consists of 10 subtests (6 measuring developmental abilities and 4 measuring maladaptive behaviors) that form three composite scores: Communication, Motor, and Maladaptive Behavior. The Caregiver Report is completed by a parent or caregiver, based on daily observations of the child. The Caregiver Report consists of two sections: (1) Child's current developmental level and (2) degree of problems in different diagnostic categories. This information can be used to aid in clinical diagnosis. The Caregiver Report contains three subtests: Problem Behaviors, Personal Self-Care, and Adaptive Behavior.

Items on the PEP-3 are scored according to scoring criteria provided in the Examiner Scoring and Summary Booklet. Normative data are provided to facilitate a normative analysis, which allows the examiner to establish adaptive/developmental levels and make comparisons of the child to other autistic children. These scores can also be used in clinical analysis and provide information on a child's passing, emerging, or failing performance on individual items, as well as appropriate, mild, or severe performance on individual Maladaptive Behavior items.

Normative scores allow examiners to compare a child's developmental age to that of a typically developing sample. The test authors state that a child identified as having an ASD characteristically has an uneven developmental profile in relation to the developmental subtests. This developmental profile can then be used for determining the child's strengths and weaknesses. Percentile ranks were determined based upon a comparison sample with ASD and are available for subtests (and composite scores for the developmental subtests). The manual provides interpretive guidelines for these scores. Percentile scores above 89 are considered to be at the adequate developmental/adaptive level, 75–89 at the mild level, 25–74 at the moderate level, and below 25 at the severe level. Percentile ranks for the Maladaptive Behavior composite can also be used in interpretation. The manual states that a score lower than the 90th percentile in this composite usually places a child on the autism spectrum. Scores on the Problem Behaviors and Adaptive Behavior subtests, as well as the Caregiver Report, can be used to reinforce this interpretation.

Description of the Comparison Group

A sample of 407 children with autism and other ASD, as well as 148 typically developing children, was used for the PEP-3 normative sample. In the group with ASD, 95% of the children were classified as having autism, 4% as having Asperger syndrome, and 1% as exhibiting a developmental delay. Children in the sample ranged from the ages of 2 to 21 years (2 years, $n = 38$; 3 years, $n = 60$; 4 years, $n = 63$; 5 years, $n = 51$; 6 years, $n = 48$; 7 years, $n = 23$; 8 years, $n = 27$; 9 years, $n = 21$; 10 years, $n = 19$; 11 years, $n = 16$; 12 years, $n = 15$; 13–21 years, $n = 26$). The sample closely matched the U.S. population with regard to geographic area, gender, race, Hispanic ethnicity, family income, and educational attainment of parents.

Individuals in the typically developing sample consisted of 148 children between the ages of 2 and 6 (2 years, $n = 27$; 3 years, $n = 33$; 4 years, $n = 36$; 5 years, $n = 27$; 6 years, $n = 26$). This sample was 53% female and 47% male. The normative population closely matched the U.S. population on the domains of geographic area, race, Hispanic heritage, family income, educational attainment, and disability status.

Reliability

Internal consistency was assessed in a sample of individuals with autism at 11 age intervals (ages 2 through 11). Average alpha coefficients for Performance subtests, Caregiver Report subtests, and composites ranged from .84 to .99. Coefficient alphas were also provided for six subgroups of individuals with autism and the normally developing sample. The six subgroups, and the range of their alpha values for the Performance Part subtests, Caregiver Report subtests, and composites, were as follows: white (.78–.99), black (.76–.99), other race (.80–.99), Hispanic (.79–.99), male (.77–.99), female (.81–.99), and the normally developing sample (.75–.97).

Test–retest reliability was also examined in a sample of 33 autistic children between the ages of 4 and 14 residing in California, Oklahoma, and Texas. The sample consisted of 28 males and 5 females, and was also broken down by race and Hispanic ethnicity (white = 24, black = 4, other race = 5, Hispanic ethnicity = 6). The correlation coefficients ranged from .94 to .99 for Performance Part subtests and Caregiver Report subtests. Correlation coefficients could not be calculated for composite scores, as raw data were used. The time lapse between the first and second test was 2 weeks.

Interrater reliability was assessed by using polychoric correlations, because items on the Caregiver Report are ordered categorical data. The sample used in this reliability study consisted of 40 individuals ages 2 through 10 from seven different states. Of the 40 participants, 33 were male and 7 were female; 1 was Hispanic, 32 were white, 6 were black, and 2 were of other races. Nine of the 40 children did not have a disability, 29 were diagnosed with autism, and 2 were diagnosed with Asperger syndrome. Two parents of each child independently completed the Caregiver Report, and polychoric correlations for the items on the Problem Behaviors, Personal Self-Care, and Adaptive Behavior subtests were computed. Polychoric correlations for the items on the Adaptive Behavior subtest ranged from .70 to .91 (mean = .85); Personal Self-Care items correlations ranged from .65 to 1.00 (mean = .90); and correlations for the Adaptive Behavior subtest items ranged from .52 to .90 (mean = .78). It should be noted that one item on the Adaptive Behavior subtest was eliminated because it had a very low correlation.

Validity

Median item discrimination coefficients were calculated by the test authors for a sample of children with autism ages 2 through 12, to assess the degree to which an item would correctly differentiate among test takers. Such coefficients were calculated for 11 age intervals for each subtest of the Performance Part and the Caregiver Report. Item difficulty coefficients were also calculated at these 11 age intervals, to determine the items that were too easy or too difficult and arrange them in order from least to most difficult.

In order to detect differential item function (DIF), a logistic regression procedure was applied to all PEP-3 subtest items. The sample of individuals with autism was used to make comparisons between these groups: male versus female, black versus nonblack, and Hispanic versus non-Hispanic. Four of these comparisons were found to illustrate DIF at the .001 significance level. However, after reviewing these items, the test authors suggested that the four items exhibited benign DIF.

Criterion prediction validity was assessed in four studies by examining the relationship between the PEP-3 and four criterion measures. First, the authors examined the relationship between the PEP-3 and the original Vineland Adaptive Behavior Scales, Expanded Form (Sparrow, Balla, & Cicchetti, 1984) for a sample of 45 children with autism between the ages of 2 and 14. In general, the correlations were high, with only a few exceptions (e.g., Vineland Motor Skills with PEP-3 Problem Behaviors). The second study ($N = 68$) examined the correlations between the CARS and the PEP-3. Significant and large correlations were found. Similarly, the third study involved the correlations of the PEP-3 with the Autism Behavior Checklist—Second Edition (Krug, Arick & Almond, 2008). The results for this sample of 316 children suggested that the two scales are highly correlated.

The test authors calculated correlations between all subtests and found that these correlations ranged from .39 to .90, with a mean of .68. The authors state that coefficients for the subtests range from moderate to very large, and that the mean coefficient falls within the large range. Because of this, they suggest that the PEP-3 subtests measure different skills or behaviors and that evidence thus exists for construct identification validity. These intercorrelations were further subjected to confirmatory factor analysis, to test the degree to which the subtests' assignment to the three composites were supported by data from the standardization sample. The results indicated that the three composites (Communication, Motor, and Maladaptive Behavior) could be considered a viable structure for this instrument.

Social Communication Questionnaire

Description

The SCQ (Rutter et al., 2003a) is a 40-item rating scale completed by parents to assess the symptoms associated with ASD. The content of the scale is the same as that of the ADI-R (Rutter at al., 2003b), reviewed above, with items worded identically, but it is administered as a parent questionnaire rather than via an extended interview. The scale uses a yes–no format and, according to the test manual, takes approximately 10 minutes to complete and 5 minutes to score. Raw scores are summed to yield a total score, which is interpreted based on the form being used and recommended cutoff scores. The SCQ has two forms: Lifetime and Current Behavior. The Lifetime form assesses the individual's entire developmental history, whereas the Current Behavior form assesses behavior in the most current three months. The Lifetime form is considered more useful for diagnosing or screening ASD, while the Current Behavior form can be beneficial for developing treatment plans.

According to the authors, the SCQ has three main uses. First, it can be used as a screening device for the presence of ASD. If a child is suspected of having an ASD after being screened, further clinical assessment should be conducted. The SCQ is an alternative to the ADI-R, for use when time does not permit a lengthy assessment, such as in screening; the questions are identical, so one or the other can be used, but not both. The subscores produced by the SCQ can also be used to match the domains of the ADI-R (Reciprocal Social Interaction; Language/Communication; Restricted, Repetitive, and Stereotyped Behaviors and Interests). Although the production of subscores can be used for interpretation, the manual warns that these subscores have not been adequately researched. A second use of the SCQ is for research purposes; it can be used with groups of children diagnosed with ASD to compare symptoms across groups. A third identified use of the SCQ is its ability to identify severity of ASD symptoms or changes in severity of symptoms over time. This is accomplished through the use of the Current Behavior form.

Description of the Comparison Group

Raw scores from the SCQ are compared to those earned by a sample of 200 children who had participated in previous studies using the ADI-R. The children in this sample had a variety of developmental disabilities: 83 had autism, 49 had atypical autism, 16 had Asperger syndrome, 7 had fragile X syndrome, 5 had Rett syndrome, 10 had conduct disorder, 7 had language delay, 15 had mental retardation, and 8 had other clinical diagnoses.

Reliability

Information is provided on the internal consistency of the SCQ as a measure of reliability. Alpha coefficients were computed in two different ways. First, a sample of 214 children with both ASD and non-spectrum diagnoses was divided into 5 different groups. These groups consisted of a "no-language" group and four "language" groups divided by age. Alpha coefficients for these groups ranged from .84 to .93. Next, internal consistency was examined by dividing the 157 children in the language group into one of three diagnostic categories: autism, other ASD, and non-spectrum. Measures of internal consistency for these groups ranged from .81 to .92.

Validity

Of the 39 items scored on the SCQ, 33 showed statistically different differentiation of children with ASD from those with other abnormalities. The items that did not show differentiation primarily concerned abnormal language features. These items had a relatively high frequency among children without ASD, but correlated with the total score (.64, .53, .45, and .57). Two items (self-injury and unusual attachment to objects) differentiated at the 7% significance level and showed more modest correlations with the total score (.37 and .27). Correlations were also calculated for the total score and domains (Reciprocal Social Interaction: Language/Communication; and Restricted, Repetitive, and Stereotyped Behaviors and Interests). All correlations were significant at the .0005 level within and across the domains and ranged from .31 to .71 (Berument et al., 1999)

Three- and four-factor solutions were explored for 39 items of the SCQ (items 2–40). Analysis suggested that a four-factor structure appeared to be an acceptable fit. Principal-component factoring with varimax rotation yielded four factors and explained 42.4% of the total variation of the SCQ data; 24.3% (eigenvalue = 9.7) was accounted for by a social interaction factor, 8.7% (eigenvalue = 3.38) by a communication factor, 5% (eigenvalue = 1.94) by an abnormal language factor, and 4.5% (eigenvalue = 1.74) by a stereotyped behavior factor. The alpha reliability was .90 for the total scale, .91 for factor 1, .71 for factor 2, .79 for factor 3, and .67 for factor 4. The individual item-to-total scores were positive and mainly substantial, with a range of .26 to .73. The four factors mapped onto the three domains that were operationalized by the ADI-R algorithm criteria. Factor 1 coincided with the Reciprocal Social Interaction domain; factor 4 coincided with the Restricted, Repetitive, and Stereotyped Behaviors and Interests domain; and the Language/Communication domain items were mainly divided between factors 2 and 3 (Berument et al., 1999).

Receiver operating characteristics (ROC) analysis and a series of t tests were used to assess the discriminative power of the SCQ (Berument et al., 1999). After examining the area under the curve (AUC), the authors reported that the SCQ was able to differentiate ASD (including autism) from non-ASD conditions, including mental retardation (AUC = .86). The SCQ also effectively differentiated between autism and non-ASD conditions other than mental retardation (AUC = .94), autism and mental retardation (AUC = .92), and autism and other ASD (AUC= .74), although this last distinction was less clear-cut.

Analyses were then repeated, using an SCQ score that did not include the six items that failed to differentiate the groups at the 5% significance level. The authors reported that some improvement in discriminative validity was obtained. However, the discriminative validity between autism and other ASD was worse. The discriminative validity of the SCQ was then compared to that of the ADI-R. AUC results were contrasted for ASD versus non-ASD conditions (AUC = .88 and .87, respectively), autism versus mental retardation (AUC = .93 and .96), and autism versus other ASD (AUC = .73 and .74).

The authors also reported that groups differed in IQ distribution, and considered that SCQ diagnostic differentiation could be due to this differentiation. In order to investigate this possibility, analyses were repeated within the identified IQ bands. Data came from various studies, and as a result, several different IQ tests were used to assess cognitive abilities. Results showed that in the comparison group the SCQ score was the lowest (8.39) in the group with an IQ above 70 and the highest in the group with severe mental retardation (14.74), and that SCQ score did not vary by IQ within the group with ASD. The diagnostic differentiation within the IQ bands was significant and clearest in the group with an IQ above 70.

Another set of analyses was conducted to examine whether individual behavioral domains of the SCQ provided better diagnostic information than that obtained with the total score. Items of the SCQ were placed in one of three domains determined by the equivalent items on the ADI-R. All three domains provided differentiation of ASD from other disorders (AUC ranged from .79 to .83), and differentiation on the total score was stronger (AUC = .90). The authors reported that the total score provided the best differentiation. This is supported by the finding that the Restricted, Repetitive, and Stereotyped Behaviors and Interests domain was not good at differentiating autism from mental retardation (AUC = .70) or autism from other ASD (AUC = .59).

The authors reported that the ROC analysis for the total SCQ suggests a score of 15 or more as the cutoff for differentiating ASD from other diagnoses (sensitivity = .85, specificity = .75, positive predictive value = .55 for the sample). The authors also suggested that other cutoffs may be desirable for general population samples or other purposes. The cutoff of 15 or more had a sensitivity of .96 and a specificity of .80 for autism versus other diagnoses, excluding mental retardation, and a sensitivity of .96 and a specificity of .67 for autism versus mental retardation. Finally, a higher cutoff of 22 or more was required to differentiate autism from other ASD with a sensitivity of .75 and a specificity of .60.

As noted earlier, the relationships between the ADI-R and SCQ were examined in a sample of children with developmental language disorders to assess concurrent validity (Bishop & Norbury, 2002). See the "Validity" section in the ADI-R for the results of that study.

The relationships between the SCQ and ADI-R total scores were reported by the test authors for 81 children involved in an international genetics study. The correlation between the SCQ and ADI-R was .78 and the intercorrelations among domains ranged from .44 to .77 ($p < .01$). The authors reported that the intercorrelations did not vary by age, gender, and IQ. When scores of 1, 2, and 3 on the ADI-R were compared with SCQ scores of 1, agreement ranged from 36.6% to 91.9%, with an average of 69.8%. When the ADI-R codes of 0 and 1 were collapsed and contrasted with scores of 2 on the SCQ, agreements were very similar and had an average of 68.5%.

Social Responsiveness Scale

Description

The Social Responsiveness Scale (SRS; Constantino & Gruber, 2005) is a 65-item questionnaire that covers various dimensions of interpersonal behavior, communication, and repetitive/stereotypical behavior. The SRS can be used with children ages 4–18 as both a screening tool and an aid to clinical diagnosis; it helps to identify autistic disorder, Asperger disorder, PDD-NOS, and schizoid personality disorder. The SRS is completed by someone familiar with the child's current behavior and developmental history. Items on the scale focus on the behavior of the child, and the rater's responses are given in a Likert format. There are separate parent and teacher forms, each of which takes approximately 15 minutes to complete and 5–10 minutes to score.

The test authors recommend that the SRS results be used in different ways, depending upon the goal of assessment. When the SRS is used as a broad screening tool for any ASD in general populations, a cutoff raw score of 70 is recommended for males and a raw score of 65 for females. When the instrument is used for screening children suspected of having social development problems, a cutoff score of 85 is recommended for both genders. When SRS scores are converted to T scores, a value of 60–70 is considered to be in the mild to moderate range and is typical of children with mild or high-functioning ASD. A T score of 76 or higher is in the severe range and indicative of a diagnosis of autism. In addition to total T scores, the SRS also yields T scores for five treatment subscales: Social Awareness, Social Cognition, Social Communication, Social Motivation, and Autistic Mannerisms. Instructions for interpretation of these scores are provided in the test manual.

Description of the Comparison Group

Subjects from five research studies were combined to produce a sample of over 1,600 children to norm the SRS. The first three groups consisted of random samples of twins identified from Missouri birth records. The fourth group was based on parent report data on 145 males and 127 females from elementary, middle, and high schools located in an economically diverse U.S. Midwestern suburban school district. The fifth sample consisted of teacher report data from 552 students taken from a large suburban school district in the Midwest and a large urban district in the West. The racial composition of this normative group was as follows: White (74%), black (11%), Hispanic (11%), Asian (2%), and other (2%). Separate norms based on these data were created for both parent and teacher versions of the SRS.

Reliability

Internal consistency, construct temporal stability, and interrater agreement data are provided by the SRS manual as assessments of reliability. Internal consistency alpha coefficients are provided for various samples of normative parent ratings, normative teacher ratings, and clinical ratings. Parent and teacher ratings were broken down by gender. The alpha coefficient for parent data for males was .94 (n = 512) and for females was .93 (n = 569). In turn, the alpha coefficient for teacher data for the male population was .97 (n = 278) and for females was .96 (n = 277). Alpha coefficients were not broken down by gender for clinical ratings, and the coefficient for a sample of 281 was .97. Alpha coefficients were also broken down by gender when construct temporal stability was reported. The coefficient for males was .85 (n = 102) and for females was .77 (n = 277). Finally, interrater reliability coefficients were provided from a sample of 63 children. Coefficients were provided for mother–father rater pairings (r = .91), mother–teacher pairings (r = .82), and father–teacher pairings (r = .75).

Validity

The test authors used three independent samples to assess the factor structure of the SRS. These samples included a teacher report from a normal school sample (Constantino, Przybeck, Friesen, & Todd, 2000), an epidemiological sample of male twins (Constantino, Davis et al., 2003), and a clinical sample involving 226 child psychiatric patients with and without pervasive developmental disorders (PDD) (Constantino et al., 2004). Results of the factor analysis of these samples failed to support the existence of independent subdomains of dysfunction in ASD. The analysis supported one factor, which resulted in disparate phenotypic manifestations across the three criterion domains for autistic disorder: social deficits, language deficits, and repetitive/stereotypical behaviors. Over 25 SRS items had factor loadings greater than .60 on this primary factor, including items representing all three DSM-IV criterion domains for autism (social deficits, language deficits, and restricted interests/stereotypical behavior).

The authors also report that ROC analysis revealed high degrees of sensitivity and specificity for both the screening and clinical cutoff scores. Although research on the SRS has identified autistic symptoms that may be attributable to a singular underlying deficiency, SRS treatment subscales were developed to aid in identifying therapeutic needs and approaches. The authors also report that a total raw score of 75 was associated with a sensitivity of .85 and specificity of .75 for any ASD as rated by expert clinicians, and a total raw score of 85 was associated with sensitivity of .70 and a specificity of .90.

The authors also describe a study conducted to evaluate the placement of the 65 SRS items into five treatment subscales: Social Awareness, Social Cognition, Social Communication, Social Motivation, and Autistic Mannerisms. Expert judges (N = 25), including counselors, social workers, psychiatrists, pediatricians, and psychologists who had experience in working with ASD and PDD, were given the 65 items and asked to sort each item into one of the five groups. Each item was given an expert assignment based on the majority of placements. In order to compare the original placements with the expert placements, nominal scale cross-tabulation was used. There was a significant result (χ^2 = 94.24, p < .001). Proportional-reduction-in-error statistics yielded Cohen's kappa of .585 and lambda = .506 (for both, p < .001).

The manual also reports that because subscales were not created as fully independent measures, there is a high degree of intercorrelation among them. Parent report data from 168 cases were used to assess the consistency between the item-to-scale assignments (Constantino et al., 2004). Alpha reliabilities were calculated for the set of items in each subscale. Values ranged from .77 in the Social Awareness subscale (8 items) to .92 for the Social Communication subscale (22 items). In addition, the correlations of items with their subscale membership versus other subscales were examined. The authors concluded that there was some support for the assignment of items to their respective scales.

The structure of the SRS was further examined in a sample of parents (N = 1,576) of randomly ascertained twins. The mean scores for males in this sample was 35.3 and for females was 27.5 (t = 7.63, p < .001). When the previously established cutoff score for males with PDD-NOS was used, 1.4% of males and 0.3% of females had scores at or above the cutoff (Fisher exact test, p = .03)(Constantino & Todd, 2003). In addition, Chakrabarti and Fombonne (2001) found the prevalence of PDD to be 0.6%, with a male-to-female ratio of 4:1.

The authors used structural equation modeling to examine the factor structure of the SRS for 232 monozygotic and dizygotic male twins. Intraclass correlations of twin–twin pairs for scores on the SRS were .73 for monozygotic twins and .37 for dizygotic twins. They reported that genetic factors accounted for approximately 76% of the total variance, and that SRS scores were not significantly influenced by age, rater bias, or rater contrast effects (Constantino & Todd, 2000). The authors also reported that the additive genetic influence on social deficits in the epidemiological sample of females was .40. In order to determine whether gender-specific genetic effects accounted for the discrepancy between males and females, the SRS was administered to the parents of 300 of opposite-sex dizygotic twins. The authors reported that genes influencing autistic traits appear to be the same for males and females (Constantino & Todd, 2003).

Data for the Child Behavior Checklist (CBCL) and SRS were also obtained for male twins (N = 219). Regression analysis indicated that scores for internalizing and externalizing behavior explained less than 5% of the variance in SRS scores. *SEM* was used to determine that the best-fitting model was one in which the majority of causal influences on SRS scores (55%; 90% confidence interval = .45–.70) were genetic influences specific to the SRS. Less than 20% of the overlap in the causal influence scores on either instrument was accounted for by overlap in phenotypic characteristics of the SRS and syndromal CBCL scores for attention problems and social problems (Constantino, Hudziak, & Todd, 2003). The authors suggested that the SRS measures a unique, genetically determined component of psychopathology independent from other domains of child psychopathology, and that subthreshold autistic differences may operate to make other psychopathology worse (Constantino & Todd, 2003). The authors further suggest that measuring subthreshold autistic differences can be helpful for predicting a clinical course and understanding influences on other child mental health problems.

In order to further assess the structural validity of the SRS, a preliminary study of the extent to which subthreshold autistic traits measured were related to familial predisposition to autism in the clinical sample (Constantino et al., 2004) was conducted. Parent report data were collected from 72 siblings of the initial clinical sample (48 siblings of participants with PDD, 24 siblings of participants with non-PDD psychiatric diagnoses). The mean SRS score for siblings with PDD (45.9) was substantially higher than that for siblings with non-PDD psychiatric diagnoses (16.8) ($t = 4.09$, $p = .0001$). According to the authors, these results indicate that autistic deficits measurable by the SRS aggregate in the siblings of patients with PDD.

Discriminant validity—the extent to which the SRS differentiates ASD from other psychiatric disorders—was assessed in psychiatric patients ($N = 158$) with and without ASD, as well as 287 randomly selected children from a St. Louis school district who participated in the initial study of the SRS (Constantino et al., 2000). High scores on the SRS were associated with the clinical diagnoses of autistic disorder, Asperger's disorder, and PDD-NOS, and not with other psychiatric conditions or with low IQ. Average SRS scores for children with various noncomorbid Axis I mood disorders were as follows: mood disorder, 59.4; conduct disorder, 48.4; psychotic disorder, 40.3; attention-deficit/hyperactivity disorder, 51.1; and PDD-NOS, 101.5. Children with PDD-NOS had significantly higher scores than children in other groups (single-factor analysis of variance [ANOVA]: $F = 11.69$, $df = 4.75$, $p < .001$).

The SRS manual also describes a study (Constantino, Davis, et al., 2003) to assess the relationships between the SRS and the ADI-R in a clinical sample of 61 child psychiatric patients. Subjects were evaluated with the SRS and the ADI-R a month apart. Participants whose SRS scores score fell within 2 SD of the mean (100) for PDD-NOS had ADI-R social deficit scores ranging from 0 to 30 (the ADI-R clinical cutoff being 10). No respondent with an ADI-R score above the clinical cutoff had an SRS score below 65, indicating the presence of symptoms that were at least mildly to moderately clinically significant. Mean scores for clinical participants without

PDD were also lower than scores for participants with PDD (single-factor ANOVA: $F = 72.95$; $df = 2.58$; $p < .0001$). Significant correlations between mothers, fathers, and teachers on quantitative assessments of autistic deficits with the SRS were found and ranged from .75 to .91. SRS scores were also found to be unrelated to IQ and exhibited a 2-year test–retest stability of .83.

CONCLUSIONS

The information summarized in this chapter provides researchers and clinicians with important characteristics of methods used to assess behaviors associated with ASD, as well as a review of the psychometric qualities that such measures should possess. Table 3.2 provides a summary of the essential aspects of these instruments. As is apparent from examination of the table and the reviews provided earlier in this chapter, the authors of these rating scales differ considerably in their approach to instrument development. For example, some of the scales are very short (e.g., the CARS has only 15 items), whereas others contain many items (e.g., 93) for the ADI-R. Some authors provide only raw scores, which make interpretation difficult, and only two scales (the ASRS and SRS) provide standard scores (*T* scores). Although these two tests provide derived scores, only the sample upon which the ASRS was based was selected to represent the normal population. Basing standard scores on a national sample is greatly preferable to basing them on a sample of individuals who may have autism.

All the scales except the ASRS and SRS use children with suspected or verified psychological disorders from either research studies or clinic settings as a comparison group. This method allows a clinician to determine whether an examinee is like other children with suspected or documented psychological problems, but comparing the score a child gets on a rating scale to the scores of other children who (1) were referred for evaluation, (2) had some diagnosis on the autism spectrum, or (3) participated in a study of autistic children has several problems. First, if an individual gets a *T* score of 50, this would mean that he or she has evidenced behaviors like those of persons who may have ASD. This is not a diagnostic statement, however, for two reasons. First, there is no evidence that the samples used to create the comparison groups for each scale are representative of children with ASD or of the U.S. population. The samples may be limited in demographic characteristics, and therefore the comparison will be affected by the variability of that sample. The sample may be restricted or very heterogeneous, either of which will (1) be undetectable and (2) have a considerable effect on the quality of the comparison. Second, because it is unknown how well such a sample represents children and adolescents with

TABLE 3.2. Comparison of Essential ASD Rating Scale Characteristics

Behavior rating scale	No. of items	Age range	Comparison sample size	Comparison sample	Representative standardization sample	Scores for total scale	Scores for scales
Autism Diagnostic Interview—Revised (ADI-R)	93	2–x years	Exact N not given	Children with and without ASD, studies conducted by authors where interviews were administered as part of routine initial clinical assessment and systematic research evaluations	No	Raw score	Summary raw scores
Autism Spectrum Rating Scale (ASRS)	80	2–5 and 6–18 years	2,000	National standardization sample of children and youth in the United States and Canada	Yes	T score	T scores
Childhood Autism Rating Scale (CARS)	15	Exact ages not given	1,600	Children who were referred to the TEACCH program (see text)	No	Raw score	None
Social Communication Questionnaire (SCQ)	40	4–x years	200	A wide variety of individuals (persons with autism, atypical autism, Asperger syndrome, fragile X syndrome, Rett syndrome, conduct disorder, language delay, mental retardation, and other clinical diagnoses)	No	Raw score	Raw scores
Social Responsiveness Scale (SRS)	65	4–18 years	1,636	Cases from five studies, combined into one sample (74% white, 11% black, 11% Hispanic, 2% Asian, 2% other)	No	T score	T scores

ASD in the particular state in which the sample was collected, or any other state, generalization to clients in other states is limited.

Using a national sample to construct a norm conversion table provides a considerable advantage, for several reasons. First, a large sample allows for reliable calibration of derived scores. Second, comparison to that sample yields an understanding of how often behaviors associated with ASD are found within the typical population. Third, the comparison of a child's or adolescent's behavior to what is expected in the typically developing population provides for greater understanding of how far an individual may be from the norm. Fourth, having a well-normed score provides a means of calibrating how much response to intervention is needed to bring the individual's behavior into a range that can be considered typical.

The most glaring shortcoming of nearly all these scales is that they do not have standard scores that are based on a national standardization sample. This poses a considerable liability for those who choose to use these measures, because it is imperative to know how different an examinee's behavior is from that of typical individuals, as well as how the behaviors compare to those of persons with ASD. The only way to know the rate at which typical children show behaviors associated with ASD is to have a national standardization group and to base norms on this sample. Clinicians can then make defensible statements about how far a child deviates from normality and to what extent the normative data support a diagnosis. Those measures that do not have a national standardization sample should be viewed with caution by clinicians, because interpretation of results across tests is made very difficult by the differences in the samples, and the stability of the norms cannot be determined. The use of well-developed, psychometrically sound assessments will greatly enhance the likelihood that accurate and valid information can be obtained.

REFERENCES

American Educational Research Association (AERA), American Psychological Association, & National Council on Measurement in Education. (1999). *Standards for educational and psychological testing*. Washington, DC: AERA.

American Psychiatric Association. (2000). *Diagnostic and statistical manual of mental disorders* (4th ed., text rev.). Washington, DC.

Anastasi, A., & Urbina, S. (1997). *Psychological testing* (7th ed.). Upper Saddle River, NJ: Prentice Hall.

Berument, S. K., Rutter, J., Lord, C., Pickles, A., & Bailey, A. (1999). Autism screening questionnaire: Diagnostic validity. *British Journal of Psychiatry, 175,* 444–451.

Bishop, D. V. M., & Norbury, C. F. (2002). Exploring the borderlands of autistic disorder and specific language impairment: A study using standardized diagnostic instruments. *Journal of Child Psychology and Psychiatry, 43,* 917–929.

Bracken, B. A., & McCallum, R. S. (1997). *Universal Nonverbal Intelligence Test.* Itasca, IL: Riverside.

Bracken, B. A. (1987). Limitations of preschool instruments and standards for minimal levels of technical adequacy. *Journal of Psychoeducational Assessment, 5,* 313–326.

Chakrabarti, S., & Fombonne, E. (2001). Pervasive developmental disorders in preschool children. *Journal of the American Medical Association, 285,* 3093–3099.

Cohen, J. (1988). *Statistical power analysis in the behavioral sciences* (2nd ed.). Hillsdale, NJ: Erlbaum.

Constantino, J. N., Przybeck, R., Friesen, D., & Todd, R. D. (2000). Reciprocal social behavior in children with and without pervasive developmental disorders. *Journal of Developmental and Behavior Pediatrics, 21,* 2–11.

Constantino, J. N., & Todd, R. D. (2003). The genetic structure of reciprocal social behavior. *American Journal of Psychiatry, 157,* 2043–2045.

Constantino, J. N., Hudziak, J. J., & Todd, R. D. (2003). Deficits in reciprocal social behavior in male twins: Evidence for a genetically independent domain of psychopathology. *Journal of the American Academy of Child and Adolescent Psychiatry, 42,* 458–467.

Constantino, J. N., & Gruber, C. P. (2005). *Social Responsiveness Scale.* Los Angeles: Western Psychological Services.

Constantino, J. N., Gruber, C. P., Davis, S., Hayes, S., Passanante, N., & Przybeck, R. (2004). The factor structure of autistic traits. *Journal of Child Psychology and Psychiatry, 45,* 719–726.

Constantino, J. N., Davis, S. A., Todd, R. D., Schindler, M. K., Gross, M. M., Brophy, S. L., et al. (2003). Validation of a brief quantitative genetic measure of autistic traits: Comparison of the Social Responsiveness Scale with the Autism Diagnostic Interview—Revised. *Journal of Autism and Developmental Disorders, 33,* 427–433.

Creek, M. (1961). Schizophrenia syndrome in childhood: Progress report of a working party. *Cerebral Palsy Bulletin, 3,* 501–504.

Crocker, L., & Algina, J. (1986). *Introduction to classical and modern test theory.* New York: Holt, Rinehart & Winston.

DiLavore, P., Lord, C., & Rutter, M. (1995). Pre-linguistic autism diagnostic Observation Schedule (PL-ADOS). *Journal of Autism and Developmental Disorders, 25,* 355–379.

Goldstein, S., & Naglieri, J. A. (2009). *Autism Spectrum Rating Scale.* Toronto: Multihealth Systems.

Gotham, K., Risi, S., Pickles, A., & Lord, C. (2007). The Autism Diagnostic Observation Schedule: Revised algorithms for improved diagnostic validity. *Journal of Autism and Developmental Disorders, 37,* 613–627.

Kanner, L. (1943). Autistic disturbances of affective contact. *Nervous Child, 2,* 217–250.

Kaufman, A. S., & Kaufman, N. L. (2004). *Kaufman Assessment Battery for*

Children—Second Edition manual. Circle Pines, MN: American Guidance Service.

Krug, D. A., Arick, J. R., & Almond, P. J. (2008). *Autism Behavior Checklist— Second Edition.* Austin, TX: PRO-ED.

Lord, C., Rutter, M., Goode, S., Heemsbergen, J., Jordan, H., Mawhood, L., et al. (1989). Autism Diagnostic Observation Schedule: A standardized observation of communicative and social behavior. *Journal of Autism and Developmental Disorders, 19,* 185–212.

Lord, C., Rutter, M., DiLavore, P. C., & Risi, S. (2002). *Autism Diagnostic Observation Schedule.* Los Angeles: Western Psychological Services.

Naglieri, J. A., & Das, J. P. (1997). *Cognitive Assessment System interpretive handbook.* Itasca, IL: Riverside.

National Society for Autistic Children. (1978). National Society for Autistic Children definition of the syndrome of autism. *Journal of Autism and Developmental Disorders, 8,* 132–137.

Nunnally, J. C., & Bernstein, I. H. (1994). *Psychometric theory.* New York: McGraw-Hill.

Rutter, M. (1978). Diagnosis and definition of childhood autism. *Journal of Autism and Developmental Disorders, 8,* 139–161.

Rutter, M., Bailey, A., & Lord, C. (2003a). *Social Communication Questionnaire.* Los Angeles: Western Psychological Services.

Rutter, M., Le Couteur, A., & Lord, C. (2003b). *Autism Diagnostic Interview— Revised.* Los Angeles: Western Psychological Services.

Schopler, E., Lansing, M. D., Reichler, R. J., & Marcus, L. M. (2005). *Psychoeducational Profile—Third Edition.* Austin, TX: PRO-ED.

Schopler, E., Reichler, R. J., & Renner, B. R. (1988). *Childhood Autism Rating Scale.* Los Angeles: Western Psychological Services.

Sparrow, S. S., Balla, D. A., & Cicchetti, D. V. (1984). *Vineland Adaptive Behavior Scales.* Circle Pines, MN: American Guidance Services.

Thorndike, R. L. (1982). *Applied psychometrics.* Boston: Houghton Mifflin.

Wechsler, D. (2003). *Wechsler Intelligence Scale for Children—Fourth Edition.* San Antonio, TX: Psychological Corporation.

CHAPTER FOUR

—

Subtyping the Autism
Spectrum Disorders
THEORETICAL, RESEARCH,
AND CLINICAL CONSIDERATIONS

Ami Klin

The pervasive developmental disorders (PDD) are early-emerging neu-rodevelopmental disorders that have an impact on most domains of social and communicative functioning, as well as on variable domains of cognitive and adaptive functioning. PDD are vastly heterogeneous in both genotype and phenotype; this heterogeneity probably reflects multiple etiologies and pathogenic courses (Volkmar, Lord, Bailey, Schutz, & Klin, 2004). Current models of genetic susceptibility predict involvement of multiple genes and gene combinations, with both *de novo* and familial origins (Zhao et al., 2007). Specific genetic etiologies have been, so far, primarily associated with small groups of individuals and their families (e.g., involving rare variant alleles) (Gupta & State, 2007). In terms of clinical presentation, individuals with PDD range from those who are profoundly intellectually disabled to those with IQs in the gifted range; from those who are non-verbal to those who are hyperverbal; from those who are extraordinarily socially isolated to those who cannot stop themselves from approaching others, albeit inappropriately; and from those whose lives are enchained by stereotypic movements or repetitive behaviors to those whose lives are dominated by learning about unusual topics (Volkmar & Klin, 2005).

These multiple levels of heterogeneity are often viewed as one of the greatest obstacles blocking the advancement of research on the causes and treatments of these disorders (Volkmar et al., 2004). Basic and clinical scientists are continually frustrated by the fact that their hypotheses are diluted in this sea of variability. Their work typically requires homogeneous samples, and systems of classification have so far failed to provide subgroupings characterized by the required level of constraints in syndrome expression.

This frustration has led to the increasing use of the term "autism spectrum disorders" (ASD), which blurs the categorical boundaries among the most common PDD—autism, Asperger syndrome, and PDD not otherwise specified (PDD-NOS)—into a hypothesized continuum of affectedness (Wing, 1986, 2000; Wing & Gould, 1979). The term "spectrum" implies that a number of meaningful dimensions could generate the full spectrum of syndrome expression (not unlike, for example, the spectrum of light). These dimensions, if validated, could be considered as factors mediating the relationship between etiology/etiologies and behavioral expressions of this family of conditions. These so-called "endophenotypes," however, are still very much works in progress, and various candidates have been proposed at multiple levels of causation—from gene(s) and gene combinations, neuroanatomical abnormalities, and disease processes to onset patterns, neurocognitive abnormalities, combinations of symptom clusters, and levels of such developmental skills as language and intellectual endowment (Dawson et al., 2002; DiCicco-Bloom et al., 2006). In light of this, the need for PDD subtyping—in terms of etiology, genotype, brain pathology, pathogenesis, behavioral expressions, skill and symptom profile, among other possibilities—is hardly a quest necessitating justification. And yet discussions of such subtyping typically focus primarily on the creation of categorical subdivisions of ASD, their validation, and their utility (Volkmar & Klin, 2005). This chapter argues for the need to expand the discussion of the "subtyping enterprise," as the establishment of meaningful research goals requires a focus on this question: *What is the subtyping for?* The answer to this question shapes the identification of relevant concepts, defines the levels of analyses, and ultimately determines the types of research programs needed to maximize chances of success.

At present, individuals with autism (or autistic disorder), the paradigmatic PDD, correspond to perhaps one-fifth of the epidemiological samples identified as having ASD, whereas those with PDD-NOS, the residual and by necessity poorly defined PDD category, correspond to the remaining four-fifths; those with Asperger syndrome, because of this category's unresolved nosological status and variable usage, fall into one camp or the other (Fombonne, 2003; Fombonne & Tidmarsh, 2003). Since the majority of individuals affected by a PDD are assigned to the NOS category (Fombonne & Tidmarsh, 2003), historically reserved in the *Diagnostic and Statistical Manual of Mental Disorders* (DSM) and *International Classi-*

fication of Diseases (ICD) systems for those who do not meet criteria for the better-defined and better-established syndrome entities, there is clearly a need for reevaluation of our classification systems.

Compounding the problems in subtyping research is the ubiquitous expectation that subtyping solutions in one domain of research or clinical practice should necessarily apply to other domains. And yet there is no reason to assume, for example, that factors underlying classification for the purpose of eligibility for educational services should be the same as those underlying classification for the purpose of etiological research. ICD-10 has addressed this issue by creating "clinical" and "research" criteria separately, although these are conceptually very similar. DSM-IV-TR requires only one set of criteria, given its formal implications for issues of medical practice, entitlements, and eligibility for school-based remediation programs. Without consideration of these various realities, subtyping research is likely to perpetuate unsatisfactory solutions. And the blurring of pertinent factors influencing this discussion can lead to sterile controversies concerning the nosological validity of this or another subcategory (Klin & Volkmar, 2003).

Classification systems are the results of (among other things) the historical origins of concepts; the work of influential clinicians; the evolving usage of concepts and their acceptance by the community of investigators and the general public; and scientific trends and discoveries (Kendler, 1990). As noted, it would be naïve to assume that classification systems could be equally relevant across various domains of research and clinical practice, from molecular genetics to educational law. This chapter provides the backdrop for discussions of research on PDD subtyping. I begin with a brief historical overview, which sets the stage for current nosological problems. I then discuss the different subtyping considerations arising from different questions in clinical practice and research programs.

HISTORICAL PERSPECTIVES

With some exceptions, the history of ASD classification reflects some uneven paradigm shifts in descriptions of early onset social disabilities. The modern history of these disorders can be traced back to some isolated descriptions of "feral children" (supposedly "growing up in the wild" without human socialization influences), and of children who presented with prodigious but circumscribed skills while being severely intellectually disabled (who were then labeled "idiot savants"). Many of these children displayed behaviors that can now be understood as consistent with autism. The period prior to the 1940s was dominated by descriptions of psychopathology in children on the basis of catchall terms such as "psychosis" (which implied an unwarranted link between autism and schizophrenia), or on the basis of theoretically derived concepts or hypothesized causative principles with origins in psychoanalytic thought and practice (Rutter, 1965; 1972). The former trend was not immediately pertinent to discussions of classification since by definition it focused on the very small number of children with savant skills. The latter discussion was so dependent on its theoretical origins that the concepts could not otherwise be codified for use in general practice while achieving some measure of standardized use and interclinician reliability.

A momentous advance occurred with Leo Kanner's original description of 11 children as having a congenital disorder of "affective contact," which he termed "autism" (Kanner, 1943). Kanner's paper has retained its relevance to this day because of his exquisite and theory-free descriptions of actual behaviors, and because of his success in contextualizing these behaviors in developmental terms. The most well-known child psychiatrist of his generation working in the United States, Kanner's "autism" became the major conceptualizing force of ASD for years to come. At about the same time, however, the Austrian pediatrician Hans Asperger published his account of a small number of children who were similar to Kanner's in some areas (e.g., their social adaptive disabilities) but distinct in others (e.g., their preserved intellectual and language abilities) (Asperger, 1944). He assigned the label of "autistic psychopathy" to these children, thus emphasizing their "autism" but failing to highlight the developmental nature of the condition (e.g., he thought that the condition might not be identified in the first 3 years of life). Asperger published his work in German, and with the moving of the center of gravity of child psychiatry from the German- to the English-speaking countries after World War II, his work never reached academic centers in the United States and United Kingdom until after his death (through the initial work of Lorna Wing, 1981). And this, of course, was after the publication of the influential third edition of DSM (DSM-III; American Psychiatric Association, 1980), which created for the first time the category of PDD. In this edition, PDD had five subtypes: infantile autism, residual infantile autism, child onset PDD, residual child onset PDD, and atypical PDD.

In the 1960s and 1970s, programmatic research began in autism with the publication of the first substantial studies in epidemiology (Lotter, 1966, 1967), genetics (Folstein & Rutter, 1977), and experimental psychology (Hermelin & O'Connor, 1970). Almost immediately, it became apparent that comparability across studies required operational definitions of autism that could be followed by any investigator wishing to study the condition. Rutter's influential codification of Kanner's prose (Rutter, 1978), combined with the work of others who wanted to include aspects of the condition that were now emerging from systematic studies, eventually led to the formal definition of autism—or "infantile autism," in DSM-III (American Psychiatric Association, 1980). The need for the residual, or subthreshold, category of atypical PDD reflected the awareness that a number of cases might not meet the full criteria for infantile autism because their symptom profile was atypical or less severe relative to the benchmark description of autism.

DSM-III-R (American Psychiatric Association, 1987) introduced the category of PDD-NOS as we know it today. It also reflected the body of work gaining momentum on the developmental nature and variability in syndrome expression of autism and the need for the criteria to be more detailed in order to better operationalize the guidelines for diagnosis. To some extent, this trend reflected the epidemiological work and advocacy of Lorna Wing, who emphasized the need for a more inclusive approach to autism, as well as for increased awareness of the important implications of formal diagnostic systems to issues of patient management and entitlements (Wing, 2000). Empirical validation of DSM-III-R criteria relative to a "gold standard" (defined as the practice of highly experienced clinicians) indicated that DSM-III-R criteria were "overly inclusive" relative to clinician-assigned diagnoses, resulting in many false positives (Volkmar, Bregman, Cohen, & Cicchetti, 1988; Volkmar, Cicchetti, Bregman, & Cohen, 1992).

This finding was addressed in DSM-IV (American Psychiatric Association, 1994) through a substantial field trial of criteria for autistic disorder, in which previous and proposed diagnostic schemes were tested relative to clinicians' practices in 19 centers around the world, involving over 1,000 children (Volkmar et al., 1994). The field trial also included a number of emerging diagnostic entities that were included as potential candidates for inclusion under the PDD category. These were Asperger syndrome (Asperger's disorder), Rett syndrome (Rett's disorder), and childhood disintegrative disorder (CDD). The inclusion of Asperger's disorder in DSM-IV syndrome reflected the proliferation of this diagnosis following Wing's (1981) report and the work of Christopher Gillberg and colleagues (e.g., Gillberg, 1989; Gillberg & Gillberg, 1989), among others. The inclusion of Rett's disorder followed advancements in behavioral and medical research related to a condition first described by Andreas Rett, an Austrian child neurologist (Rett, 1966; see also van Acker, Loncola, & van Acker, 2005). And the inclusion of CDD followed the corroboration that autism could indeed develop in children who had exhibited normal development for several years. This condition was first described by Theodore Heller, an Austrian special educator (Heller, 1908; see also Volkmar, Koenig, & State, 2005).

Results of the DSM-IV field trial by and large determined the text finally formalized in DSM-IV. The DSM criteria for PDD have generated some controversies that are still unresolved to date:

1. The criteria for autistic disorder became more "narrow" than in DSM-III-R. It is therefore not surprising that the residual category of PDD-NOS became more heavily populated (Volkmar et al., 1994).

2. The DSM-IV criteria for Asperger's disorder were modeled closely after those for autistic disorder, resulting in extensive overlap, with a distinction between the two focused primarily on onset patterns and developmental skills (e.g., the typical onset and preservation of formal language skills and intellectual functioning in Asperger's disorder). This issue and the tentative status of Asperger's disorder resulted in the "precedence rule," by which cases should be given the diagnosis of autistic disorder rather than Asperger's disorder if they appear to meet criteria for both. That notwithstanding, the stage was set for a highly problematic literature focused on whether these two conditions are "the same or different." To some extent, this situation came about because (a) until recently, data on onset patterns were by and large retrospective; (b) criteria were not included to operationalize differences between prototypical cases of the two conditions; and (c) there were (and continue to be) several widespread diagnostic schemes and clinical/research practices already in use (e.g., considering Asperger syndrome a form of autism without accompanying intellectual or language impairment regardless of onset patterns; separating the two conditions on the basis of presence–absence of fundamental language delays, such as the emergence of first words or phrase speech, in the first 2 or 3 years of life) (Klin, McPartland, & Volkmar, 2005a).

3. Rett's disorder was included in DSM-IV primarily because of the potential for error in the diagnosis of girls with this syndrome who typically also exhibit symptoms, at least for a period of time, similar to those seen in children with autism (Rutter, 1994; van Acker et al., 2005). There were concerns, however, later substantiated, that this is a genetic syndrome of mental retardation—not unlike, for example, fragile X syndrome, which is not a PDD (Ropers & Jamel, 2005).

4. Despite capturing an exceedingly small number of cases, CDD was included with the other PDD in DSM-IV because of its potential for elucidating causative mechanisms involved in autism (Volkmar et al., 2005).

The next update of the DSM system came with DSM-IV-TR, the text revision of DSM-IV (American Psychiatric Association, 2000). This version included only updates and changes in accompanying text and correction of important typos. Actual criteria were not changed in any of the PDD subtypes. For example, an attempt was made to ensure that the diagnosis of PDD-NOS would be used only in cases of early-emerging social disabilities (children with this diagnosis have to meet criteria in the social cluster and in the communication *or* stereotypic behavior cluster). Also, additional guidelines (but only heuristic, not formal) were provided for the distinction between autistic disorder and Asperger's disorder.

It is important to note that despite the practical importance of DSM-IV, this system is but a collection of briefly described symptoms and hierarchical rules for diagnostic decision making. It is supposed to be the repository of nosological research and to guide future research studies by setting standards for inclusion of subjects in studies. In practice, however, with the advent of large genetic research consortia involving countries around the globe, the need for further standardization of diagnostic procedures across vastly different clinical and research settings, in different countries and cultures, has become all too apparent. Similar pressure has come from epidemiological studies, which are extremely susceptible to variation in the definition and/or use of diagnostic criteria and procedures. Thus various diagnostic instruments have appeared, which provide more rigorous, comprehensive, and operationalized procedures for obtaining clinical data and for making diagnostic decisions (Lord & Corsello, 2005). Chief among these are the Autism Diagnostic Interview—Revised (ADI-R; Rutter, Le Couteur, & Lord, 2003) and the Autism Diagnostic Observation Schedule (ADOS; Lord, Rutter, DiLavore, & Risi, 1999), both of which are keyed to DSM-IV criteria and provide the benchmark for the diagnosis of autism. Training and achievement of interrater reliability on these instruments are prerequisites for their use, as is a level of clinical experience with individuals with ASD across the lifespan. However, neither instrument includes Asperger's disorder; they make distinctions only between autism/ASD and not-ASD. Thus the nosological status of Asperger's disorder remains uncertain as the field now gears up toward DSM-V.

There are yet other issues left untouched by the current DSM system. Some of these reflect the emergence of new fields of research activities, whereas others reflect increasingly widespread patterns of use of diagnostic labels or changes in the overall perception of autism and related disorders resulting from increased public awareness of the ASD. First, despite autism's being defined as an early-emerging neurodevelopmental disorder, data on children under the age of 2 or 3 years are only beginning to emerge—as a result of (among other things) prospective studies of siblings of children with autism (Zwaigenbaum et al., 2007). Very few children under the age of 3 years were included in the DSM-IV field trial; therefore, the criteria included in DSM-IV did not include this group in any meaningful way (Volkmar et al., 1994). Studies of the applicability of DSM-IV criteria to this age group, as well as studies of their validity, reliability, and stability (over time), have not yet resulted in established guidelines, despite the fact that the numbers of such referrals have increased exponentially in the past 10 years or so (Chawarska, Klin, Paul, & Volkmar, 2007; Zwaigenbaum et al., 2005). Second, many clinicians and investigators alike appear to have ignored DSM-IV by (1) opting to use the term "ASD" for all PDD subtypes (though typically individuals with Rett's disorder and CDD are studied separately); (2) making a distinction only between autism and other ASD (combining cases of Asperger's disorder and PDD-NOS, and ignoring any overlap between autistic disorder and Asperger's disorder); (3) using the term "Asperger syndrome" for any case of ASD with IQ in the normative range or above; or (4) using the term "Asperger syndrome" for any person with ASD who is relatively "higher-functioning" (variably defined), or who has a "milder" form of the condition, or is no longer a child (i.e., an adult) (Klin et al., 2005a). Third, more and more cases who were not identified in childhood are now being referred (often self-referred) for diagnostic evaluation. This is a natural development resulting from increased public awareness, coupled with the fact that the global notion of Asperger syndrome (and milder forms of autism) were not available, or were not truly accepted as autism-like conditions, until the mid-1990s. Many individuals who were born in the 1970s or earlier were therefore not recognized as having a social disability within the autistic spectrum. For some of these individuals, their early history is not easily or reliably obtained, presenting a vexing problem for clinicians who need to make diagnostic judgments about the quintessential family of neurodevelopmental disorders with origins in infancy. The fact that social disabilities or difficulties can also result from combinations of other Axis I and/or Axis II disorders creates problems that have not as yet been adequately addressed in clinical investigations (Klin, Mayes, Volkmar, & Cohen, 1995a; Tantam, 2003).

Finally, it is important to note that the utility of the "gold standard" criterion for nosological studies—venerably encapsulated by the senior and highly experienced clinician—is now being called into question, given the inherent discrepancy between individuals seen in tertiary specialized clinics (e.g., more "prototypical," impaired, and challenged) and those included in population-based studies (which are not equally influenced by such a referral bias). Historically, criteria were created and operationalized on the basis of the former. With increased public awareness of the ASD, those nonprototypical or "milder" cases that were only identified in population-based studies are becoming current clinical referrals. In other words, the "gold standard" image of autism is also changing. This is an inevitable but not fully acknowledged development. For example, the shift in the intellectual distribution of people assigned the generic label of autism or ASD has been tremendous: Whereas about 80% were thought to have intellectual disabilities some two or three decades ago (Lockyer & Rutter, 1969), a new epidemiological study of the Centers for Disease Control and Prevention (2007) revealed that only 54% of the identified population had mental retardation. Of course, the former related primarily to prototypical individuals with autism, whereas the latter adopted a much broader view of autism and related disorders. In the past, the work in the clinics shaped the perception of autism in the community; nowadays, the work in clinical science is being influenced by knowledge originating in the community.

SUBTYPING FOR CLINICAL MANAGEMENT

In many ways, subtyping for clinical management is probably the least problematic form of subtyping. Whereas research stumbles on heterogeneity, variability of profiles is the very stuff of clinical management (Klin, Saulnier, Tsatsanis, & Volkmar, 2005c). Best-practice parameters establish that programs of treatment and intervention are not created on the basis of diagnostic labels but on the basis of individualized profiles of strengths and weaknesses, couched in terms of both autistic symptoms (e.g., social and communication disabilities) and developmental skills (e.g., intellectual and language levels) (National Research Council, 2001). Other factors are the child's age, behavioral challenges, psychiatric comorbidities, and anything else that either helps or hinders the child in profiting from behavioral and educational interventions. Adequate programming is thus defined as a comprehensive and intensive package of services and supports that addresses the child's needs while capitalizing on the child's assets.

This consideration builds on the principle that clinical management—from the diagnostic evaluation through the process of securing eligibility for services and implementing individualized education programs—does not necessarily require the assignment of a PDD subtype (Klin et al., 2005c). Clearly, there are practical considerations that vary widely from educational system to educational system (within states, around the United States, and around the world). For example, autism is often considered a diagnosis that connotes more disability (and provides more leverage in securing services) than PDD-NOS, Asperger syndrome, or ASD. However, individuals with any of these conditions should be entitled to an individual education plan, regardless of PDD subtype. This process should be entirely based on the principle of maximizing a positive outcome, which in turn has to be determined case by case. Even in regard to psychopharmacological treatment, symptom profiles and behavioral challenges are much more important considerations than PDD subtyping (Scahill & Martin, 2005).

Of course, this directive may change in the future if studies begin to indicate that membership in a given PDD subtype predicts (1) response to specific treatments, (2) future challenges that can be avoided or minimized, or (3) resilience-related factors or assets that can be fostered and capitalized upon. To date, however, research comparing individuals with different PDD subtypes have not led to generalizable conclusions on the basis of such subgrouping. For example, considerations at the level of an individual's profile exceed (by far) in importance differences in treatment prescriptions on the basis of labels such as "[higher-functioning] autism," "PDD-NOS," or "Asperger syndrome." No current studies suggest that different PDD subtypes require different treatments. The most powerful predictors of outcome are still the individual child's levels of cognitive functioning and communicative speech (Howlin, 2005).

SUBTYPING FOR CLINICAL RESEARCH

The delineation of a behavioral syndrome carries the hope that a given subtype will facilitate discoveries related to its causes, be they neurobiological, genetic, environmental, or a combination thereof (Rutter & Schopler, 1992). Among the PDD, only Rett syndrome has fulfilled this promise to date, with the discovery of mutations in the X-linked MECP2 gene in over 80% of affected girls (Amir et al., 1999). Although some believe that this advancement will benefit research on autism because of behavioral commonalities (at least for a period of the development of girls with Rett syndrome), others are more circumspect: They point out the vast number of X-linked forms of mental retardation (Ropers & Hamel, 2005), the most prevalent of which is fragile X syndrome. And although there are social disabilities associated with fragile X syndrome (and other genetic syndromes of mental retardation), it is still unknown whether the behavioral commonalities with autism are of the same nature to justify the hope for shared etiology (Dykens & Hodapp, 2001). Underlying this discussion is the question of whether it is legitimate to consider behavioral symptoms in isolation from the clinical "gestalt" internalized by experienced clinicians. For example, many diagnostic criteria for autism refer to the "absence of" or "marked impairment in" a given skill—say, eye contact or facial expressiveness. It is possible that the same behavioral observation—lack of eye contact or lack of facial expressiveness in individuals with different conditions—could be the behavioral endpoint of different immediate causes (e.g., social anxiety and facial paralysis, respectively, in individuals with fragile X syndrome and Mobius syndrome). This would be very different from what is presumed to be the case in autism. Given that such similarities are often presented as justification for shared programs of etiological research, this issue should become an important topic for systematic discussion and study.

From a nosological standpoint, one can also make the converse argument. If the case is made for inclusion of Rett syndrome as a form of PDD, it is unclear why we should not also include fragile X syndrome, or maybe even other forms of mental retardation associated with some autism-like features. There have been striking advances in genetic research on mental retardation syndromes since the early 1990s, when Rett's disorder was first included in the DSM-IV class of PDD. These developments have not yet been assimilated in nosological research.

In this respect, however, there is some tension between clinicians and nonclinician basic science researchers. Whereas the former are more likely to draw lines of separation between the ASD and mental retardation syndromes, the latter are more likely to argue for capitalizing on exciting new molecular genetic and neurobiological findings emerging from research on fragile X syndrome, Rett syndrome, and others. And yet the ascertainment of cases of ASD is still very much a clinical endeavor and very much dependent on the use of standardized diagnostic instruments. In this regard, differential level of experience of the examiner may lead to differences in ascertainment, which in turn can bias sample compositions. For example, it is not entirely clear as yet what the rate of autistic disorder is in individuals with fragile X syndrome, and estimates vary widely (Volkmar et al., 2004). Almost invariably, however, the rates of fragile X syndrome in individuals with ASD are lower. And it is important to note that in contrast with these mental retardation syndromes, intellectual disabilities are present in only about half of ASD cases, and that intellectual impairment does not seem to be familial (Volkmar & Pauls, 2003). Complicating these connections further, whereas in Rett syndrome fewer than 1% of cases are inherited, genetic research in autism has revealed strong familial factors (as well as a considerable proportion of sporadic cases), and fragile X syndrome is the most common form of inherited mental retardation (Feinstein & Singh, 2007). All of these issues await more systematic discussions and studies. The status quo of the DSM system, which appears to mix behavioral syndromes anchored by autism (ASD) with one syndrome of mental retardation (Rett's disorder), but not others, is not sustainable. DSM-V will need to address this conceptual issue, and to consider a fast-approaching future in which a behavioral syndrome (or symptoms) may be associated with multiple etiologies.

More traditionally, discussion of nosological classification has focused on the "utility" of diagnostic categories, or the extent to which different subtypes can predict differential patterns of developmental course, response to treatment, and outcome (Szatmari, 2000). In this regard, only CDD (or Heller syndrome) can be considered a success story among the PDD. Indeed, the late onset of autism following a prolonged period of truly normative development (2 or 3 years) is associated with more severe autistic symptoms, more severe intellectual impairment, and more seriously compromised outcome. True cases of CDD are very rare, although some underreporting was likely in the past, and no medical or other causes have been discovered as yet for the dramatic developmental regression followed by stability without significant recovery. Developmental gains are limited, while motor skills and medical health are not compromised (Volkmar et al., 2005).

These various issues notwithstanding, the vast majority of research studies involving individuals with ASD do not include subjects with Rett syndrome or other syndromes with known etiology, or CDD. The prevalence rates for these conditions are quite low (e.g., 1 in every 10,000 to 15,000 females for Rett syndrome; van Acker et al., 2005). Thus, at least from the standpoint of sheer numbers of individuals involved, subtyping research needs to be focused on the three other categories of PDD—autism, Asperger syndrome, and PDD-NOS. As noted, the term "ASD" is often applied to individuals with these conditions who do not have significant intellectual impairment. Those with intellectual impairment are much more likely to be "prototypically" autistic and more homogeneous as a group. Thus the greatest nosological challenges are associated with the "higher-functioning" or less severely affected individuals with ASD.

Close to two decades of studies focused on phenomenological, neurocognitive, and neurobiological differences among these three groups—autism unaccompanied by mental retardation, or higher-functioning autism; Asperger syndrome; and PDD-NOS—have failed to yield solid conclusions as to whether they should be kept separate or be combined (Klin et al., 2005; Miller & Ozonoff, 2000). Although inconsistent findings across studies have often been considered strong arguments for eliminating these subcategories of PDD (or eliminating Asperger syndrome while retaining autism and PDD-NOS) and moving formally to the concept of ASD, these studies have been fraught with methodological problems—including inconsistent definitions, inconsistent operationalization of concepts, and circular reasoning, among others (Klin et al., 2005). Comparability of findings is virtually impossible, as many studies share only the inclusion of the term Asperger syndrome in their title; the concept is operationalized (explicitly or not at all) in multiple ways, so as to render any clear sense of subject samples very difficult indeed. To exemplify this fact, one study compared the impact of variable definitions of Asperger syndrome on the diagnostic composition of a large group of individuals with higher-functioning ASD. Three widespread definitions were used. By necessity, these different definitions not only alter the number of subjects meeting criteria for Asperger syndrome, but also the number of subjects assigned the label "autism" or "PDD-NOS," since the operationalization of the former changes the operationalization of the latter. Agreement among the three systems for diagnostic assignment to a given subject was 44%. Thus 56% of subjects received at least two different diagnoses, depending on the different diagnostic scheme (Klin, Pauls, Schultz, & Volkmar, 2005b).

Typically, studies using very detailed symptom descriptions supplementing DSM-IV criteria (e.g., adding differential patterns of onset and more "prototypical" positive symptoms) find some differences in cognitive profiles, comorbid psychopathology, and genetic liability—all of which, however, are of modest effect sizes (e.g., Klin, Volkmar, Sparrow, Cicchetti, & Rourke, 1995b; Ehlers, Nyden, Gillberg, & Dahlgren Sandberg, 1997). In contrast, studies differentiating higher-functioning autism from Asperger syndrome on the basis of single variables (e.g., presence–absence of speech by 2 or 3 years) do not (e.g., Gilchrist et al., 2001; Szatmari, Bartolucci, & Bremner, 1989). And some studies using DSM-IV criteria have failed to find significant differences in independently ascertained factors, such as neuropsychology (Miller & Ozonoff, 2000). More problematic is the fact that DSM-IV criteria are mostly ignored; even if they are followed, they are not operationalized, or sufficient details are not provided (e.g., the number of subjects with Asperger's disorder who would also meet criteria for autistic disorder). And concerns abound as to the very viability of DSM-IV criteria for Asperger's disorder (Mayes, Calhoun, & Crites, 2001; Miller & Ozonoff, 1997). Still more frequent is the situation in which the term "Asperger's disorder" is used with no operationalization at all, as a synonym for higher-functioning ASD.

Clearly, this problem could only be systematically tackled if there were some agreement on a set of criteria, comprehensively detailed and uniformly utilized according to standardized ascertainment procedures. But at the root of this problem is the fact that the all-important onset criteria have universally been ascertained retrospectively, often many years after the subjects' early childhood. It is possible that the advent of prospective studies will answer some of these questions. For example, meaningful differential patterns of onset can be used as independent variables, whereas diagnostic assignment later in life can be analyzed as dependent variables; this will enable researchers to explore the range of diagnostic outcomes associated with clusters of early symptoms or developmental profiles (e.g., language, joint attention skills, communication, nonverbal and verbal problem-solving skills, gross and fine motor skills).

But this solution hints at the possibility that the answer to this quandary lies in asking a different question. A more productive research program might focus on bidirectional analyses of developmental and current data of prospective cohorts, systematically mapping developmental factors on trajectories and eventual outcomes. In this way, researchers may avoid the rather circular reification of definitions, moving instead to a developmentally based and empirically derived nosology of higher-functioning ASD. Such studies are under way, and there is some hope that they will be available prior to DSM-V. In their absence, a new round of arbitrary decisions affecting the definition of Asperger disorder is very likely; the field may eventually adopt the concept of "usage validity" (i.e., most popular patterns of use) (Klin et al., 2005).

Finally, the concept of PDD-NOS continues to be highly problematic (Towbin, 2005). It is the most prevalent among the PDD, but the "residual" nature of its definition perpetuates a sense of nosological ignorance in the field. Clearly, this is an extremely important concept for practical reasons. Without it, hundreds of thousands of children would not receive services. But the hope throughout has been that the size of this amorphous group would be reduced gradually through the discovery of new subtypes or new syndromes. Indeed, there have been many candidates, but all have failed the test of time. Some concepts originated from discipline-specific definitions, such as "nonverbal learning disabilities" (NLD; neuropsychology) (Rourke, 1989) and "semantic–pragmatic disorder" (psycholinguistics) (Bishop, 2000; Rapin & Allen, 1983). Others were hybrids of symptom clusters and neuropsychological deficits, such as "deficits in attention, motor control and perception" (Gillberg, 2003). Still others, such as "multiplex developmental disorder" (MDD), resulted from consideration of comorbid psychopathology (e.g., anxiety and thought disorder) as core defining features (Cohen, Paul, & Volkmar, 1986). There were several reasons why these concepts have failed to spur research more widely, but chief among these is the fact that the concepts were often defined according to nosological criteria other than the staples of the DSM system—namely, developmental behavioral history and current behavioral presentation. For example, NLD are defined in terms of neuropsychological assets and deficits. Although they are associated with significant social vulnerabilities (Rourke, Young, & Leenaars, 1989), they are found in a number of psychiatric, genetic, and neurological conditions (Rourke, 1995). This creates the problem that concepts originating from different nosologies cannot be easily evaluated against one another because they are not mutually exclusive (e.g., a person may have *both* Asperger syndrome and NLD).

And yet all of these concepts have made heuristic contributions to the discussion of PDD subtyping. For example, the developmental modeling of NLD (which predicts a set of primary, secondary, and tertiary symptoms following developmental progression) (Klin & Volkmar, 1996; Rourke, 1989) points to the need to consider developmental trajectories in PDD subtyping, including learning profiles and their implications for adaptation. The focus on psychiatric comorbidity of MDD (Klin et al., 1995a) points to the need to take into account factors other than core autistic features that complicate and alter the expression of social and communicative symptoms. To illustrate this point, one study comparing profiles of psychiatric comorbidity and their familial loading in a sample of individuals with higher-functioning autism, Asperger syndrome, and PDD-NOS showed that these were more prevalent in individuals with PDD-NOS and their families than in individuals with higher-functioning autism or Asperger syndrome and their families (Klin et al., 2005b). Such conceptualization raises the possibility that for some individuals with ASD, the "autism" is the driving force of their social disabilities, whereas for others the accumulation of serious psychiatric disorders is what results in their socially disabled presentation. This is a key question, now that so many undiagnosed adults for whom developmental history is not available, or cannot be considered reliable or sufficiently detailed, are coming to clinical attention with a differential diagnosis of ASD.

Subtyping for Epidemiological Research

The need for a discussion of subtyping for epidemiological studies stems from the alarming increase in prevalence rates of ASD revealed in epidemiological studies since the early 1990s (Fombonne, 2005). Interestingly, it seems that rates for more "prototypical" individuals with autism (who, coincidentally, were those more likely to be identified in older epidemiological studies) have remained relatively stable, whereas those with nonautistic ASD (essentially, individuals with PDD-NOS) have increased dramatically (Fombonne & Tidmarsh, 2003).

Epidemiological studies are extremely dependent upon definitions of disorders and ascertainment procedures. Behind the increased rates of ASD, there may be a number of hints about the evolution of the term "PDD-NOS," as well as about specific patterns and profiles of developmental skills, autistic symptomatology, and psychiatric comorbidity. It is possible, therefore, that changes in nosological classification and more advanced understanding of ascertainment practices related to the concept of PDD-NOS may have a sizeable impact on rates of ASD in future epidemiological studies. Given the enormous public policy implications, as well as the proliferation of causative hypotheses of autism on the basis of gene–environment interactions, immunological factors, and environmental variables, there is an urgent need for increasingly detailed characterization of identified individuals beyond their "affected" status. Thus epidemiological research ought to become more hypothesis-driven in the future.

Dimensional Subtyping

Because of their defining algorithms, the ASD are typically ranked as more to less severe as one moves from autism to Asperger syndrome to PDD-NOS. Nevertheless, categorical diagnoses do not lend themselves to quantitative analysis of affectedness. And no diagnostic instrument has been designed with the explicit goal of quantifying the severity of ASD. The major problem with such a goal relates to the fact that symptoms are not distributed normally. Nevertheless, the summary scores of the ADOS are often used in experimental studies for correlational analyses between results on a given experimental paradigm and level of autistic symptomatology in the various domains (communication, social functioning, repetitive behaviors). But the ADOS was not designed for this purpose, nor does it result in a dimensional scale of affectedness (Lord & Corsello, 2005). Rather, it quantifies the presence of certain symptoms and their severity; as such, it can differentiate highly disparate levels of severity, but not in a quantifiable manner. The quantification in the instrument was primarily designed to add rigor to the categorical diagnostic decisions to which it is keyed. And there are some complexities, such as the fact that verbal children may receive higher scores on the ADOS (suggesting greater severity of impairment) than those who are nonverbal, because individuals with language can be scored on more items than those without language. Recently an analysis of 1,630 cases was performed, and some of these issues were addressed through modification of diagnostic algorithms, with a view to increasing their predictive value (Gotham, Risi, Pickles, & Lord, 2007). With the new algorithms, the ADOS is now likely to yield a more valid index of severity.

Truly dimensional clinical instruments are possible when the focus is on a normative skill, such as level of adaptive functioning, communication, or sociability. The two most researched instruments used in this fashion have been the Vineland Adaptive Behavior Scales (Sparrow, Balla, & Cicchetti, 1984) and the Social Responsiveness Scale (Constantino & Todd, 2003). Initial studies of the Vineland in autism showed its utility in differentiating patterns of results across the various domains (Communication, Daily Living Skills, Socialization, and Motor Skills) relative to other populations (Volkmar et al., 1987). Regression equations were derived that predict a diagnosis of autism on the basis of scatter of results across domains (Volkmar, Carter, Sparrow, & Cicchetti, 1993). And standard scores were made available that are specific to the population of children with autism (Carter et al., 1998). Indeed, Vineland scores work well in quantifying these children's level of adaptive ability, particularly in the Socialization domain. However, most of the earlier work in this area involved children with a degree of intellectual impairment. More recent work looking at the distribution of Communication and Socialization scores for normative-IQ (or higher-functioning) individuals with ASD (across the three diagnostic categories) revealed a more limited distribution, with individuals across all three categories scoring quite low, particularly in the Socialization domain (Klin et al., 2007; Saulnier & Klin, 2007). Thus, for this group of children (especially the older ones), the Vineland is less helpful in creating the dimensionality necessary to characterize children with different PDD diagnoses (or individuals within a diagnosis) along a widely distributed scale. In the recent revision of the Vineland (Sparrow, Cicchetti, & Balla, 2005) a great effort has been made to expand the number of adaptive behaviors so as to address some of these issues, particularly in the Socialization domain, and with a special focus on the first 3 years of life. The new Vineland, therefore, may create the dimensionality needed to subtype the population of young children with ASD along the all-important concept of real-life adaptation, which is critical for clinical management and measurement of both response to treatment and global progress. It remains to be seen whether this promise applies to all domains of adaptive functioning.

The Social Responsiveness Scale was conceived from the outset as an instrument to screen and quantify a normative "quantitative trait" in genetic studies of large samples of twins (Constantino & Todd, 2003). Although it contains various domains of behavior, its focus is on social reciprocity. Despite its various clinical applications, its uniqueness lies in the fact that it measures sociability along a normative dimension that applies to the whole population, typical or disabled. In this way it makes possible the creation of a normative distribution, with empirically derived cutoffs designating affected individuals (or samples). This process empowers genetic analyses, since dimensional (in contrast to categorical) approaches not only embrace populations of "affected" and "nonaffected" individuals together, but also capture a dimension of affectedness in individuals with subclinical traits of the disorder that are presumed to be genetically associated—for example, in nonaffected family members (Constantino et al., 2004; Constantino & Todd, 2005). This is particularly important, given the emergence of the concept of the "broader autism phenotype," which needs to be characterized and identified for a fuller picture of genetic liability in a given family (Bailey et al., 1995; Bailey, Palferman, Heavey, & Le Couteur, 1998; Le Couteur, Bailey, Goode, & Pickles, 1996).

A historically older attempt at dimensional subtyping is related to the fact that IQ and language are powerful predictors of outcome. There have been suggestions that subtyping should combine a categorical diagnosis and a dimensional axis listing IQ or language levels. This is, of course, done routinely during clinical assessments. The suggestion here was to formalize this procedure, incorporating it into the actual subtyping directives defined by the DSM system. This is likely to be one of the possibilities addressed in DSM-V. The utility of this suggestion lies in the fact that talents and challenges, as well as opportunities in life and vulnerability for forms of psychopathology (among other factors), are qualitatively different for individuals with great versus no intellectual impairment.

SUBTYPING FOR BRAIN RESEARCH

General intellectual level and specific neuropsychological constructs (e.g., handedness) are of greater importance in structural and functional brain imaging research than comparisons across ASD subtypes (Schultz, Romanski, & Tsatsanis, 2000). Data on the utility of the latter are still limited. A much more promising form of clinical subtyping is emerging in association with research indicating accelerated brain growth in the infancy period of children with ASD (Courschene et al., 2001). Although at present this is still a group phenomenon, the full potential of this finding will depend to some extent on quantified evaluation of the behavioral correlates of accelerated brain growth. Given the suggestion of a specific (though variable) timetable for onset and course of the atypical brain growth patterns (Hazlett et al., 2005), a critical form of subtyping required in this research enterprise is a much more exact and quantified phenotype, based on onset of autistic symptomatology and changes of growth curves of developmental skills. If such a correlation is established, it will provide sorely needed evidence for the utility of brain growth patterns as endophenotypes for genetic and outcome studies of ASD.

Such an advancement would also add a critical tool for early identification of vulnerability for ASD. This is now an exciting possibility, given the recent formation and funding of consortia focused on brain imaging of infant siblings of children with autism followed prospectively from birth.

SUBTYPING FOR GENETIC RESEARCH

In no other field is ASD heterogeneity more baffling to investigators than in genetic research. Linkage studies performed on the basis of ASD subtypes or symptom clusters have not led to major discoveries of genes, nor have they added substantially to the identification of susceptibility regions. Hence there is a great need for identification of endophenotypes or quantitative traits, the use of which may generate more homogeneous samples for genetic studies (Geschwind & Alarcón, 2006).

A large number of candidates have been proposed, although application of these potential endophenotypes is still lacking. Some of these relate to neurocognitive concepts (e.g., face-processing deficits, theory-of-mind skills, executive functions, local/configural learning styles). Others relate to structural and functional neuroimaging variables (Dawson et al., 2002). In the better examples, the case for the endophenotype is made in terms of the familiality of the concept or measure, in that the deficit is present in both the affected and the nonaffected family members. Although this approach is exciting, there is still little evidence establishing that these candidates mediate the expression of the disorder. One step in this direction would be to show a stronger relationship between the quantitative trait and core features of the disorder (either the expression of symptoms or the developmental vulnerabilities typically associated with ASD).

One challenge in this regard is that, with one exception (Alarcón, Yonan, Gilliam, Cantor, & Geschwind, 2005), the candidates so far have not been developmental in nature. ASD are essentially neurodevelopmental disorders leading to a cascade of effects that then interact with nongenetic factors, such as treatment and individual-specific environmental and experiential variables. In fact, given the early onset of these conditions, the greater the distance in developmental time at which the endophenotype is measured, the more complex the process of disentangling genetic liabilities from confounding or extraneous factors becomes—and the hypothesized effect on syndrome expression is thus diluted.

FUTURE DIRECTIONS

A theme emphasized throughout this chapter is the need to redouble our efforts to understand, in greater detail and in a quantitative approach, the first 2–3 years of life of children with ASD. It is critical to consider the full range of implications following from the fact that autism and related disorders are early-onset neurodevelopmental disorders, and that virtually all aspects of interest in investigations and clinical practice are affected by developmental psychopathology processes (Klin et al., 2003). Two parallel sets of advancements bode well for this field. First, our knowledge of normative processes in child development has increased dramatically since the early 1990s, although autism research has been slow in fully assimilating new investigative paradigms, technologies, and concepts (Volkmar et al., 2004). Second, the advent of prospective studies of large cohorts of genetically at-risk infants, a proportion of whom will develop autism, carries the promise of shedding light on this critical period of pathogenesis; hitherto, our knowledge of this period has been confined to retrospective accounts or less-than-ideal methods of infancy research (Zwaigenbaum et al., 2007). As knowledge accrues from these efforts, it is very likely that a great deal of what we know about ASD (e.g., genetic mechanisms, brain structure and function, neurocognitive course, socialization trajectories) will have to be reappraised and updated, if not fully modified.

In regard to nosology and classification of ASD, prospective work singling out relevant patterns of onset and examining the range of associated symptomatic expressions over time is likely to systematize the search for empirically defined subtypes. This should allow for an examination of their utility in terms of response to treatment and outcomes. This process has begun with the identification of earlier- and later-onset autism (Landa, Holman, & Garrett-Mayer, 2007), and possibly the existence of regressive subtypes (Lord, Shulman, & DiLavore, 2004; Siperstein & Volkmar, 2004; Werner & Dawson, 2005). It is possible, however, that these distinctions are still too crude, to be remediated only by more detailed and quantified analyses of infancy data than those performed to date.

The same point applies to the critical elucidation of what accelerated brain growth means insofar as syndrome onset and expression are concerned, as well as a better assessment of the utility of neuropathological hypotheses that could underlie the abnormal brain growth (e.g., abnormalities associated with brain growth factors). A multimethod, multilevel approach to investigating causes of ASD may result in mutually constrained hypotheses whereby gene–brain relationships are elucidated. However, for this to happen, the processes, timing, and patterns of pathogenesis need to be further mapped, quantified, and correlated with the measures underlying the hypothesized causative factors.

It is in this context that a surprising puzzle emerges in the current state of ASD research. This family of conditions is by most accounts caused by a plethora of etiologies (e.g., genotypically). And yet they are still very much a unitary set of syndromes. Although interclinician reliability for the diagnosis of ASD subtypes is poor, the distinction between ASD and non-ASD conditions is solidly established. How can such multicausal syndromes result in a clearly delineated cluster of symptoms and adaptive profiles?

Although some common genetic or neuropathological process cannot be ruled out, it is equally possible that the final common pathway is not within the causative factors themselves, but in the processes that they disrupt (Klin et al., 2003). Humans are born in a much more fragile state than most other species are. Survival depends on an infant's caregiver and on the mutually reinforcing relationship between infant and caregiver, which launches the process of socialization. The child development literature on phases and stages of accomplishments and qualitative leaps in infancy sets a timetable by which we may judge the effects of disruption any time in the first 2 years of life (Johnson, 2001). Variable onset patterns may result in "hits" varying in developmental time and course. The derailment of the socialization process may be the common factor, whereas the timing of disruption may be the dimension generating variability in syndrome expression. Such a developmental endophenotype will need to be explored, as it is unrealistic to expect that different timings of syndrome onset (say, at 2 months of age and at 14 months of age) will have similar results. Several predictions may follow from this hypothesis. We should expect (rather as in embryonic maturation) that the earlier the disruption, the more severe the impact of this derailment should be for the acquisition of sociability and communicative skills. If so, autism or autistic symptoms may be seen as the result of the disruption, having little direct, causative relationship to etiological factors.

REFERENCES

Alarcón, M., Yonan, A. L., Gilliam, T. C., Cantor, R. M., & Geschwind, D. H. (2005). Quantitative genome scan and ordered-subtests analysis of autism endophenotypes support language QTLs. *Molecular Psychiatry, 10,* 747–757.

American Psychiatric Association. (1980). *Diagnostic and statistical manual of mental disorders* (3rd ed.). Washington, DC: Author.

American Psychiatric Association. (1987). *Diagnostic and statistical manual of mental disorders* (3rd ed., rev.). Washington, DC: Author.

American Psychiatric Association. (1994). *Diagnostic and statistical manual of mental disorders* (4th ed.). Washington, DC: Author.

American Psychiatric Association. (2000). *Diagnostic and statistical manual of mental disorders* (4th ed., text rev.). Washington, DC: Author.

Amir, R. E., Van den Veyver, I. B., Wan, M., Tran, C. Q., Francke, U., & Zoghbi, H. Y. (1999). Rett syndrome is caused by mutations in X-linked MECP2, encoding methyl-CpG-binding protein 2. *Nature Genetics, 23,* 185–188.

Asperger, H. (1944). Die 'Autistischen Psychopathen' im Kindesalter. *Archiv für Psychiatrie und Nervenkrankheiten, 117,* 76–136.

Bailey, A., Palferman, S., Heavey, L., & Le Couteur, A. (1998). Autism: The phenotype in relatives. *Journal of Autism and Developmental Disorders, 28,* 369–392.

Bailey, A., Le Couteur, A., Gottesman, I., Bolton, P., Simonoff, E., Yuzda, E., et al. (1995). Autism as a strongly genetic disorder: Evidence from a British twin study. *Psychological Medicine, 25,* 63–77.

Bishop, D. V. M. (2000). What's so special about Asperger syndrome?: The need for further exploration of the borderlands of autism. In A. Klin, F. R. Volkmar, & S. S. Sparrow (Eds.), *Asperger syndrome* (pp. 278–308). New York: Guilford Press.

Carter, A. S., Volkmar, F. R., Sparrow, S. S., Wang, J., Lord, C., Dawson, G., et al. (1998). The Vineland Adaptive Behavior Scales: Supplementary norms for individuals with autism. *Journal of Autism and Developmental Disorders, 28*(4), 287–302.

Centers for Disease Control and Prevention. (2007, February 8). *Prevalence of the autism spectrum disorders in multiple areas of the United States, surveillance years 2000 and 2002: A report from the Autism and Developmental Disabilities Monitoring (ADDM) Network.* Atlanta, GA: Author.

Chawarska, K., Klin, A., Paul, R., & Volkmar, F. R. (2007). Autism spectrum disorders in the second year: Stability and change in syndrome expression. *Journal of Child Psychology and Psychiatry, 48*(2), 128–138.

Cohen, D. J., Paul, R., & Volkmar, F. R. (1986). Issues in the classification of pervasive developmental disorders: Toward DSM-IV. *Journal of the American Academy of Child Psychiatry, 25*(2), 213–220.

Constantino, J. N., Gruber, C. P., Davis, S., Hayes, S., Passanante, N., & Przybeck, T. (2004). The factor structure of autistic traits. *Journal of Child Psychology and Psychiatry, 45,* 719–726.

Constantino, J., & Todd, R. D. (2003). Autistic traits in the general population: A twin study. *Archives of General Psychiatry, 60*(5), 524–530.

Constantino, J. N., & Todd, R. D. (2005). Intergenerational transmission of subthreshold autistic traits in the general population. *Biological Psychiatry, 57,*655–660.

Courschene, E., Karns, C. M., Davis, H. R., Ziccardi, R., Carper, R. A., Tigue, Z. D., et al. (2001). Unusual brain growth patterns in early life in patients with autism disorder: An MRI study. *Neurology, 57,* 245–254.

Dawson, G., Webb, S., Schellenberg, G. D., Dager, S., Friedman, S., Aylward, E., et al. (2002). Defining the broader phenotype of autism: Genetic, brain, and behavioral perspectives. *Development and Psychopathology, 14,* 581–611.

DiCicco-Bloom, E., Lord, C., Zwaigenbaum, L., Courchesne, E., Dager, S. R., Schmitz, C., et al. (2006). The developmental neurobiology of autism spectrum disorder. *Journal of Neuroscience, 26*(26), 6897–6906.

Dykens, E. M., & Hodapp, R. M. (2001). Research in mental retardation: Toward an etiologic approach. *Journal of Child Psychology and Psychiatry, 42*(1), 49–71.

Ehlers, S., Nyden, A., Gillberg, C., & Dahlgren Sandberg, A. (1997). Asperger syndrome, autism and attention disorders: A comparative study of the cognitive profiles of 120 children. *Journal of Child Psychology and Psychiatry, 38*(2), 207–217.

Feinstein, C., & Singh, S. (2007). Social phenotypes in neurogenetic syndromes. *Child and Adolescent Psychiatric Clinics of North America, 16*(3), 631–647.

Folstein, S., & Rutter, M. (1977). Genetic influences and infantile autism. *Nature, 265*(5596), 726–728.

Fombonne, E. (2003). The prevalence of autism. *Journal of the American Medical Association, 289*(1), 87–89.

Fombonne, E. (2005). Epidemiological studies of pervasive developmental disorders. In F. R. Volkmar, R. Paul, A. Klin, & D. J. Cohen (Eds.), *Handbook of autism and pervasive developmental disorders* (3rd ed., Vol. 1, pp. 42–69). Hoboken, NJ: Wiley.

Fombonne, E., & Tidmarsh, L. (2003). Epidemiologic data on Asperger disorder. *Child and Adolescent Psychiatric Clinics of North America, 12,* 15–22.

Geschwind, D. H., & Alarcón, M. (2006). Finding genes in spite of heterogeneity: Endophenotypes, QTL mapping, and expression profiling in autism. In S. O. Moldin & J. L. R. Rubenstein (Eds.), *Understanding autism: From basic neuroscience to treatment* (pp. 75–93). New York: Taylor & Francis.

Gilchrist, A., Green, J., Cox, A., Burton, D., Rutter, M., & Le Couteur, A. (2001), Development and current functioning in adolescents with Asperger syndrome: A comparative study. *Journal of Child Psychology and Psychiatry, 42,* 227–240.

Gillberg, C. (1989). Asperger syndrome in 23 Swedish children. *Developmental Medicine and Child Neurology, 31,* 520–531.

Gillberg, C. (2003). Deficits in attention, motor control, and perception: A brief review. *Archives of Diseases in Childhood, 88*(10), 904–910.

Gillberg, I. C., & Gillberg, C. (1989). Asperger syndrome: Some epidemiological considerations. *Journal of Child Psychology and Psychiatry, 30,* 631–638.

Gotham, K., Risi, S., Pickles, A., & Lord, C. (2007). The Autism Diagnostic Observation Schedule: Revised algorithms for improved diagnostic validity. *Journal of Autism and Developmental Disorders, 37*(4), 613–627.

Gupta, A. R., & State, M. W. (2007). Recent advances in the genetics of autism. *Biological Psychiatry, 61*(4), 429–437.

Hazlett, H. C., Poe, M. D., Gerig, G., Smith, R. G., Provenzale, J., Ross, A., et al. (2005). An MRI and head circumference study of brain size in autism: Birth through age two years. *Archives of General Psychiatry, 62,* 1366–1376.

Heller, T. (1908). Dementia infantilis. *Zeitschrift für die Erforschung und Behandlung des Jugenlichen Schwachsinns, 2,* 141–165.

Hermelin, B., & O'Connor, N. (1970). *Psychological experiments with autistic children.* Oxford: Pergamon Press.

Howlin, P. (2005). Outcomes in autism spectrum disorders. In F. R. Volkmar, R. Paul, A. Klin, & D. J. Cohen (Eds.), *Handbook of autism and pervasive developmental disorders* (3rd ed., pp. 201–221). Hoboken, NJ: Wiley.

Johnson, M. (2001). Functional brain development in humans. *Nature Reviews Neuroscience, 2,* 475–483.

Kanner, L. (1943). Autistic disturbances of affective contact. *Nervous Child, 2,* 217–253.

Kendler, K. S. (1990). Toward a scientific psychiatric nosology: Strengths and limitations. *Archives of General Psychiatry, 47*(10), 969–973.

Klin, A., Jones, W., Schultz, R. T., & Volkmar, F. R. (2003). The enactive mind—from actions to cognition: Lessons from autism. *Philosophical Transactions of the Royal Society. Series B, Biological Sciences, 358,* 345–360.

Klin, A., Mayes, L. C., Volkmar, F. R., & Cohen, D. J. (1995a). Multiplex developmental disorder. *Journal of Developmental and Behavioral Pediatrics, 16*(3), S7–S11.

Klin, A., McPartland, J., & Volkmar, F. R. (2005a). Asperger syndrome. In F. R. Volkmar, R. Paul, A. Klin, & D. J. Cohen (Eds.), *Handbook of autism and pervasive developmental disorders* (3rd ed., pp. 88–125). Hoboken, NJ: Wiley.

Klin, A., Pauls, D., Schultz, R., & Volkmar, F. R. (2005b). Three diagnostic approaches to Asperger syndrome: Implications for research. *Journal of Autism and Developmental Disorders, 35*(2), 221–234.

Klin, A., Saulnier, C., Tsatsanis, K., & Volkmar, F. R. (2005c). Clinical evaluation in autism spectrum disorders: Psychological assessment within a transdisciplinary framework. In F. R. Volkmar, R. Paul, A. Klin, & D. J. Cohen (Eds.), *Handbook of autism and pervasive developmental disorders* (3rd ed., pp. 772–798). Hoboken, NJ: Wiley.

Klin, A., Saulnier, C. A., Sparrow, S. S., Cicchetti, D. V., Volkmar, F. R., & Lord, C. (2007). Social and communication abilities and disabilities in higher functioning individuals with autism spectrum disorders. *Journal of Autism and Developmental Disorders, 37*(4), 748–759.

Klin, A., & Volkmar, F. R. (1996). The pervasive developmental disorders: Nosology and profiles of development. In S. Luthar, J. Burack, D. Cicchetti, & J. Wiesz (Eds.), *Developmental perspectives on risk and psychopathology* (pp. 208–226). New York: Cambridge University Press.

Klin, A., & Volkmar, F. R. (Eds.). (2003). Asperger syndrome. *Child and Adolescent Psychiatric Clinics of North America, 12*(1).

Klin, A., Volkmar, F. R., Sparrow, S. S., Cicchetti, D. V., & Rourke, B. P. (1995b). Validity and neuropsychological characterization of Asperger syndrome. *Journal of Child Psychology and Psychiatry, 36*(7), 1127–1140.

Landa, R. J., Holman, K. C., & Garrett-Mayer, E. (2007). Social and communication development in toddlers with early and later diagnosis of autism spectrum disorders. *Archives of General Psychiatry, 64*(7), 853–864.

Le Couteur, A., Bailey, A., Goode, S., & Pickles, A. (1996). A broader phenotype of autism: The clinical spectrum in twins. *Journal of Child Psychology and Psychiatry, 37*(7), 785–801.

Lockyer, L., & Rutter, M. (1969). A five to fifteen year follow-up study of infantile psychosis: III. Psychological aspects. *British Journal of Psychiatry, 115,* 865–882.

Lord, C., & Corsello, C. (2005). Diagnostic instruments in autism spectrum disorders. In F. R. Volkmar, R. Paul, A. Klin, & D. J. Cohen (Eds.), *Handbook of autism and pervasive developmental disorders* (3rd ed., pp. 730–771). Hoboken, NJ: Wiley.

Lord, C., Rutter, M., DiLavore, P. C., & Risi, S. (1999). *Autism Diagnostic Observation Schedule—WPS (ADOS-WPS)*. Los Angeles: Western Psychological Services.

Lord, C., Shulman, C., & DiLavore, P. (2004). Regression and word loss in autistic spectrum disorders. *Journal of Child Psychology and Psychiatry, 45*(5), 936–955.

Lotter, V. (1966). Epidemiology of autistic conditions in young children: I. Prevalence. *Social Psychiatry, 1,* 124–137.

Lotter, V. (1967). Epidemiology of autistic conditions in young children: II. Some characteristics of the parents and children. *Social Psychiatry, 1,* 163–173.

Mayes, S. D., Calhoun, S. L., & Crites, D. L. (2001). Does DSM-IV Asperger's disorder exist? *Journal of Abnormal Child Psychology, 29,* 263–271.

Miller, J. N., & Ozonoff, S. (1997). Did Asperger's cases have Asperger disorder?: A research note. *Journal of Child Psychology and Psychiatry, 38*(2), 247–251.

Miller, J. N., & Ozonoff, S. (2000). The external validity of Asperger disorder: Lack of evidence from the domain of neuropsychology. *Journal of Abnormal Child Psychology, 109,*227–238

National Research Council. (2001). *Educating children with autism.* Washington, DC: National Academy Press.

Rapin, I., & Allen, D. (1983). Developmental language disorders. In U. Kirk (Ed.), *Neuropsychology of language, reading and spelling* (pp. 101–134). New York: Academic Press.

Rett, A. (1966). Uber ein eigenartiges hirnatrophisches Syndrome bei Hyperammonamie im Kindesalter. *Wien Medizinische Wochenschrift, 116,* 723–738.

Ropers, H.-H., & Jamel, C. J. (2005). X-linked mental retardation. *Nature Reviews Genetics, 6,* 46–57.

Rourke, B. (1989). *Nonverbal learning disabilities: The syndrome and the model.* New York: Guilford Press.

Rourke, B. (Ed.). (1995). *Syndrome of nonverbal learning disabilities: Neurodevelopmental manifestations.* New York: Guilford Press.

Rourke, B., Young, G. C., & Leenaars, A. A. (1989). A childhood learning disability that predisposes those afflicted to adolescent and adult depression and suicide risk. *Journal of Learning Disabilities, 22,* 169–185.

Rutter, M. (1965). Classification and categorization in child psychiatry. *Journal of Child Psychology and Psychiatry, 6*(2), 71–83.

Rutter, M. (1972). Childhood schizophrenia reconsidered. *Journal of Autism and Childhood Schizophrenia, 2*(4), 315–337.

Rutter, M. (1978). Diagnosis and definition of childhood autism. *Journal of Autism and Childhood Schizophrenia, 8*(2), 139–161.

Rutter, M. (1994). Debate and argument: There are connections between brain and mind and it is important that Rett syndrome be classified somewhere. *Journal of Child Psychology and Psychiatry, 35*(2), 379–381.

Rutter, M., Le Couteur, A., & Lord, C. (2003). *Autism Diagnostic Interview—Revised (ADI-R).* Los Angeles: Western Psychological Services.

Rutter, M., & Schopler, E. (1992). Classification of pervasive developmental disorders: Some concepts and practical considerations. *Journal of Autism and Developmental Disorders, 22*(4), 459–482.

Saulnier, C. A., & Klin, A. (2007). Social and communication abilities and disabilities in higher functioning individuals with autism and Asperger syndrome. *Journal of Autism and Developmental Disorders, 37*(4), 788–793.

Scahill, S., & Martin, A. (2005). Psychopharmacology. In F. R. Volkmar, R. Paul, A. Klin, & D. J. Cohen (Eds.), *Handbook of autism and pervasive developmental disorders* (3rd ed., pp. 1102–1121). Hoboken, NJ: Wiley.

Schultz, R. T., Romanski, L. M., & Tsatsanis, K. D. (2000). Neurofunctional models of autistic disorder and Asperger syndrome: Clues from neuroimaging. In A. Klin, F. R. Volkmar, & S. S. Sparrow (Eds.), *Asperger syndrome* (pp. 172–209). New York: Guilford Press.

Siperstein, R., & Volkmar, F. (2004). Brief report: Parental reporting of regression in children with pervasive developmental disorders. *Journal of Autism and Developmental Disorders, 34*(6), 731–734.

Sparrow, S. S., Balla, D. A., & Cicchetti, D. V. (1984). *Vineland Adaptive Behavior Scales.* Circle Pines, MN: American Guidance Service.

Sparrow, S. S., Cicchetti, D. V., & Balla, D. A. (2005). *Vineland Adaptive Behavior Scales, Second Edition (Vineland-II).* Circle Pines, MN: American Guidance Service.

Szatmari, P. (2000). Perspectives on the classification of Asperger syndrome. In A. Klin, F. R. Volkmar, & S. S. Sparrow (Eds.), *Asperger syndrome* (pp. 403–417). New York: Guilford Press.

Szatmari, P., Bartolucci, G., & Bremner, R. (1989). Asperger's syndrome and autism: Comparison of early history and outcome. *Developmental Medicine and Child Neurology, 31*(6), 709–720.

Tantam, D. (2003). The challenge of adolescents and adults with Asperger syndrome. *Child and Adolescent Psychiatric Clinics of North America, 12*(1), 143–163.

Towbin, K. E. (2005). Pervasive developmental disorder not otherwise specified. In F. R. Volkmar, R. Paul, A. Klin, & D. J. Cohen (Eds.), *Handbook of autism and pervasive developmental disorders* (3rd ed., pp. 165–200). Hoboken, NJ: Wiley.

van Acker, R., Loncola, J. A., & van Acker, E. Y. (2005). Rett syndrome: A pervasive developmental disorder. In F. R. Volkmar, R. Paul, A. Klin, & D. J. Cohen (Eds.), *Handbook of autism and pervasive developmental disorders* (3rd ed., pp. 126–164). Hoboken, NJ: Wiley.

Volkmar, F. R., Bregman, J., Cohen, D. J., & Cicchetti, D. V. (1988). DSM-III and DSM-III-R diagnoses of autism. *American Journal of Psychiatry, 145*(11), 1404–1408.

Volkmar, F. R., Carter, A., Sparrow, S. S., & Cicchetti, D. V. (1993). Quantifying social development of autism. *Journal of the American Academy of Child and Adolescent Psychiatry, 32,* 627–632.

Volkmar, F. R., Cicchetti, D. V., Bregman, J., & Cohen, D. J. (1992). Brief report: Developmental aspects of DSM-III-R criteria for autism. *Journal of Autism and Developmental Disorders, 22*(4), 657–662.

Volkmar, F. R., & Klin, A. (2005). Issues in the classification of autism and related conditions. In F. R. Volkmar, R. Paul, A. Klin, & D. J. Cohen (Eds.), *Handbook of autism and pervasive developmental disorders* (3rd ed., pp. 5–41). Hoboken, NJ: Wiley.

Volkmar, F. R., Klin, A., Siegel, B., Szatmari, P., Lord, C., Campbell, M., et al. (1994). DSM-IV autism/pervasive developmental disorder field trial. *American Journal of Psychiatry, 151*, 1361–1367.

Volkmar, F. R., Koenig, K., & State, M. (2005). Childhood disintegrative disorder. In F. R. Volkmar, R. Paul, A. Klin, & D. J. Cohen (Eds.), *Handbook of autism and pervasive developmental disorders* (3rd ed., pp. 70–87). Hoboken, NJ: Wiley.

Volkmar, F. R., Lord, C., Bailey, A., Schultz, R. T., & Klin, A. (2004). Autism and pervasive developmental disorders. *Journal of Child Psychology and Psychiatry, 45*(1), 135–170.

Volkmar, F. R., & Pauls, D. (2003). Autism. *Lancet, 362*(9390), 1133–1141.

Volkmar, F. R., Sparrow, S. A., Goudreau, D., Cicchetti, D. V., Paul, R., & Cohen, D. J. (1987). Social deficits in autism: An operational approach using the Vineland Adaptive Behavior Scales. *Journal of the American Academy of Child and Adolescent Psychiatry, 26*, 156–161.

Werner, E., & Dawson, G. (2005). Validation of the phenomenon of autistic regression using home videotapes. *Archives of General Psychiatry, 62*(8), 889–895.

Wing, L. (1981). Asperger's syndrome: A clinical account. *Psychological Medicine, 11*, 115–129.

Wing, L. (1986). Clarification on Asperger's syndrome [Letter to the editor]. *Journal of Autism and Developmental Disorders, 16*(4), 513–515.

Wing, L. (2000). Past and future of research on Asperger syndrome. In A. Klin, F. R. Volkmar, & S. S. Sparrow (Eds.), *Asperger syndrome* (pp. 418–432). New York: Guilford Press.

Wing, L., & Gould, J. (1979). Severe impairments of social interaction and associated abnormalities in children: Epidemiology and classification. *Journal of Autism and Developmental Disorders, 9*, 11–29.

Zhao, X., Leotta, A., Kustanovich, V., Lajonchere, C., Geschwind, D. H., Law, P., et al. (2007). A unified genetic theory for sporadic and inherited autism. *Proceedings of the National Academy of Sciences USA, 104*(31), 12831–12836.

Zwaigenbaum, L., Bryson, S., Rogers, T., Roberts, W., Brian, J., & Szatmari, P. (2005). Behavioral manifestations of autism in the first year of life. *International Journal of Developmental Neuroscience, 23*(2–3), 143–152.

Zwaigenbaum, L., Thurm, A., Stone, W., Baranek, G., Bryson, S., Iverson, J., et al. (2007). Studying the emergence of autism spectrum disorders in high-risk infants: Methodological and practical issues. *Journal of Autism and Developmental Disorders, 37*(3), 466–480.

CHAPTER FIVE

Age-Related Issues in the Assessment of Autism Spectrum Disorders

Victoria Shea
Gary B. Mesibov

Although the universal goal of assessing autism spectrum disorders (ASD) is obtaining information that will in some way benefit each individual and his or her family, the specific focus and tools for assessment of ASD vary markedly, depending on the age of the person being assessed. In this chapter, we discuss age-related issues in ASD assessment in five developmental stages: early childhood (up to age 3 years); preschool (ages 3–5 years); elementary school (ages 6–11 years); middle school and high school (ages 12–17 years); and adulthood (ages 18 years and beyond).

Many assessments for ASD take place through local developmental clinics or agencies, public schools, small teams, or individual clinicians. The assessment models described by most researchers—involving large university-based interdisciplinary teams, analysis of videotapes, multiple assessment sessions, home visits, or observation of the target child with other children—may not be available or affordable for many families. Nevertheless, given the increasing availability of good assessment tools for diagnosis and skill measurement, along with training in ASD, it is possible for clinicians in a variety of settings to perform meaningful, appropriate evaluations for individuals across the age range (Ozonoff, Goodlin-Jones, & Solomon, 2005).

Focus of Assessment
at Different Developmental Stages

We begin with a discussion of the ways the focus and nature of assessment change, depending on the individual's age. As a general rule, assessments of young children tend to focus on establishing a diagnosis, whereas assessments at later ages tend to focus on measuring skills.

Early Childhood and Preschool Age

At present in the United States and other developed countries, a child's first assessment for an ASD often (but not always) takes place before elementary school (Centers for Disease Control and Prevention, 2007; Howlin & Asgharian, 1999; Howlin & Moore, 1997; Mandell, Listerud, Levy, & Pinto-Martin, 2002). The typical focus of assessment at these stages is on answering these underlying questions: "Is it autism?" and then "What can be done to help the child?"

Many parents come to the assessment having observed, suspected, or been told by someone that their child's development is delayed or disordered—but some parents of a child with high-functioning autism/Asperger syndrome are stunned by a diagnosis at this age, having thought that their child, although somewhat socially immature, was developmentally precocious or gifted. Some parents have had to wait and worry for months before the assessment appointment—but sometimes the initial use of an ASD diagnosis comes unexpectedly at a medical appointment or a well-baby checkup.

Many parents are devastated by hearing an ASD diagnosis for the first time. Professionals who tell parents that their child has an ASD, and perhaps mental retardation as well, must be both honest and compassionate as they present information and answer questions (Mesibov, Shea, & Schopler, 2005). Accurate diagnostic terms should be used and explained, and questions about the child's future developmental course should be answered as fully as possible, given the research literature, a professional's experience, and the profile of the child's disabilities. Emotional support, kindness, and empathy are also essential during such sessions with the parents.

As discussed by Hogan and Marcus in Chapter 11 of this volume, information about educational and treatment options should usually be part of the initial diagnostic assessment. Parents may or may not be ready to hear details about local programs, theories of intervention, or the like; however, making basic recommendations (such as good books and websites about ASD), providing contact information for the early intervention system, and offering suggestions for handling pressing behavioral concerns are often the most meaningful outcomes of assessment at this stage of development.

Elementary School Age

Assessments (which are often reassessments) for children of elementary school age occasionally focus on making or confirming the diagnosis of ASD, but are more likely to focus on the underlying question "Will he or she be able to . . . ?" Assessments during this stage thus move away from diagnostic issues to periodic evaluation of a child's skills. During the elementary school years, the child's intellectual, language, academic, and adaptive skills and potential typically become clear, based on increased cooperation with standardized testing procedures, trends in test scores over the years, and reports of the child's response to stimulation and instruction.

Because an important function of assessment at this stage is to support a wide range of interventions, scores on standardized tests in isolation are not very useful, although they may indicate specific instructional needs. In addition to needs in the areas of cognitive, language, and academic instruction, however, many youngsters with ASD have significant problems with activities of daily living and social skills, both at school and at home; these often require qualitative assessment.

School-based skills and behaviors that may need instruction and intervention include behavior on the school bus, making transitions throughout the school day, and remaining calm and engaged during activities in high-stress locations such as the cafeteria and gym. Various home-based daily living skills may also need assessment and intervention: aspects of getting ready for school in the morning (e.g., dressing, eating breakfast, brushing teeth, and leaving home on time) and after-school routines (e.g., doing homework or playing constructively, eating dinner, bathing, brushing teeth, and going to bed on time).

For students at this age with significant mental retardation, aspects of toilet training may still require assessment and intervention, both at home and at school. For more cognitively capable students, assessment-based support is often needed with the homework cycle of writing down assignments, taking materials home, completing the work, taking the work back to school, and turning it in to the teacher. Also, assessment of social skills is important for ascertaining children's intervention needs in terms of playing near or with other children (including siblings), sharing materials, taking turns, initiating and accepting social bids to and from peers, and beginning to learn social behaviors through observation and imitation (see Gamliel & Yirmiya, Chapter 6, this volume).

Some students with high-functioning autism/Asperger syndrome at elementary school age have not yet been identified as having special needs, or at least as having ASD. These students often have strong academic skills, particularly in math, science, and aspects of reading, so that they may not be considered by school systems to need special services (although in the later years of elementary school, difficulties with such school-related skills as organization of materials, time management, handwriting, and inferential reading usually become evident, even if they are misinterpreted). When parents seek assessments that yield a diagnosis of high-functioning autism/ Asperger syndrome at this age, they sometimes ask, "Should we tell the school?" As a general principle, we believe that providing accurate and complete information to school systems is the most effective way to obtain appropriate supports and services. Rather than not disclosing the diagnosis because of stereotypes (such as "All students with ASD are mentally retarded or nonverbal") or inappropriate tracking (such as "All students with ASD are placed in self-contained special education classrooms"), it is almost always preferable to share information with the school system and individualized education program (IEP) team (with additional professional and advocacy support as needed), and then to work collaboratively to design an individualized program of supports and services based on the student's assessed needs.

Middle School and High School Age

Reassessments for youngsters of middle school and high school age may focus on several related questions: "What does he or she need now in the way of instruction or supports?", "What services and supports may be needed in the future?", and "For what services is he or she eligible?" Assessment thus typically includes both developing school-based programs and helping develop plans for adulthood. For youngsters with ASD and significant cognitive impairments, assessment may be needed as part of the application process for publicly funded programs, such as Medicaid and Medicaid waiver programs (*www.cms.hhs.gov/MedicaidEligibility, www.cms.hhs.gov/MedicaidStWaivProgDemoPGI/02_ConsumerInformation.asp*), Supplemental Security Income (*www.ssa.gov/ssi/*) and vocational rehabilitation services administered by each state (*www.jan.wvu.edu/SBSES/VOCREHAB.HTM*). For youngsters with high-functioning autism/Asperger syndrome, assessment of ASD-related special needs may be used as part of the process of selecting and applying to colleges (Palmer, 2006), including obtaining modified administration of college admissions tests (*www.collegeboard.com/ssd/student/index.html*).

Parents of a youngster who arrives at middle school or high school without a diagnosis of high-functioning autism/Asperger syndrome have typically experienced years of academic and social difficulties, emotional distress, and diagnostic confusion by the time of the ASD assessment and diagnosis. Their underlying question is often a frustrated "What's wrong with him or her?", and their reaction to the diagnosis may be, in effect, a relieved "Aha, so that's it!" Even though the diagnosis of an ASD may be hard to hear, at this stage parents are often grateful to have an explanation for the difficulties they have lived with, and to receive recommendations for addressing behavioral and social problems and obtaining appropriate accommodations in the youngster's school program. They may or may not want to tell the youngster about the diagnosis, and doing so may or may not be advisable at this age, given the combination of sensitivity to criticism and lack of insight that many adolescents with ASD exhibit.

Adulthood

Reassessment for the purpose of answering the multifaceted question "What public services and funds are available for him or her?" continues to be typical for adults with ASD, who may need such supports as supplemental income, room and board, supervision and instruction in self-care and community living skills, job training and supported employment, medical care, and transportation. These and other publicly funded services have specific guidelines in terms of assessment tools and documentation of functional deficits (*www.govbenefits.gov/govbenefits_en.portal*).

Individuals whose first assessment for ASD comes at adulthood usually fall into two categories: those with severe developmental delays who are screened for autism in institutional settings, and those with very high-functioning autism/Asperger syndrome. These latter individuals may refer themselves for assessment because of employment-related difficulties and/or social/interpersonal problems; they may have come to suspect their diagnosis in conjunction with the ASD assessment of one of their children; or they may be assessed in forensic or outpatient psychiatric settings (Nylander & Gillberg, 2001; Murrie, Warren, Kristiansson, & Dietz, 2002).

AGE-BASED TOOLS FOR DIAGNOSTIC ASSESSMENT

Because the behavioral characteristics of ASD differ over the course of development, different approaches to assessment for the purpose of diagnosis are needed at various ages.

Early Childhood: First Year

There is currently a great deal of research interest in identifying characteristics of ASD in children below the age of 12 months (Werner, Dawson, Munson, & Osterling, 2005; Zwaigenbaum et al., 2007). This research has generally used retrospective parent reports (Werner et al., 2005; Young, Brewer, & Pattison, 2003) and analysis of family movies and videotapes

(Palomo, Belinchon, & Ozonoff, 2006). In addition, several standardized assessment tools are currently under development, including the Autism Observation Scale for Infants (Bryson, McDermott, Rombough, Brian, & Zwaigenbaum, in press), which is a semistructured play-based measure, and the First Year Inventory (Resnick, Baranek, Reavis, Watson, & Crais, 2007; Watson et al., 2007), which is a parent report instrument.

Using these and other measures, several research groups have identified a large number of behaviors or characteristics that differentiate *groups* of very young children who are eventually diagnosed with ASD from control groups of children with either typical development or various other types of developmental disabilities; however, no assessment tools are yet available for *individual* diagnosis of children younger than 12 months of age. Behaviors in the first year of life that have been reported to be strongly associated with later diagnoses of autism include decreased social responsiveness (e.g., responding to name, looking at people, joint attention behaviors) and atypical sensory-regulatory behaviors (e.g., increased mouthing of objects, unusual visual attention patterns, increased irritability; Bryson et al., in press; Chawarska & Volkmar, 2005; Polomo et al., 2006; Reznick et al., 2007; Zwaigenbaum et al., 2005). Other standardized assessment tools that have been used to differentiate a group of children 1 year of age or less are the MacArthur–Bates Communicative Development Inventories— Infant Form and the Mullen Early Learning Scales. Zwaigenbaum et al. (2005) reported that on the MacArthur–Bates Infant Form at 12 months of age, a group of youngsters later diagnosed with autism used significantly fewer gestures and understood fewer phrases than controls; Landa and Garrett-Mayer (2006) reported that such children had significantly lower scores than control group children on all subscales of the Mullen except Visual Reception.

Early Childhood: Second Year

The "gold standard" direct observation measure for diagnosis of *some* children beginning in the second year of life is the Autism Diagnostic Observation Schedule (ADOS; Lord, Rutter, DiLavore, & Risi, 1999). According to its authors, the ADOS can be used with children who have a nonverbal developmental age of at least 12 months and who are able to walk independently, although scores should be interpreted with caution below a developmental age of 18 months (*portal.wpspublish.com/portal/ page?_pageid=53,84992&_dad=portal&_schema=PORTAL*). The ADOS is widely acknowledged to be the most sophisticated and psychometrically sound direct observation tool for ASD; however, it is expensive to purchase and time-consuming to learn, administer, and score. An additional limitation of the ADOS in early childhood is that it overidentifies ASD in children with significant mental retardation (Lord & Corsello, 2005; Risi et al., 2006).

An alternative assessment instrument for this age group is the Communication and Symbolic Behavior Scales Developmental Profile (Wetherby & Prizant, 2002), which consists of a brief parent report checklist, a follow-up parent questionnaire, and standardized activities with the child, which are videotaped and later analyzed and scored. Using this measure, Wetherby et al. (2004) reported that nine behaviors differentiated children later diagnosed with ASD from children with other developmental disabilities: (1) aversion to social touch or proximity; (2) lack of appropriate gaze; (3) lack of warm, joyful expressions with directed gaze; (4) lack of sharing interest or enjoyment; (5) lack of response to name; (6) lack of coordination of gaze, facial expression, gestures, and sounds; (7) lack of showing objects; (8) repetitive movements or body posturing; and (9) repetitive movements with objects. In addition, four behaviors differentiated the group with ASD from children with typical development, thus reflecting developmental delay that is not specific to ASD. Although there is not an empirically validated cutoff score on this measure, the authors suggested that failing the majority of the 13 "red flag" items indicates the need for further evaluation for ASD.

Screening tools for ASD beginning in the second year of life include both Level 1 screens (screening for ASD or other developmental problems in the general population of young children) and Level 2 screens (screening for ASD in groups of children for whom developmental concerns have already been raised). Setting a cutoff score on a screening test involves weighing the importance of sensitivity (low rate of false negatives) vs. specificity (low rate of false positives); the lower the cutoff score, the higher the sensitivity but the lower the specificity, and vice versa (Coonrod & Stone, 2005). Sensitivity rates of ASD screening tests for young children are lowered both by the phenomenon of regression that occurs in some children after the age of screening, and also by the difficulty of identifying children with mild and high-functioning ASD. Specificity rates are affected by the overlap of ASD with other developmental disabilities, particularly mental retardation and developmental language disorders (Coonrod & Stone, 2005; Eaves, Wingert, & Ho, 2006a; Scambler, Hepburn, & Rogers, 2006).

The Early Screening of Autistic Traits Questionnaire is a screening tool for 14- to 15-month-old children that was developed in the Netherlands but is available in English (Dietz, Swinkels, van Daalen, van Engeland, & Buitelaar, 2006; Swinkels et al., 2006). Screening with this tool takes place in two stages: a 4-item questionnaire involving play behavior, reactions to sensory stimuli, and whether the child's emotional reactions are understandable to parents; then a 14-item questionnaire for the children who fail the 4-item screen. Questions on the 14-item screen that were found to be the most predictive of a later diagnosis of ASD involved interest in people, smiling, and reacting when spoken to. However, Watson et al. (2007) have indicated that the sensitivity and specificity of this measure may be limited.

For children ages 18–24 months, several screening assessments for ASD are either published in the professional literature or commercially available. The first ASD screening tool developed for this age was the Checklist for Autism in Toddlers (CHAT; Baron-Cohen, Allen, & Gillberg, 1992; Baron-Cohen et al., 1996), which was eventually found to have low sensitivity, meaning that many children with ASD passed the screen (Baird et al., 2000). Two modifications of the CHAT have since been developed: the Modified CHAT (M-CHAT; Robins, Fein, Barton, & Green, 2001; Robins & Dumont-Mathieu, 2006) and the Denver Criteria for the CHAT (Scambler et al., 2006). Other well-known screening instruments for children at this age are the Screening Tool for Autism in Two-Year-Olds (STAT; Stone, Coonrod, & Ousley, 2000) and the Pervasive Developmental Disorders Screening Test–II (PDDST-II; Siegel, 2004).

Behaviors on these instruments that are most often associated with a later diagnosis of ASD include absence or limited frequency of responding to name, following a point or a gaze, pointing for reasons other than making a request, and engaging in pretend play (Charwarska & Volkmar, 2005; Scambler et al., 2006; Ventola et al., 2007). Each screening test has one or more limitations at its current stage of development: low sensitivity (CHAT); as yet incomplete information about sensitivity and specificity rates in population samples (Denver Criteria for the CHAT, M-CHAT, PDDST-II); or limited availability thus far for clinical use (STAT) (Bryson, Rogers, & Fombonne, 2003).

Early Childhood: Ages 2–3 Years

There is a substantial research literature about assessment tools and diagnostic stability beginning at age 2 years (e.g., Charman et al., 2005; Chawarska, Klin, Paul, & Volkmar, 2007; Lord et al., 2006; Turner, Stone, Pozdol, & Coonrod, 2006). The ADOS continues to be the "gold standard" observational instrument for both clinical and research purposes at this age. An alternative observational measure beginning at age 2 years that is less expensive and less complicated than the ADOS is the Childhood Autism Rating Scale (CARS; Schopler, Reichler, & Renner, 1988), which has strong psychometric properties (Lord & Corsello, 2005; Perry, Condillac, Freeman, Dunn-Geier, & Belair, 2005). Lord (1995) indicated that in a sample of 3-year-olds, raising the CARS cutoff score from 30 to 32 increased the association between CARS results and clinical diagnosis (Coonrod & Stone, 2005).

Some of the screening tools designed for younger children have also been used for children in this age range or older (Eaves et al., 2006a; Scambler, Hepburn, Hagerman, & Rogers, 2007; Ventola et al., 2007). In addition, a psychometrically strong screening tool for autism among people from 2 to 55 years of age with mental retardation is the Pervasive Developmental Disorder in Mental Retardation Scale (Kraijer & de Bildt, 2005).

The "gold standard" parent report measure for diagnosis beginning at developmental age 2 years is the Autism Diagnostic Interview—Revised (ADI-R; Rutter, Le Couteur, & Lord, 2003). Although the ADI-R is not particularly expensive, its administration time is approximately 2 hours (Lord & Corsello, 2005), which makes it cumbersome to use in many clinical settings. However, alternative parent interview measures for diagnosis are limited: The Diagnostic Interview for Social and Communication Disorders (DISCO; Leekam, Libby, Wing, Gould, & Taylor, 2002; Wing, Leekam, Libby, Gould, & Larcombe, 2002) was developed in England, and training in its use is not available in the United States (J. Gould, personal communication, 2007); and the Parent Interview for Autism (Stone & Hogan, 1993; Stone, Coonrod, Pozdol, & Turner, 2003) is an information-gathering tool for preschool children that does not yield a cutoff score for diagnostic purposes (Coonrod & Stone, 2005).

Trillinsgaard, Sørensen, Němec, and Jørgensen (2005) reported that experienced professionals could distinguish 2- and 3-year-old children later diagnosed with ASD from those later diagnosed with other developmental disorders, based on lower rates of the following: smiling in response to a smile, responding to name, following a point, initiating a request verbally or nonverbally, joining into play with an adult, or looking to the adult's face when "cheated." Similarly, Chawarska et al. (2007) indicated that the following ADOS items were markedly abnormal in 2-year-olds with autism: responding to name, eye contact, pointing, responding to joint attention bids, and both functional and symbolic play. In that study, 2-year-olds with pervasive developmental disorder not otherwise specified (PDD-NOS) were less socially impaired than children with autism, and had fewer unusual sensory interests and repetitive motor movements. Charman et al. (2005) found that various standardized test instruments at age 2 years did not predict diagnostic status at age 7 years, but that the mean rate of nonverbal communication acts at age 2 years was significantly correlated with age 7 scores on measures of nonverbal IQ, receptive and expressive language, and, negatively, with the Reciprocal Social Interactions Domain on the ADI-R.

At age 2 years, most studies indicate that a diagnosis of ASD based on the clinical judgment of an experienced professional is the best single predictor of later diagnostic status, although Lord et al. (2006) demonstrated that the ADOS and the ADI-R make additional important contributions to diagnosis, particularly in the direction of increasing sensitivity (i.e., reducing false negatives). In general, diagnoses of autism at age 2 years are more stable than diagnoses of PDD-NOS, although any ASD diagnosis at age 2 is highly likely to be associated with some form of developmental disorder in later years (Charman & Baird, 2002; Eaves & Ho, 2004; Moore & Goodson, 2006; Sutera et al., 2007).

Preschool Age

For preschool children, the ADOS, ADI-R, CARS, and DISCO continue to be the standard measures for diagnosis. Most studies indicate that a diagnosis of ASD made at age 3 is very stable (Charman & Baird, 2002; Jónsdóttir et al., 2007; Turner et al., 2006).

Fein et al. (1999) reported that the original Vineland Adaptive Behavior Scales (Sparrow, Balla, & Cicchetti, 1984), particularly the socialization domain, made additional contributions to prognosis beginning at this age, with a socialization standard score of 61 or higher suggesting better outcome.

For screening and research beginning at age 4 years (except for children with severe or profound mental retardation), the Social Communication Questionnaire (SCQ; Rutter et al., 2003) can be used (Eaves, Wingert, & Ho, 2006a; Eaves, Wingert, Ho, & Mickelson, 2006b; Howlin & Karpf, 2004; Wetherby, Watt, Morgan, & Shumway, 2007). The SCQ is a 40-item parent report measure using the items from the ADI-R that were found to be most discriminative of ASD. Because of its questionnaire format and brevity compared to the full ADI-R, it is more practical than the ADI-R for use in typical clinical settings.

Elementary School Age

As previously noted, most children with classic autism are now diagnosed before elementary school age; however, many youngsters with milder or higher-functioning forms of broad ASD are not yet identified as preschoolers (McConachie, LeCouteur, & Honey, 2005). In addition to the standard autism assessment tools previously mentioned (i.e., the ADOS, ADI-R, CARS, and DISCO), several assessment tools for mild or high-functioning autism and/or Asperger syndrome beginning at elementary age have been developed in the past decade. These include the following, in alphabetical order:

Asperger Syndrome Diagnostic Scale (Myles, Bock, & Simpson, 2001)
Autism Spectrum Screening Questionnaire (ASSQ; Ehlers, Gillberg, & Wing, 1999)

Childhood Asperger Syndrome Test (CAST; Scott, Baron-Cohen, Bol-
ton, & Brayne, 2002)
Gilliam Asperger Disorder Scale (Gilliam, 2001)
Krug Asperger's Disorder Index (KADI; Krug & Arick, 2003)

According to reviews of the psychometric properties of these scales
(Campbell, 2005; Goldstein, 2002), the tools with the fewest psychometric
weaknesses are the ASSQ and KADI. In addition, the Children's Social
Behavior Questionnaire (Hartman, Luteijn, Serra, & Minderaa, 2006) is
under development as a measure of various characteristics of milder forms
of ASD, and the Social Responsiveness Scale (SRS; Constantino & Gruber,
2005) has strengths as a measure of the social deficits associated with ASD
in youngsters ages 4–18 years (an adaptation of the SRS for 3-year-olds is
also under development; Pine, Luby, Abbacchi, & Constantino, 2006).

Middle School and High School Age

The assessment tools just discussed for elementary school children can
also be used for middle and high school students (with the exception of
the CAST, which was designed for youngsters up to age 11). A study of
the CARS with a group of adolescents found that mean scores were lower
(reflecting improvement) than the youngsters' earlier scores, and suggested
a lower cutoff score for the autism spectrum (27 instead of 30; Mesibov,
Schopler, Schaffer, & Michal, 1989). For youngsters ages 10–15 years
with average intelligence, a self-report measure is under development (the
Autism-Spectrum Quotient [AQ]—Adolescent Version; Baron-Cohen,
Hoekstra, Knickmeyer, & Wheelwright, 2006).

Adulthood

For individuals who can report on their own experiences, the adult version of the AQ (Baron-Cohen, Wheelwright, Skinner, Martin, & Clubley,
2001a, 2001b) can be used alone or as part of the Adult Asperger Assessment method (Baron-Cohen, Wheelwright, Robinson, & Woodbury-Smith,
2005), which also includes a clinical interview and a self-report measure
called the Empathy Quotient (Baron-Cohen & Wheelwright, 2004).

AGE-RELATED ISSUES IN SKILL ASSESSMENT

As discussed in the preceding section, diagnoses of ASD made at or after 2
years of age by experienced professionals using clinical judgment and standardized diagnostic tools are generally stable. Skills on developmental tests,

on the other hand, are more variable over time. The most obvious factor accounting for this is that all children develop and learn new skills as they age. In addition to this universal upward trajectory, the developmental trajectory of children with autism is particularly variable. Low scores on developmental tests at age 2 are *not* stable or predictive in many cases (Charman et al., 2005; Turner et al., 2006), with significant numbers of children either making marked developmental progress or cooperating better with testing (or both) during the preschool years (Rapin, 2003). In general, after that age mean Verbal IQ scores of groups tend either to remain stable or to increase, and behavioral symptoms decrease through childhood, adolescence, and even adulthood, particularly for individuals without mental retardation (Howlin, 2005; McGovern & Sigman, 2005; Sigman & Ruskin, 1999; Shattuck et al., 2007). However, group means may mask *individual* differences: Some people make marked progress, while others' cognitive scores and general functioning decline in adolescence or adulthood (Shea & Mesibov, 2005). Furthermore, academic and vocational skills and independence in daily life often do not develop to the same extent as IQ and language skills, so that in adulthood the majority of individuals diagnosed with ASD as children require some combination of family support and social services (Howlin, 2005; Klin et al., 2007; Seltzer et al., 2004).

Specific age-related aspects of assessing the skills of individuals with ASD are discussed below.

Early Childhood

Before the age of 3 years, skill assessment generally does not require intentional cooperation on the part of a child with ASD; it relies instead on observation of the child's exploration of standardized materials and reactions to events in the assessment setting. Commonly used developmental tests at this age (many recently revised) are the Bayley Scales of Infant and Toddler Development, Third Edition (Bayley-III; Bayley, 2005), the Mullen Scales of Early Learning: AGS Edition (Mullen, 1995), and the Psychoeducational Profile—Third Edition (Schopler, Lansing, Reichler, & Marcus, 2005). Parent report measures often used at this age include the MacArthur–Bates Communicative Development Inventories, Second Edition (Fenson et al., 2007) and the Vineland Adaptive Behavior Scales, Second Edition (Vineland-II; Sparrow, Cicchetti, & Balla, 2005).

Preschool Age

Evaluations of preschool-age children with both ASD and significant developmental delays must continue to rely on the observational and parent report techniques used with younger children, but some children at this age can cooperate with requests to perform tasks with standardized test materials (such as those described by Paul & Wilson in Chapter 7 [language and communication], by Klinger, O'Kelley, & Mussey in Chapter 8 [intelligence], and by Corbett, Carmean, & Fein in Chapter 9 [neuropsychological functions]). When test items become too difficult, however, behaviors such as leaving the table, having tantrums, or giving perseverative answers are often seen. Returning to developmentally earlier items is a useful method for assessing whether the behavioral difficulties are related to the developmental level of the tasks.

Accurate assessment requires engaging a child's attention and motivation to demonstrate his or her skills (Koegel, Koegel, & Smith, 1997; Ozonoff, Rogers, & Hendren, 2003). One way to do this is to use visual structure that shows the child how many tasks he or she will be asked to complete before receiving a small reward. For example, a word-processing program can be used to create rows of blank boxes, with a shaded box at the end of each row to represent a treat (see Figure 5.1). Each blank box represents one test item; when the child attempts or completes it, the examiner says something like "Good job. Check," and puts a check in the box. This procedure is used for *each* question or test item, regardless of the child's success, so that the reward reflects cooperation, not correct performance. The child can see that he or she is making progress along each row toward the shaded box, as well as progress down the page. When the examiner senses that the child needs a break, a special line or the word "Break" can be written at the end of a row. Multiple pages may be needed for testing with many items; it is advisable to have more than enough pages prepared and visible to the child since it is better to end early than to present additional test items that the child is not expecting.

Elementary School Age

Most elementary-school-age children with ASD can cooperate with testing requests (as long as test items are not too developmentally challenging)—but sometimes children are older than norms of tests at their functioning level, so test results must be reported carefully (see Klinger et al., Chapter 8). For delayed students, the grid in Figure 5.1 can still be used. More developmentally advanced students can typically work for longer periods (i.e., with more columns before the column of reward boxes), and some may like to choose a reward from options that are written in each shaded box. These more advanced students may also benefit from seeing a list of subtests checked off.

(Item 1)	(Item 2)	(Item 3)	(Item 4)	
(Item 5)	(Item 6)	(Item 7)	(Item 8)	
(Etc.)				

FIGURE 5.1. Sample of visual support sheet for standardized testing. The shaded box at the end of each row represents a treat as a reward for cooperation.

Middle School Age, High School Age, and Adulthood

For higher-functioning individuals at older ages, checking off a list of subtests, though not absolutely necessary, may reduce anxiety about how long testing will last and what it will consist of.

CONCLUDING COMMENTS

Accurately diagnosing ASD and assessing skills and behaviors are central to providing good services. Assessment should be an ongoing, carefully designed process, although it is sometimes taken for granted or not implemented with the rigor that it requires.

Individuals with ASD differ greatly from one another in terms of their cognitive skills, communication ability, interests, behaviors, and social understanding, among other factors. Assessment enables professionals to understand each person as an individual and to develop appropriate intervention strategies and programs. Furthermore, in addition to individual differences, developmental changes occur as each person with ASD grows and matures. At different ages, there are different skills to be taught and different challenges to be addressed. For this reason, assessment strategies and instruments change as people with ASD move through the lifespan.

Although the field of ASD includes a wide variety of theories and treatment strategies, it is universally agreed that the population is enormously varied in terms of skills, interests, and behaviors. The implementation of age-appropriate diagnostic and skills assessment strategies is essential for any theoretical approach to working with these students to be effective. Our goal in writing this chapter has been to contribute to the understanding, strategies, and instruments that will advance this process for individuals with ASD at different ages.

REFERENCES

Baird, G., Charman, T., Baron-Cohen, S., Cox, A., Swettenham, J., Wheelwright, S., et al. (2000). A screening instrument for autism at 18 months of age: A 6-year follow-up study. *Journal of the American Academy of Child and Adolescent Psychiatry, 39,* 694–702.

Baron-Cohen, S., Allen, J., & Gillberg, C. (1992). Can autism be detected at 18 months?: The needle, the haystack, and the CHAT. *British Journal of Psychiatry, 161,* 839–843.

Baron-Cohen, S., Cox, A., Baird, G., Swettenham, J., Nightengale, N., Morgan, K., et al. (1996). Psychological markers in the detection of autism in infancy in a large population. *British Journal of Psychiatry, 168,* 158–163.

Baron-Cohen, S., Hoekstra, R. A., Knickmeyer, R., & Wheelwright, S. (2006). The Autism-Spectrum Quotient (AQ)—Adolescent Version. *Journal of Autism and Developmental Disorders, 36,* 343–350.

Baron-Cohen, S., & Wheelwright, S. (2004). The Empathy Quotient: An investigation of adults with Asperger syndrome or high functioning autism, and normal sex differences. *Journal of Autism and Developmental Disorders, 34,* 163–175.

Baron-Cohen, S., Wheelwright, S., Robinson, J., & Woodbury-Smith, M. (2005). The Adult Asperger Assessment (AAA): A diagnostic method. *Journal of Autism and Developmental Disorders, 35,* 807–819.

Baron-Cohen, S., Wheelwright, S., Skinner, R., Martin, J., & Clubley, E. (2001a). The Autism-Spectrum Quotient: Evidence from Asperger syndrome/high functioning autism, males and females, scientists and mathematicians. *Journal of Autism and Developmental Disorders, 31,* 5–17.

Baron-Cohen, S., Wheelwright, S., Skinner, R., Martin, J., & Clubley, E. (2001b). Errata. *Journal of Autism and Developmental Disorders, 31,* 603.

Bayley, N. (2005). *Bayley Scales of Infant and Toddler Development, Third Edition (Bayley-III).* San Antonio, TX: Harcourt Assessment.

Bryson, S. E., McDermott, C., Rombough, V., Brian, J., & Zwaigenbaum, L. (in press). The Autism Observation Scale for Infants: Scale development and reliability data. *Journal of Autism and Developmental Disorders.*

Bryson, S. E., Rogers, S. J., & Fombonne, E. (2003). Autism spectrum disorders: Early detection, intervention, education, and psychopharmacological management. *Canadian Journal of Psychiatry. 48,* 506–516.

Campbell, J. M. (2005). Diagnostic assessment of Asperger's disorder: A review of five third-party rating scales. *Journal of Autism and Developmental Disorders, 35,* 25–35.

Centers for Disease Control and Prevention. (2007). Prevalence of autism spectrum disorders—Autism and Developmental Disabilities Monitoring Network, six sites, United States, 2000. *MMWR Surveillance Summaries, 56*(SS01), 1–11. (Retrieved from *www.cdc.gov/mmwr/preview/mmwrhtml/ss5601a1.htm*)

Charman, T., & Baird, G. (2002). Practitioner review: Diagnosis of autism spectrum disorder in 2- and 3-year-old children. *Journal of Child Psychology and Psychiatry, 43,* 289–305.

Charman, T., Taylor, E., Drew, A., Cockerill, H., Brown, J., & Baird, G. (2005). Outcome at 7 years of children diagnosed with autism at age 2: Predictive validity of assessments conducted at 2 and 3 years of age and pattern of symptom change over time. *Journal of Child Psychology and Psychiatry, 46,* 500–513.

Chawarska, K., Klin, A., Paul, R., & Volkmar, F. R. (2007). Autism spectrum disorders in the second year: Stability and change in syndrome expression. *Journal of Child Psychology and Psychiatry, 48*(2), 128–138.

Chawarska, K., & Volkmar, F. R. (2005). Autism in infancy and early childhood. In F. R. Volkmar, R. Paul, A. Klin, & D. Cohen (Eds.), *Handbook of autism and pervasive developmental disorders* (3rd ed., Vol. 1, pp. 223–246). Hoboken, NJ: Wiley.

Constantino, J. N., & Gruber, C. P. (2005). *Social Responsiveness Scale (SRS).* Los Angeles: Western Psychological Services.

Coonrod, E. E., & Stone, W. L. (2005). Screening for autism in young children. In F. R. Volkmar, R. Paul, A. Klin, & D. Cohen (Eds.), *Handbook of autism and pervasive developmental disorders* (3rd ed., Vol. 2, pp. 707–729). Hoboken, NJ: Wiley.

Dietz, C., Swinkels, S., van Daalen, E., van Engeland, H., & Buitelaar, J. K. (2006). Screening for autistic spectrum disorder in children aged 14–15 months: II. Population screening with the Early Screening of Autistic Traits Questionnaire (ESAT): Design and general findings. *Journal of Autism and Developmental Disorders, 36,* 713–722.

Eaves, L. C., & Ho, H. H. (2004). The very early identification of autism: Outcome to age 4½–5. *Journal of Autism and Developmental Disorders, 34,* 367–378.

Eaves, L. C., Wingert, H., & Ho, H. H. (2006a). Screening for autism: Agreement with diagnosis. *Autism, 10,* 229–242.

Eaves, L. C., Wingert, H., Ho, H. H., & Mickelson, E. C. R. (2006b). Screening for autism spectrum disorders with the Social Communication Questionnaire. *Journal of Developmental and Behavioral Pediatrics, 27*(Suppl. 2), S95–S103.

Ehlers, S., Gillberg., C., & Wing, L. (1999). A screening questionnaire for Asperger syndrome and other high-functioning autism spectrum disorders in school age children. *Journal of Autism and Developmental Disorders, 29,* 129–141.

Fein, D., Stevens, M., Dunn, M., Waterhouse, L., Allen, D., Rapin, I., et al. (1999). Subtypes of pervasive developmental disorder: Clinical characteristics. *Child Neuropsychology, 5,* 1–23.

Fenson, L., Marchman, V. A., Thal, D. J., Dale, P. S., Reznick, J. S., & Bates, E. (2007). *MacArthur–Bates Communicative Development Inventories (CDIs),* Second Edition. Baltimore: Brookes.

Gilliam, J. E. (2001). *Gilliam Asperger Disorder Scale.* Austin, TX: PRO-ED.

Goldstein, S. (2002). Review of the Asperger Syndrome Diagnostic Scale. *Journal of Autism and Developmental Disorders, 32,* 611–614.

Hartman, C. A., Luteijn, E., Serra, M., & Minderaa, R. (2006). Refinement of the Children's Social Behavior Questionnaire (CSBQ): An instrument that describes the diverse problems seen in milder forms of PDD. *Journal of Autism and Developmental Disorders, 36,* 325–342.

Howlin, P. (2005). Outcomes in autism spectrum disorders. In F. R. Volkmar, R. Paul, A. Klin, & D. Cohen (Eds.), *Handbook of autism and pervasive developmental disorders* (3rd ed., Vol. 1, pp. 201–230). Hoboken, NJ: Wiley.

Howlin, P., & Asgharian, A. (1999). The diagnosis of autism and Asperger syndrome: Findings from a survey of 770 families. *Developmental Medicine and Child Neurology, 41,* 834–839.

Howlin, P., & Karpf, J. (2004). Using the Social Communication Questionnaire to identify 'autism spectrum' disorders associated with other genetic conditions: Findings from a study of individuals with Cohen syndrome. *Autism, 8,* 175–182.

Howlin, P., & Moore, A. (1997). Diagnosis in autism: A survey of over 1200 patients in the UK. *Autism, 1,* 135–162.

Jónsdóttir, S. L., Saemundsen, E., Ásmundsdóttir, G., Hjartardóttir, S., Ásgeirsdóttir, B., Smaradóttir, H. H., et al. (2007). Follow-up of children diagnosed with pervasive developmental disorders: Stability and change during the preschool years. *Journal of Autism and Developmental Disorders, 37,* 1361–1374.

Klin, A., Saulnier, C. A., Sparrow, S. S., Cicchetti, D. V., Volkmar, F. R., & Lord, C. (2007). Social and communication abilities and disabilities in higher functioning individuals with autism spectrum disorders: The Vineland and the ADOS. *Journal of Autism and Developmental Disorders, 37,* 748–759.

Koegel, L. K., Koegel, R., & Smith, A. (1997). Variables related to differences in standardized test outcomes for children with autism. *Journal of Autism and Developmental Disorders, 27,* 233–243.

Kraijer, D., & de Bildt, A. (2005). The PDD-MRS: An instrument for identification of autism spectrum disorders in persons with mental retardation. *Journal of Autism and Developmental Disorders. 35,* 499–513.

Krug, D. J., & Arick, J. R. (2003). *Krug Asperger's Disorder Index.* Austin, TX: PRO-ED.

Landa, R., & Garrett-Mayer, E. (2006). Development in infants with autism spectrum disorders: A prospective study. *Journal of Child Psychology and Psychiatry, 47,* 629–638.

Leekham, S., Libby, S., Wing, L., Gould, J., & Taylor, C. (2002). Diagnostic Interview for Social and Communication Disorders: Algorithms for ICD-10 childhood autism and Wing and Gould autistic spectrum disorder. *Journal of Child Psychology and Psychiatry, 43,* 327–342.

Lord, C. (1995). Follow-up of two-year-olds referred for possible autism. *Journal of Child Psychology and Psychiatry, 36,* 1365–1382.

Lord, C., & Corsello, C. (2005). Diagnostic instruments in autistic spectrum disorders. In F. R. Volkmar, R. Paul, A. Klin, & D. Cohen (Eds.), *Handbook of autism and pervasive developmental disorders* (3rd ed., Vol. 2, pp. 730–771). Hoboken, NJ: Wiley.

Lord, C., Risi, S., DiLavore, P., Shulman, C., Thurm, A., & Pickles, A. (2006). Autism from 2 to 9 years of age. *Archives of General Psychiatry, 63,* 694–701.

Lord, C., Rutter, M., DiLavore, P., & Risi, S. (1999). *Autism Diagnostic Observation Schedule—WPS Edition*. Los Angeles: Western Psychological Services.

Mandell, D. S., Listerud, J., Levy, S. E., & Pinto-Martin, J. (2002). Race differences in the age at diagnosis among Medicaid-eligible children with autism. *Journal of the American Academy of Child and Adolescent Psychiatry, 41,* 1447–1453.

McConachie, H., Le Couteur, A., & Honey, E. (2005). Can a diagnosis of Asperger syndrome be made in very young children with suspected autism spectrum disorder? *Journal of Autism and Developmental Disorders, 35,* 167–176.

McGovern, C. W., & Sigman, M.. (2005). Continuity and change from early childhood to adolescence in autism. *Journal of Child Psychology and Psychiatry, 46,* 401–408.

Mesibov, G. B., Schopler, E., Schaffer, B., & Michal, N. (1989). Use of the Childhood Autism Rating Scale with autistic adolescents and adults. *Journal of the American Academy of Child and Adolescent Psychiatry, 28,* 538–541.

Mesibov, G. B., Shea, V., & Schopler, E. (with Adams, L., Burgess, S., Chapman, S. M., et al.). (2005). *The TEACCH approach to autism spectrum disorders.* New York: Kluwer Academic/Plenum.

Moore, V., & Goodson, S. (2006). How well does early diagnosis of autism stand the test of time?: Follow-up study of children assessed for autism at age 2 and development of an early diagnostic service. *Autism, 7,* 47–63.

Mullen, E. M. (1995). *Mullen Scales of Early Learning: AGS edition.* Circle Pines, MN: American Guidance Service.

Murrie, D. M., Warren, J. I., Kristiansson, M., & Dietz, P. E. (2002). Asperger syndrome in forensic settings. *International Journal of Forensic Mental Health, 1,* 59–70.

Myles, B., Bock, S., & Simpson, R. (2001). *Asperger Syndrome Diagnostic Scale.* Austin, TX: PRO-ED.

Nylander, L., & Gillberg, C. (2001). Screening for autism spectrum disorders in adult psychiatric out-patients: A preliminary report. *Acta Psychiatrica Scandinavica, 103,* 428–434.

Ozonoff, S., Goodlin-Jones, B. L., & Solomon, M. (2005). Evidence-based assessment of autism spectrum disorders in children and adolescents. *Journal of Clinical Child and Adolescent Psychology, 34,* 523–540.

Ozonoff, S., Rogers, S.J., & Hendren, R.L. (2003). *Autism spectrum disorders: A research review for practitioners.* Washington, DC: American Psychiatric Publishing.

Palmer, A. (2006). *Realizing the college dream with autism or Asperger syndrome.* London: Jessica Kingsley.

Palomo, R., Belinchon, M., & Ozonoff, S. (2006). Autism and family home movies: A comprehensive review. *Journal of Developmental and Behavioral Pediatrics, 27*(Suppl. 2), S59–S68.

Perry, A., Condillac, R. A., Freeman, N. L., Dunn-Geier, J., & Belair, J. (2005). Multi-site study of the Childhood Autism Rating Scale (CARS) in five clinical groups of young children. *Journal of Autism and Developmental Disorders, 35,* 625–634.

Pine, E., Luby, J., Abbacchi, A., & Constantino, J. N. (2006). Quantitative assessment of autistic symptomatology in preschoolers. *Autism, 10,* 344–352.

Rapin, I. (2003). Value and limitations of preschool cognitive tests, with an emphasis on longitudinal study of children on the autistic spectrum. *Brain and Development, 25,* 546–548.

Resnick, J. S., Baranek, G. T., Reavis, S., Watson, L. R., & Crais, E. R (2007). A parent-report instrument for identifying one-year-olds at risk for an eventual diagnosis of autism: The First Year Inventory. *Journal of Autism and Developmental Disorders, 37,* 1691–1710.

Risi, S., Lord, C., Gotham, K., Corsello, C., Chrysler, C., Szatmari, P., et al. (2006). Combining information from multiple sources in the diagnosis of autism spectrum disorders. *Journal of the American Academy of Child and Adolescent Psychiatry, 45,* 1094–1103.

Robins, D. L., & Dumont-Mathieu, T. M. (2006). Early screening for autism spectrum disorders: Update on the Modified Checklist for Autism in Toddlers. *Journal of Developmental and Behavioral Pediatrics, 27*(Suppl. 2), S111–S119.

Robins, D. L., Fein, D., Barton, M. L., & Green, J. A. (2001). The Modified Checklist for Autism in Toddlers: An initial study investigating the early detection of autism and pervasive developmental disorders. *Journal of Autism and Developmental Disorders, 31,* 131–144.

Rutter, M., Le Couteur, A., & Lord, C. (2003). *The Autism Diagnostic Interview— Revised: WPS Edition.* Los Angeles: Western Psychological Services.

Schopler, E., Lansing, M. D., Reichler, R. J., & Marcus, L. M. (2005). *Psychoeducational Profile—Third Edition (PEP-3).* Austin, TX: PRO-ED.

Schopler, E., Reichler, R. J., & Renner, B. R. (1988) *The Childhood Autism Rating Scale (CARS).* Austin, TX: PRO-ED.

Scott, F. J., Baron-Cohen, S., Bolton, P., & Brayne, C. (2002). The CAST (Childhood Asperger Syndrome Test). *Autism, 6,* 9–31.

Scambler, D. J., Hepburn, S. L., Hagerman, R. J., & Rogers, S. J. (2007). A preliminary study of screening for risk of autism in children with fragile X syndrome: Testing two risk cut-offs for the Checklinst for Autism in Toddlers. *Journal of Intellectual Disability Research, 51,* 269–276.

Scambler, D. J., Hepburn, S. L., & Rogers, S. J. (2006). A two-year follow-up on risk status identified by the Checklist for Autism in Toddlers. *Journal of Developmental and Behavioral Pediatrics, 27*(Suppl. 2), S104–S110.

Seltzer, M. M., Shattuck, P., Abbeduto, L., & Greenberg, J. S. (2004). Trajectory of development in adolescents and adults with autism. *Mental Retardation and Developmental Disabilities Research Reviews, 10,* 234–247.

Shattuck, P., Seltzer, M. M., Greenberg, J. S., Orsmond, G., Bolt, D., Kring, S., et al. (2007). Change in autism symptoms and maladaptive behaviors in adolescents and adults with an autism spectrum disorder. *Journal of Autism and Developmental Disorders, 37,* 1735–1747.

Siegel, B. (2004). *Pervasive Developmental Disorders Screening Test–II (PDDST-II).* San Antonio, TX: Harcourt Assessment.

Shea, V., & Mesibov, G. B. (2005). Adolescents and adults with autism. In F. R.

Volkmar, R. Paul, A. Klin, & D. Cohen (Eds.), *Handbook of autism and pervasive developmental disorders* (3rd ed., Vol. 1, pp. 288–311). Hoboken, NJ: Wiley.

Sigman, M., & Ruskin, E. (1999). Continuity and change in the social competence of children with autism, Down syndrome, and developmental delays. *Monographs of the Society for Research in Child Development, 64*(1, Serial No. 256).

Sparrow, S. S., Balla, D., & Cicchetti, D. (1984). *Vineland Adaptive Behavior Scales*. Circle Pines, MN: American Guidance Service.

Sparrow, S. S., Cicchetti, D., & Balla, D. (2005). *Vineland Adaptive Behavior Scales, Second Edition (Vineland-II)*. Circle Pines, MN: American Guidance Service.

Stone, W. L., Coonrod, E. E., & Ousley, O. Y. (2000). Screening Tool for Autism in Two-Year-Olds (STAT): Development and preliminary data. *Journal of Autism and Developmental Disorders, 30*, 607–612.

Stone, W. L., Coonrod, E. E., Pozdol, S. L., & Turner, L. M. (2003). The Parent Interview for Autism—Clinical Version (PIA-CV): A measure of behavioral change for young children with autism. *Autism, 7*, 9–30.

Stone, W. L., & Hogan, K. L. (1993). A structured parent interview for identifying young children with autism. *Journal of Autism and Developmental Disorders, 23*, 639–652.

Sutera, S., Pandey, J., Esser, E.L., Rosenthal, M. A., Wilson, L. B., Barton, M., et al. (2007). Predictors of optimal outcome in toddlers diagnosed with autism spectrum disorders. *Journal of Autism and Developmental Disorders, 37*, 98–107.

Swinkels, S. H. N., Dietz, C., van Daalen, E., Kerkhof, I. H. G. M., van Engeland, H., & Buitelaar., J. K. (2006). Screening for autistic spectrum disorder in children aged 14–15 months. I: The Development of the Early Screening of Autistic Traits Questionnaire (ESAT). *Journal of Autism and Developmental Disorders, 36*, 723–732.

Trillingsgaard, A., Sørensen, E. U., Němec, G., & Jørgensen, M. (2005). What distinguishes autism spectrum disorders from other developmental disorders before the age of four years? *European Child and Adolescent Psychiatry, 14*, 65–72.

Turner, L. M., Stone, W. L., Pozdol, S. L., & Coonrod, E. E. (2006). Follow-up of children with autism spectrum disorders from age 2 to age 9. *Autism, 10*, 243–265.

Ventola, P., Kleinman, J., Pandey, J., Wilson, L., Esser, E., Boorstein, H., et al. (2007). Differentiating between autism spectrum disorders and other developmental disabilities in children who failed a screening instrument for ASD. *Journal of Autism and Developmental Disorders, 37*, 425–436.

Watson, L. R., Baranek, G. T., Crais, E. R., Reznick, J. S., Dykstra, J., & Perryman, T. (2007). The First Year Inventory: Retrospective parent responses to a questionnaire designed to identify one-year-olds at risk for autism. *Journal of Autism and Developmental Disorders, 37*, 49–61.

Werner, E., Dawson, G., Munson, J., & Osterling, J. (2005). Variation in early developmental course of autism and its relation with behavioral outcome at 3–4 years of age. *Journal of Autism and Developmental Disorders, 35,* 337–350.

Wetherby, A. M., & Prizant, B. M. (2002). *Communication and symbolic behavior scales developmental profile.* Baltimore: Brookes.

Wetherby, A. M., Watt, N., Morgan, L., & Shumway, S. (2007). Social communication profiles of children with autism spectrum disorders late in the second year of life. *Journal of Autism and Developmental Disorders, 37,* 960–975.

Wetherby, A. M., Woods, J., Allen, L., Cleary, J., Dickinson, H., & Lord, C. (2004). Early indicators of autism spectrum disorders in the second year of life. *Journal of Autism and Developmental Disorders, 34,* 473–493.

Wing, L., Leekham, S. R., Libby, S. J., Gould, J., & Larcombe, M. (2002). The Diagnostic Interview for Social and Communication Disorders: Background, inter-rater reliability and clinical use. *Journal of Child Psychology and Psychiatry, 43,* 307–325.

Young, R. L., Brewer, N., & Pattison, C. (2003). Parental identification of early behavioural abnormalities in children with autistic disorder. *Autism, 7,* 125–143.

Zwaigenbaum, L., Bryson, S., Rogers, T., Roberts, W., Brian, J., & Szatmari, P. (2005). Behavioral manifestations of autism in the first year of life. *International Journal of Developmental Neuroscience, 23,* 143–152.

Zwaigenbaum, L., Thurm, A., Stone, W., Baranek, G., Bryson, S., Iverson, J., et al. (2007). Studying the emergence of autism spectrum disorders in high-risk infants: Methodological and practical issues. *Journal of Autism and Developmental Disorders, 37,* 466–480.

CHAPTER SIX

Assessment of Social Behavior in Autism Spectrum Disorders

Ifat Gamliel

Nurit Yirmiya

The diathesis–stress or transactional model of development suggests that genetic and environmental regulators of behavior transact continuously over time and thus constantly mutually influence each other (Sameroff, 2000). Typically developing infants are born with the genetic predisposition or preparedness that endows them to learn and acquire certain behaviors quite easily (Seligman, 1970). In typical development, for example, infants become social very early. They identify their mothers by 1 week of age, and by 3 months they recognize photographs of their mothers and prefer them over photographs of strangers (Barrera & Maurer, 1981; Pascalis, de Schonen, Morton, Deruelle, & Fabre-Grenet, 1995). They also begin very early to imitate, which is a powerful mechanism for learning. Some researchers have suggested that even newborns at 2 days of age are able to imitate adults' facial movements, such as tongue protrusion and mouth opening (Meltzoff & Moore, 1977, 1999); most researchers agree that by 1 year of age, infants are able to use imitation to learn new behaviors quite easily and flawlessly. Thus typically developing infants engage in nonverbal social-communicative behaviors and are able to synchronize or attune their affective and arousal states to those of their partners from a very early period (Feldman, 2007). The intact newborn develops normatively and progresses through major developmental cornerstones in all realms of development, including the social realm. These achievements are attributed to biological maturational processes and to a good enough environmental experience, as suggested by the transactional diathesis–stress model.

In contrast to typically developing children, children diagnosed with autism spectrum disorders (ASD), and some children even prior to receiving such diagnoses, experience difficulties in achieving milestones and displaying behaviors easily achieved by their typically developing peers. A major area of these difficulties is social: The social behavior of children, adolescents, and adults with ASD differs qualitatively from that of their typically developing agemates. Indeed, impairments in social behavior constitute one of the three general areas of impairments required for an ASD diagnosis.

For example, the diagnostic criteria for autistic disorder in the *Diagnostic and Statistical Manual for Mental Disorders,* fourth edition, text revision (DSM-IV-TR; American Psychiatric Association, 2000) and the *International Classification of Diseases,* 10th revision (ICD-10; World Health Organization, 1992) describe behaviors and impairments in three domains, one of which pertains to the focus of the current chapter: qualitative impairments in reciprocal social interaction. According to the *DSM-IV-TR* (American Psychiatric Association, 2000, p. 75), the diagnostic criteria for the social impairment domain are as follows:

(1) qualitative impairment in social interaction, as manifested by at least two of the following:

(a) marked impairment in the use of multiple nonverbal behaviors such as eye-to-eye gaze, facial expression, body postures, and gestures to regulate social interaction
(b) failure to develop peer relationships appropriate to developmental level
(c) a lack of spontaneous seeking to share enjoyment, interests, or achievements with other people (e.g., by a lack of showing, bringing, or pointing out objects of interest)
(d) lack of social or emotional reciprocity

The other two domains comprise impairments in communication, and restricted, repetitive, and stereotyped patterns of behavior, interests, and activities.

In this chapter, adopting a developmental framework, we review the cardinal findings and assessment measures pertaining to social behavior in children and adolescents with ASD.

IDENTIFYING SOCIAL DIFFICULTIES
IN THE EARLY YEARS

The earliest evidence for social difficulties of children later diagnosed with ASD comes from two lines of research. The first consists of retrospective investigations, such as retrospective parental interviews or the investigation of home movies videotaped during the first year of life (or soon after) of children who later receive an ASD diagnosis. The second comprises prospective studies of infants who are at risk for ASD.

The early ontogeny of autism has often been examined via retrospective analyses of home videos of infants who were later diagnosed with the disorder (e.g., Adrien et al., 1991, 1993; Baranek, 1999; Clifford & Dissanayake, 2008; Clifford, Young, & Williamson, 2007; Losche, 1990; Maestro et al., 2002, 2005; Osterling & Dawson, 1994; Osterling, Dawson, & Munson, 2002; Werner, Dawson, Osterling, & Dinno, 2000). This body of literature has revealed evidence of early impairments in social engagement among such infants. For example, in comparison to a group of typically developing children, infants who were later diagnosed with autism revealed impairments in sensory–motor development, joint social activities, and symbolic play (Losche, 1990); impairments in social interaction, social smiling, and facial expressions, combined with hypoactivity and poor attention (Adrien et al., 1993); and significantly less eye contact and less responsiveness to their names being called (Osterling & Dawson, 1994). Comparing children later diagnosed with autism to children later diagnosed with developmental delays, Baranek (1999) validated that only the children who were later diagnosed with autism demonstrated impairments in response to their names and in orientation to visual stimuli, as well as aversion to touch. Clifford and Dissanayake (2008) also investigated early development of infants later diagnosed with autism during the first 2 years of life, by using retrospective parental interviews and analyses of home videos. They suggested that abnormalities in dyadic behaviors, such as poor quality of eye contact, impairment in the use of smiling, and inappropriate affect, may be detected in home videos even before the first birthday.

In contrast to retrospective studies with children who were later diagnosed with ASD, the strategy of prospective studies has been to employ groups of children known to be at risk for ASD, and to follow their development from close to birth until they reach the age of 2 or 3 years or older, at which time their outcome diagnosis of ASD or non-ASD becomes known (Yirmiya & Ozonoff, 2007). Researchers working with at-risk samples employ various observations and screening measures, as well as experimental methods. Great effort has been invested in producing predictive measures for ASD and for related difficulties among young infants. Some of these screening measures are designed as "Level 1" screeners—that is, brief instruments used to identify children at risk for ASD in the general population, and administered mostly by primary care physicians and general practitioners. In contrast, "Level 2" screeners are used to identify risk for ASD versus other types of developmental delays among selected groups of children who are already considered as being at risk (e.g., younger siblings of children with ASD, or children referred with various developmental concerns and delays). These latter screeners are usually more time-consuming instruments, and are administered more often by trained professionals other than general practitioners (Robins & Dumont-Mathieu, 2006).

In the next section, we describe instruments that involve parental reports, observations and testing by health care professionals, or both, as these pertain to the assessment of social behavior in young infants and toddlers and early identification of ASD, as well as to the assessment of social behavior in older children, adolescents, and adults. We present these measures chronologically, from those that are suitable for the youngest of infants to those relevant for toddlers, older children, adolescents and adults. It is important to note that different measures are used for different purposes. Some measures are most appropriate for developmental surveillance or Level 1 screening, some for Level 2 screening, and some for diagnosis and/or research. Although a clinician should never base a formal diagnosis of an ASD on any of this set of measures alone, especially without actually seeing a child, some of the assessments described in this next section do provide cost-effective means of achieving a current perspective on a child's difficulties at any particular time. (For further information about diagnosis vs. screening, see Naglieri, Chapter 3, this volume.)

ASSESSMENT AND DIAGNOSTIC MEASURES FOR SOCIAL BEHAVIOR

The Autism Observation Scale for Infants (AOSI; Bryson, McDermott, Rombough, Brian, & Zwaigenbaum, 2000), as its name indicates, is a short observational assessment designed to detect and monitor putative signs of ASD in infants ages 6–18 months. After a short interaction and observation, the attending professional uses a checklist for 18 specific behavioral risk markers for autism, including visual attention and attention disengagement, coordination of eye gaze with action, imitation, affect, behavioral reactivity, social-communicative behaviors, and sensory–motor development. Using the AOSI, Zwaigenbaum et al. (2005) compared a group of high-risk infants (siblings of children with autism) to a group of low-risk infants, and found that several behaviors observed at 12 (but not at 6) months predicted a future Autism Diagnostic Observation Schedule

(ADOS) classification of autism at 24 months for the high-risk group. At 12 months, these behaviors included impairments in eye contact, visual tracking, disengagement of visual attention, orienting to name, imitation, social smiling, reactivity, social interest, and sensory-oriented behaviors. Bryson, Zwaigenbaum, McDermott, Rombough, and Brian (2007) reported good to excellent reliability and called for further investigation of the AOSI's ability to discriminate high-risk infants who will eventually develop ASD.

In contrast to the AOSI, which is administered and coded by a trained professional, the First Year Inventory (FYI; Reznick, Baranek, Reavis, Watson, & Crais, 2007) is a questionnaire administered to infants' caregivers to identify 12-month-olds in the general population who are at risk for atypical development in general, but with a special focus on infants whose risk patterns are most predictive of a future ASD diagnosis. The target behaviors depicted by the various items are based on retrospective and prospective studies that suggested risk markers in infancy for an eventual diagnosis of autism. In this 63-item checklist, parents are asked to describe their children on two major domains: Social and Communicative Behaviors (i.e., social orienting, receptive communication, social affective engagement, imitation, and expressive communication) and Sensory and Regulatory Behaviors (i.e., sensory processing, regulatory patterns, reactivity, and repetitive behavior). A retrospective version of the FYI was administered to parents of preschool children with ASD, children with other developmental disabilities, and children with typical development, to strengthen the validity of the FYI and to improve its utility for prospective screening of both infants from the general population and infants at risk (Watson et al., 2007).

The Early Screening for Autistic Traits Questionnaire (ESAT; Swinkels et al., 2006), designed as a general population screener for 14- to 15-month-old infants, is a two-stage, 14-item questionnaire administered to health practitioners and caregivers. Four items were identified as having good discriminability for ASD: readability of emotions; reaction to sensory stimuli; and two play behaviors—interest in different toys and varied play. The authors suggest that these four items could be used as a quick prescreening instrument, to limit the number of children who need to be further screened with the full version of the ESAT (Swinkels et al., 2006). In a large population study (Dietz, Swinkels, van Daalen, van Engeland, & Buitelaar, 2006), 14- to 15-month-old infants were prescreened by physicians using these four items. Infants with positive results on the prescreening were then evaluated at home by a trained professional using the full ESAT, and were also invited for a complete psychiatric examination as well as for follow-up examinations at 24 and 42 months. Dietz et al. (2006) underscored the large number of false-positive results in both the prescreening (first stage) and the administration of the ESAT (second stage) for a later diagnosis of ASD; therefore, this screener should be used with caution. However, it can assist clinicians who are considering referrals for more comprehensive diagnostic evaluation of ASD.

The Communication and Symbolic Behavior Scales (CSBS; Wetherby & Prizant, 1993) and its shortened version, the Communication and Symbolic Behavior Scales Developmental Profile (CSBS-DP; Wetherby & Prizant, 2002), are standardized tools designed as evaluation procedures for early identification of communication disorders in children between 12 and 24 months of age. The CSBS-DP actually consists of three measures: the Infant–Toddler Checklist, which is a 14-item screening questionnaire that can be completed quickly by a parent at the physician's office; a Caregiver Questionnaire; and a Behavior Sample, which is a semistructured observation of the child interacting with a parent and clinician, when the child is being presented with a series of "communication temptations" such as interesting toys and other play opportunities. Three composites may be derived from the Infant–Toddler Checklist and Behavior Sample: Social (emotion, eye gaze, and communication); Speech (sounds and words); and Symbolic (understanding and object use). The CSBS-DP has been standardized to have a mean of 10 and standard deviation of 3 for each composite, and a mean of 100 and standard deviation of 15 for the total score. Good evidence for reliability and validity supports the use of the Infant–Toddler Checklist and Behavior Sample as appropriate screening and evaluation tools for identifying young children with developmental delays at 12–24 months of age (Wetherby, Allen, Cleary, Kublin, & Goldstein, 2002; Wetherby, Goldstein, Cleary, Allen, & Kublin, 2003), with promising results regarding the identification of later ASD as well (Wetherby et al., 2004).

The CSBS-DP has also been used as a standardized measure for assessing social, communication, and play behavior of 14- to 24-month-old infants with high and low risk for autism, in a prospective longitudinal study investigating developmental trajectories of children with early and later diagnosis of ASD (Landa, Holman, & Garrett-Mayer, 2007). In Wetherby et al.'s (2004) prospective longitudinal study of a large population-based sample of children between 12 and 24 months of age, the CSBS-DP was utilized to detect early indicators of ASD ("red flags") in the second year of life, which could differentiate children later diagnosed with ASD from children diagnosed with developmental delays and children with typical development. Some of these "red flags" included indicators of atypical early social development, such as lack of sharing enjoyment or interest and lack of response to name. Furthermore, Wetherby, Watt, Morgan, and Shumway (2007) investigated the "social communication phenotype" late in the second year of life among children later diagnosed with ASD. Their research highlighted five pivotal social communication skills detected by the CSBS-DP: communicative intentions, conventional behaviors, representation, social referencing, and rate of communication.

The Checklist for Autism in Toddlers (CHAT; Baron-Cohen, Allen, & Gillberg, 1992) is one of the first screening measures designed to identify toddlers from the general population who are at risk for ASD, by detecting abnormalities in early social orienting behaviors such as joint attention and pretend play. The CHAT is a 14-item yes–no checklist completed by both parents and a home health visitor. Five key items describing protodeclarative pointing, gaze monitoring, and pretend play were found to have the best discriminability as early as 18 months for a later diagnosis of autism (Baird et al., 2000; Baron-Cohen et al., 1996). The Modified CHAT (M-CHAT; Robins, Fein, Barton, & Green, 2001) omits the CHAT's observational section but includes additional parent report items, for a total of 23 items. It may be administered to parents as well as to pediatricians and family practitioners to detect early features of autism in children ages 16–30 months. A follow-up interview is administered to parents of children who obtain positive results on the M-CHAT to review their answers on all failed items, before the children are referred for full ASD evaluation. Items regarding early social development include "Does your child enjoy playing peek-a-boo/hide-and-seek?" and "Does your child look at your face to check your reaction when faced with something unfamiliar?" Six critical items of the M-CHAT were identified as offering the best discriminability for ASD: taking interest in other children; using index finger to point and to indicate interest in something; bringing objects over to show the parent; imitating; responding to name when called; and following pointing across the room.

Robins et al. (2001) suggested that M-CHAT screening with 24-month-olds rather than 18-month-olds improves the instrument's sensitivity and acceptability to health care providers. In a replication study, Kleinman et al. (2008) confirmed the validity of the M-CHAT in detecting possible ASD in low-risk and high-risk samples of children ages 16–30 months. Furthermore, along with other screening measures, the M-CHAT was used successfully as a screener for possible ASD in a group of children with the genetic syndrome of molecularly confirmed 22q11.2 deletions (Fine et al., 2005).

The Screening Tool for Autism in Two-Year-Olds (STAT; Stone & Ousley, 1997) is a Level 2 screener designed to differentiate young children with ASD from other children already identified as being at risk (i.e., children with language and/or developmental delays), ranging in age from 24 through 35 months. The STAT is an observational measure consisting of a 20-minute play-based interactive session that provides a standard context for eliciting and observing early social-communicative behaviors. Twelve items assess behaviors in four social-communicative domains: Play,

Requesting, Directing Attention, and Motor Imitation. Reports on the STAT's psychometric properties indicate high sensitivity, specificity, and predictive values, as well as acceptable levels of reliability and concurrent validity with the ADOS (Stone, Coonrod, Turner, & Pozdol, 2004). Using the STAT, McDuffie, Yoder, and Stone (2005) investigated the associations between early prelinguistic social-communicative behaviors in 2- and 3-year-old children with ASD (i.e., attention–following, motor imitation, commenting, and requesting) and later language development. Surprisingly, commenting behavior predicted language comprehension, and both commenting and motor imitation of actions without objects predicted language production, thus suggesting their important potential as intervention targets (McDuffie et al., 2005).

In contrast to the aforementioned observations and screeners, the Early Social Communication Scales (ESCS; Mundy, Hogan, & Doehring, 1996; Seibert, Hogan, & Mundy, 1982) is a research-based procedure that enables assessment of children's initiating and responding to nonverbal communication acts, including joint attention behaviors, social play behaviors, and requesting behaviors. This 20-minute structured observation is appropriate for typically developing children between the ages of 6 and 30 months; it is commonly used for children with ASD who do not speak yet, to assess their nonverbal social-communicative abilities. A set of eliciting play and interactive situations using turn-taking tasks, social games, and interesting toys is presented to encourage social interaction between child and adult. The ESCS yields frequency-of-behavior scores in five categories: Initiating Social Interaction, Responding to Social Interaction, Initiating Joint Attention, Responding to Joint Attention, and Initiating Behavior Requests. Children with ASD show significant delays in their joint attention and requesting behaviors on the ESCS, compared to participants without ASD (Mundy, Sigman, Ungerer, & Sherman, 1986). Furthermore, performance on the ESCS in the preschool years has been found to predict language acquisition in middle childhood for children with ASD (Mundy & Gomes, 1998; Mundy, Sigman, & Kasari, 1990; Sigman & Ruskin, 1999).

As diagnoses of ASD become more stable during the third year of life and thereafter, we next describe the common diagnostic battery for children suspected of having ASD. This diagnostic battery typically involves standardized assessments specific to ASD, plus a developmental or intelligence test and a language test (language assessments are more fully discussed by Paul & Wilson, Chapter 7, this volume) based on a child's age and abilities, as well as an assessment of daily living skills. The two gold standard diagnostic systems for research purposes are the Autism Diagnostic Interview—Revised (ADI-R; Rutter, LeCouteur, & Lord, 2003b) and the Autism Diagnostic Observation Schedule (ADOS; Lord, Rutter, DiLavore, & Risi, 2002), which are based on DSM-IV (American Psychiatric

Association, 1994) and ICD-10 (World Health Organization, 1992) criteria for ASD, including specific items relating to social abilities.

The ADI-R is a semistructured interview that is completed with a child's caregivers. The Reciprocal Social Interactions items of the ADI-R include questions regarding peer relationships (e.g., imaginative play/group play with peers, interest in/response to other children), sharing enjoyment (e.g., showing and directing attention, offering/seeking to share), and social-emotional reciprocity (e.g., quality of social overtures, offering comfort). Due to its considerable length and training requirements, the ADI-R is not an ideal measure for use in clinical settings; but as stated above, it is primarily for research.

The ADOS is a semistructured, standardized observational assessment that provides a number of opportunities for interaction (e.g., play, turn-taking games, looking at books, etc.). The Reciprocal Social Interactions items of the ADOS include such behaviors as unusual eye contact; deficit in directing facial expression to others; accompanying spoken language with nonverbal communication (e.g., gaze, facial expression, gesture); showing shared enjoinment in the interaction; communicating affect; and understanding of others' emotions.

A cognitive and developmental evaluation is an essential component of the diagnostic process for ASD. Most IQ tests include at least some subscales that assess social understanding. For example, the Wechsler Intelligence Scale for Children—Third Edition (WISC-III; Wechsler, 1991) contains the Picture Arrangement subtest, in which children are asked to arrange pictures (some of which depict social situations) in the correct order, and the Comprehension subtest, in which children are asked to explain their understanding of various social situations. Individuals with autism are notorious for their low scores on WISC-III subtests (and subtests of other IQ tests) that pertain to social understanding and behavior (i.e., Ehlers et al., 1997; Happé, 1994; Mayes & Calhoun, 2003, 2004; Siegel, Minshew, & Goldstein, 1996). In all of these studies, the mean WISC-III Comprehension subtest score was lower than the mean scores on the other subtests that compose the Verbal Comprehension Index.

The Vineland Adaptive Behavior Scales, Second Edition (Vineland-II; Sparrow, Cicchetti, & Balla, 2005), a well-known instrument assessing daily living skills, is used in clinical, educational, and research settings. It assesses four broad adaptive behavior domains: Communication, Daily Living Skills, Socialization, and Motor Skills. The Vineland-II is administered as an interview or a rating scale for parents/caregivers and teachers; it was designed to assess daily functioning of individuals with a variety of disorders and disabilities, such as mental retardation, ASD, and other developmental delays. The four domain composite scores are all standard scores with a mean of 100 and a standard deviation of 15. Together, they make up the Adaptive Behavior Composite score. Furthermore, the Vineland-II may yield scaled scores for subdomains (a mean of 15 and a standard deviation of 3), percentile ranks, and age equivalents. The Socialization domain comprises three subdomains: Interpersonal Relationships (e.g., "meets with friends regularly"), Play and Leisure Time (e.g., "takes turns without being asked"), and Coping Skills (e.g., "chooses not to taunt, tease, or bully").

The Vineland-II manual describes the typically expected profile for individuals with autism: (1) a low score on the Socialization domain, including low scores on its three subdomains; (2) a low score on the Expressive subdomain of the Communication domain; and (3) significant discrepancies between domain scores.

Research on social abilities as measured by the original Vineland revealed that individuals with autism obtained lower scores on interpersonal skills than either individuals with Down syndrome (Rodrigue, Morgan, & Geffken, 1991) or individuals with developmental delays matched on chronological age, gender, and IQ (Volkmar et al., 1987). Researchers have also investigated Vineland scores associated with diagnostic procedures, age, and IQ. Tomanik, Pearson, Loveland, Lane, and Shaw (2007) have suggested that assessment of an individual's adaptive functioning using the original Vineland (including the Socialization domain score) may improve ASD diagnostic accuracy, especially when the ADI-R and ADOS classifications are not congruent. Klin et al. (2007) demonstrated that levels of social ability in high-functioning individuals with ASD (as measured by the Vineland Socialization domain) decreased markedly with age, suggesting that these high-functioning individuals become increasingly socially impaired relative to their agemates through later childhood and into adolescence. Interestingly, verbal IQ scores as well as social difficulties as measured by the ADOS were unrelated to the Vineland Socialization domain score, thus suggesting that cognitive competency and/or fewer social disabilities may not contribute to functioning in the real world (Klin et al., 2007).

Another instrument specifically designed to assess the social domain is the Social Responsiveness Scale (SRS; Constantino & Todd, 2005). This instrument was developed as a general measure of social responsiveness and is applicable to a wide continuum of people, including those who are not diagnosed with ASD. The SRS is a 65-item rating scale administered to caregivers that focuses on a child's ability to engage in emotionally appropriate reciprocal social interaction and communication. It measures the severity of ASD symptoms as they occur in natural social settings (i.e., social awareness, social information processing, capacity for reciprocal social communication, social anxiety/avoidance, and autistic preoccupations and traits). In addition to a total score, the SRS generates scores for five subscales: Receptive, Cognitive, Expressive, and Motivational aspects of social behavior, as well as Autistic Preoccupations. The SRS has also been used to investigate the social endophenotype in siblings of children with autism (Constantino et al., 2006), and in families with two or more probands with autism (Duvall et al., 2007), as well as in other populations at risk, and in the general population (Constantino et al., 2004; Reiersen, Constantino, Volk, & Todd, 2007). Furthermore, the SRS has been used in evaluating responses to intervention programs in children with ASD (Pine, Luby, Abbacchi, & Constantino, 2006).

The Childhood Autism Rating Scale (CARS; Schopler, Reichler, DeVellis, & Daly, 1980) is a 15-item checklist designed to measure the presence and severity of ASD in children ages 24 months and above. The clinician who examines a child rates each item based on observation of the child's behavior throughout the testing session, as well as on the parent's report. The CARS includes 15 items on socialization, communication, emotional responses, and sensory sensitivities. Using a 7-point scale, the clinician indicates the degree to which the child's behavior deviates from that of a typical child of the same age. Children who score above the cutoff can be classified with severe autism or with mild to moderate autism. Classification of autism with the CARS has shown good agreement with other diagnostic measures and classifications, such as the ADI-R (Reciprocal Social Interactions and Language/Communication domains), clinical judgment (Cox et al., 1999; Saemundsen, Magnusson, Smari, & Sigurdardottir, 2003), DSM-IV criteria (American Psychiatric Association, 1994), and the ADOS (Ventola et al., 2006).

The Social Communication Questionnaire (SCQ; Rutter, Bailey, & Lord, 2003a), formerly the Autism Screening Questionnaire (ASQ; Berument, Rutter, Lord, Pickles, & Bailey, 1999), designed as a screening instrument for children age 4 years and above to evaluate autism spectrum symptoms, has a cutoff score that can be used to indicate the likelihood that a child has an ASD. The SCQ is made up of 40 items from the ADI-R (Rutter et al., 2003b). It offers two algorithms: a lifetime diagnosis, which refers to behavior throughout the child's lifetime, and a current algorithm, which focuses on the most recent 3-month period. Social items include questions such as "Does she/he have any particular friends or a best friend?" or "Does she/he ever try to comfort you when you are sad or hurt?" The SCQ has good discriminative validity with respect to the separation of ASD from non-ASD diagnoses at all IQ levels (Berument et al., 1999). However, other researchers have suggested different cutoff points for different populations (i.e., younger vs. older children, verbal vs. nonverbal children, clinical vs. nonclinical populations) and pointed to the importance of adjusting cutoff scores depending on research or screening goals (Baird et al., 2006; Corsello et al., 2007; Eaves, Wingert, & Ho, 2006a; Eaves, Wingert, Ho, & Mickelson, 2006b; Lee, David, Rusyniak, Landa, & Newschaffer, 2007).

Additional instruments have been specifically developed to measure symptom severity in individuals with high-functioning autism and individuals with Asperger syndrome. For example, the Childhood Asperger Syndrome Test (CAST; Scott, Baron-Cohen, Bolton, & Brayne, 2002) was designed as a screening questionnaire to identify children at risk for Asperger syndrome and related conditions from a general population. Caregivers rate their children on 37 items describing behaviors on the autism continuum, and a cutoff of 15 reflects possible risk for Asperger syndrome and other ASD. Social items include questions regarding peer relationships (i.e., "Does s/he join in playing games with other children easily?") and play activities (i.e., "Does s/he prefer imaginative activities such as play-acting or story telling, rather than numbers or lists of facts"?). The CAST has shown good to moderate test–retest reliability in various samples (i.e., nonclinical, high-scoring) (Allison et al., 2007; Williams et al., 2006), and good specificity and sensitivity (Scott et al., 2002; Williams et al., 2005). It was also used to measure autism-like traits in a nonclinical twin study (Dworzynski et al., 2007; Ronald et al., 2006a; Ronald, Happé, Price, Baron-Cohen, & Plomin, 2006b).

Another screening measure for individuals with high-functioning autism and individuals with Asperger syndrome is the Asperger Syndrome Screening Questionnaire (ASSQ; Ehlers, Gillberg, & Wing, 1999), designed to identify symptom characteristics of Asperger syndrome and other high-functioning ASD in school-age children. The ASSQ has been used in relatively small population samples and in clinical settings. Campbell (2005) reviewed the psychometric characteristics of several available screening instruments such as the ASSQ and suggested that despite their incomplete psychometric data to date, they hold promise as clinical instruments.

Some rating scales have also been designed to detect autism-like traits, which are useful in assessing the broad phenotype of autism in at-risk samples or in other populations of interest, and which address the social domain as well. For example, the Autism-Spectrum Quotient (AQ; Baron-Cohen, Wheelwright, Skinner, Martin, & Clubley, 2001) is a self-administered questionnaire designed to measure the degree to which an adult with normal intelligence has traits associated with autism in five domains: Social Skills, Attention Switching, Attention to Detail, Communication, and Imagination. The AQ was found to have good discriminative validity in differentiating a group with high-functioning ASD from randomly selected controls (Baron-Cohen et al., 2001; Woodbury-Smith, Robinson, Wheelwright, & Baron-Cohen, 2005), but results regarding cross-cultural reliability have been mixed (Ketelaars et al., 2008; Kurita, Koyama, & Osada, 2005; Wakabayashi, Baron-Cohen, Wheelwright, & Tojo, 2006). Furthermore, gender differences were detected on the AQ (i.e., where men scored higher than women in a nonclinical sample; Austin,

2005), and the examination of parents of children with autism revealed no significant differences from parents of children with typical development (Scheeren & Stauder, 2008).

Similarly, the Broader Phenotype Autism Symptoms Scale (BPASS; Dawson et al., 2007) is a new instrument for assessing autism-related traits in children and adults with ASD, as well as in parents and nonaffected siblings. This measure assesses such traits not only through informant interview, but also through the observation made during the interaction with a clinical examiner, thus enabling the direct assessment of social behaviors characteristic to autism. The BPASS measures four separate domains of autism-related traits: Social Motivation, Social Expressiveness, Conversational Skills, and Repetitive/Restricted Behaviors.

The Friendship Questionnaire (FQ; Baron-Cohen & Wheelwright, 2003) is a self-report questionnaire designed to assess an individual's ability to enjoy close, empathic, and supportive friendships and interest in interacting with others. Baron-Cohen and Wheelwright (2003) reported that women scored significantly higher on the FQ than men, and that adults with Asperger syndrome or high-functioning autism scored significantly lower than both men and women with typical development. Thus the FQ may reflect sex differences in the style of friendship in the general population and "may help us understand conditions like autism or [Asperger Syndrome] not as qualitatively different from anything else we are familiar with but, instead, simply as an extreme of the normal quantitative variation we see in any sample" (Baron-Cohen & Wheelwright, 2003, p. 514).

As the present review has made clear, social impairment—one of the three hallmarks of ASD—is indeed assessed in every screening and diagnostic instrument for possible ASD. The social difficulties inherent in ASD are also evident in the relationships that individuals with ASD have with other people in their daily lives. In the next two sections, we discuss the social relationships that children with ASD have with significant others in their lives—their attachment to parents and their friendships with agemates. We end this chapter with a short presentation of the deficits in "theory of mind" and the recently discovered dysfunction in mirror neurons that are associated with the social deficits in ASD.

ATTACHMENT

Both the ill-conceived notion that children with autism do not differentiate between their caregivers and other adults, and Kanner's (1949) claim that autism has a psychogenic origin, led to scanty research regarding the attachment patterns of children with autism (Yirmiya & Sigman, 2001).

More recently, however, researchers within the fields of both autism and attachment have begun to revive interest in parent–child interactions in general, and in attachment in particular, among families of children with autism. "Attachment" is defined as the affectional bond that an infant forms between him/herself and his or her caregiver (Ainsworth, Blehar, Waters, & Wall, 1978), and it is thought to be fundamental for later development of social relationships and cognitive skills (Weinfield, Sroufe, Egeland, & Carlson, 1999). Behaviors that maintain proximity and contact between the child and caregiver are defined as "attachment behaviors" (Bowlby, 1969). Ainsworth and her colleagues (Ainsworth, 1979; Ainsworth et al., 1978) designed the Strange Situation paradigm as a working model to assess the attachment patterns of children between the ages of 12 and 18 months. This paradigm involves an unfamiliar setting in which the child can play in the presence of his or her mother, and includes 3-minute-long separations from the mother in the presence of an unfamiliar woman. The child's reactions to the separation from the mother, and especially to the reunion with her, are coded for the child's pattern of attachment. This pattern may be classified as indicative of secure attachment or of one of three insecure attachment categories: ambivalent, avoidant, or disorganized.

A child with a secure attachment pattern of behavior is one for whom the mother presents a secure base for investigating the unfamiliar surroundings and new toys, while maintaining eye contact with her. When the mother leaves the room, the secure child typically shows signs of distress; when she returns, the child clearly shows joy and relief, and then quickly returns to exploration and play. A child with an insecure-ambivalent pattern of attachment tends to remain close to the mother and is less willing to explore the unfamiliar room. When the mother leaves, the child tends to cry bitterly, showing extensive signs of distress. When the mother returns, the child typically rejects her attempts at reassurance—for instance, by rejecting the mother's attempts to pick him or her up. A child with an insecure-avoidant pattern of attachment shows apparent signs of ignoring the mother, both during the play session in her presence and when she leaves the room. The child also shows no apparent awareness of her return, but physiological measurement has clearly revealed that these children experience the greatest amount of stress in the Strange Situation (Ainsworth, 1979). Finally, the disorganized pattern of insecure attachment is characteristic of a child who does not show a consistent pattern of behavior in the Strange Situation, but exhibits a confused and even contradictory array of responses (Main & Solomon, 1990).

Bowlby's (1969) description of attachment behaviors suggests that the development of attachment can be disrupted by various conditions that limit or impair the child's behavior. Most important, the different patterns of attachment are considered to be responses to the behaviors of the caregivers. Mothers of children classified as securely attached were shown to display more sensitive caregiving behaviors toward their children than mothers of children classified as insecurely attached (e.g., Weinfield et al., 1999).

Several groups of researchers have investigated attachment patterns in children with autism (Dissanayake & Crossley, 1996, 1997; Oppenheim, Koren-Karie, Dolev, & Yirmiya, in press; Rogers, Ozonoff, & Maslin-Cole, 1991, 1993; Shapiro, Sherman, Calamari, & Koch, 1987; Sigman & Mundy, 1989; Sigman & Ungerer, 1984; van IJzendoorn et al., 2007; Yirmiya & Sigman, 2001). Most of these studies suggest that the majority of children with ASD form secure attachments with their mothers. In contrast, Rutgers, Bakermans-Kranenburg, van IJzendoorn, and van Berckelaer-Onnes (2004), using both a narrative approach and a meta-analytic approach, examined two questions: whether children with autism have the same chance as children without autism to form a secure attachment relationship with their parents, and whether security of attachment is correlated with mental development and chronological age. Furthermore, these researchers were interested in exploring possible differences in attachment security between children diagnosed with pervasive developmental disorder not otherwise specified (PDD-NOS) and those diagnosed with autistic disorder. In contrast to previous findings and a previous narrative summary (Yirmiya & Sigman, 2001), which suggested that children with autism do form secure attachments to their parents, Rutgers et al.'s meta-analysis revealed that when all studies were pooled together by meta-analytic procedures, (1) children with autism scored about one-half of a standard deviation lower on attachment security than did children without autism (with other diagnoses or with typical development); and (2) low-functioning children with autism showed less security in their attachment than higher-functioning children with autism. These authors suggested that children with autism experience difficulties in their relationship with their parents from very early on.

The same research group (van IJzendoorn et al., 2007) examined parental sensitivity and attachment in a group of children with ASD and concluded that these children showed more attachment disorganization and were less involved with their parents than the other groups of children studied. Several methodological and analytic issues may limit the generalizability of these results, however. First, due to power-related issues, the authors compared the attachment security of the children with ASD to that of *all* other study participants (typically developing children and those with developmental delays were combined in one group). In addition, analyses were uncorrected for multiple comparisons; group differences were marginally significant (e.g., p's = .04 to .08); and effect sizes were low. These researchers concluded, in sharp contrast to the authors of previous studies, that children with ASD are less securely attached than are other children. Further investigation and replication are needed to confirm this conclusion. At the present time, based on the great majority of empirical studies, we suggest that most children with ASD, just like most children with other diagnoses or most typically developing children, are securely attached to their parents; however, we urge the field to continue to explore this important area.

SOCIAL INTERACTIONS WITH PEERS

Following Kanner's (1943) description that the principal deficit of autistic disorder was social, or in his words "extreme autistic aloneness" (p. 242) and/or "the inability to relate themselves in the ordinary way to people and situations," (p. 242) persons with autism have been characterized as exhibiting withdrawal, aloofness, indifference, passivity, lack of cooperation, and lack of engagement in the activities of others. Such social deficits are clearly displayed: From a young age, individuals with autism reveal an inability and/or lack of desire to interact with peers, poor appreciation of social cues, and socially and emotionally inappropriate responses. These characteristics may vary in such individuals, on a continuum from total withdrawal to the ability to communicate and socialize actively (but awkwardly).

In research regarding social interactions with peers, assessments have mainly targeted school-age children with autism, with some tests measuring perceived social relationships and others measuring interactions more directly (Sigman & Ruskin, 1999; Travis & Sigman, 1998). Studies using self-reports, interviews, and projective tests of children's general perceptions of friendship and loneliness, as well as the children's specific perception of their own personal social relationships, demonstrated that higher rates of loneliness were reported by high-functioning children with autism than by children with typical development (Bauminger & Kasari, 2000; Bauminger, Shulman, & Agam, 2003, 2004). Furthermore, high-functioning children with autism who perceived their social relationship with a friend as close, safe, and supportive also perceived themselves as less lonely, similarly to typically developing children (Bauminger et al., 2004).

Other studies using more naturalistic observations of children with autism in their everyday peer relations, during school activities such as free play or mealtime, detected very few interactions with peers in group settings. The few interactions that did occur were characterized as awkward and unsuccessful, and the children exhibited difficulties in both initiating and responding to the initiations of other children (Hauck, Fein, Waterhouse, & Feinstein, 1995; Stone & Caro-Martinez, 1990; Travis & Sigman, 1998). Sigman and Ruskin (1999) investigated the social interactions with peers of several groups of children with developmental disabilities, including children with autism; they used observations in natural settings (more and less structured), and such measures as the Peer Play Scale (Howes, 1980), as well as teacher reports. Sigman and Ruskin reported that the children with autism were less socially engaged, and more infrequently initiated and accepted play bids with classmates, than either children with Down syndrome or children with developmental delays. Furthermore, using a longitudinal design to detect predictors and correlates of peer competence among individuals with autism, Sigman and Ruskin found that early language and cognitive development, especially joint attention, play, and emotional responsiveness, were associated with later social development and peer interactions.

Cooperative social behavior, fairness, and other interpersonal strategies displayed by individuals with autism have been investigated in various settings and with various procedures. In one study, children with autism did not differ significantly from other groups of children without autism (youngsters with attention-deficit/hyperactivity disorder, oppositional defiant disorder, and typical development) in their cooperative behavior, level of emotional understanding, and aloof behavior (Downs & Smith, 2004). However, the group with autism did show deficits in identifying emotions and displaying socially appropriate behavior (Downs & Smith, 2004; Sally & Hill, 2006). A possible explanation for the null findings was that the participants with autism may have received social skills training, thus making it more difficult to distinguish them from the other groups.

Several studies have investigated social problem-solving ability, considered to be associated with the social difficulties in everyday lives of individuals with ASD. Cognitive processes such as executive functions and theory-of-mind abilities (see below), as well as real-life experiences, contribute to everyday problem solving. Such problem-solving capacities include the ability to identify appropriate goals, generate potential courses of action, and make reasoned comparative judgments by looking ahead and evaluating the potential future consequences. Social problem-solving ability can be assessed by using short stories that describe a problem and then ask for possible resolutions of the problem situation. The solutions produced by individuals with Asperger syndrome in this task were shorter and less detailed, as well as less effective, than those of controls without ASD (Goddard, Howlin, Dritschel, & Patel, 2007). Furthermore, adolescents with Asperger syndrome who attempted a novel problem-solving task (videotaped scenarios of awkward everyday situations) had more difficulties in retrieving and recounting pertinent facts and in selecting preferred and efficient solutions than typically developing adolescents did; these findings thus suggested impairment in social appropriateness (Channon, Charman, Heap, Crawford, & Rios, 2001).

Empathy is essential for the ability to socialize and interact adequately, and several reports have highlighted difficulties in empathy as part of the impairment in the social-emotional domain in autism. In one study, children with high-functioning autism performed less well than typically developing children on empathy measures; however, their performance was surprisingly better than expected (Yirmiya, Sigman, Kasari, & Mundy, 1992). Empathy was measured by using videotaped stories about children experiencing different events and emotions; children were asked about their own feelings after watching each story. In more recent research, the empathic ability of high-functioning adults with autism did not significantly differ from that of typically developing participants, as measured during a conversation with a typically developing stranger (Ponnet, Buysse, Roeyers, & De Corte, 2005). In this naturalistic task of dyadic interaction, assessments of empathy tapped both the partner's overt behavioral characteristics (i.e., verbalizations, gazes, positive affect, gestures, and interpersonal distance) and the partner's covert thoughts and feelings (i.e., self-reported unexpressed thoughts and affects). Both groups revealed similar levels of empathic accuracy in inferring the thoughts and feelings of the interaction partner.

Baron-Cohen and Wheelwright (2004) designed the Empathy Quotient (EQ), a 60-item self-report scale including such items as "It is hard for me to see why some things upset people so much" or "I find it easy to put myself in somebody else's shoes." These authors found that adults with Asperger syndrome or high-functioning autism scored significantly lower on the EQ than individuals with typical development matched for age and gender; in the typical development group, women scored significantly higher than men. Lawrence, Shaw, Baker, Baron-Cohen, and David (2004) reported on the EQ's psychometric properties. The EQ was inversely correlated with two domains of the AQ (Baron-Cohen et al., 2001): Social Sensitivity and Sensitive Communication, both of which require empathy. Furthermore, the EQ was positively correlated with the FQ (Baron-Cohen & Wheelwright, 2003), which assesses empathy in the context of close relationships, thus suggesting concurrent validity support for the instrument. Lawrence et al. (2004) indicated the need for future exploration of the EQ's sensitivity and specificity.

The suggestion that the social impairments in individuals with ASD result from an inability to know about the inner world of other people is one of the leading hypotheses regarding the core deficits of autism, termed difficulties in "theory of mind." In the next section, we briefly touch upon this topic.

THEORY OF MIND

One of the current hypotheses about the etiology of autism is that cognitive deficits in "theory of mind" (hereafter abbreviated as ToM) affect the understanding of the social world. ToM abilities refer to the awareness that human behaviors result from implicit mental states (i.e., thoughts, beliefs, memories, intents, and emotions), which are not always compatible with objective reality (Wellman, 1990). This awareness is required in social interactions as a guide to reciprocal behavior and all social interactions, from simple communication to more sophisticated behaviors such as deception, empathy, and humor. Many individuals with autism have difficulties in the ability to attribute mental states both to themselves and to others, as well as the ability to utilize these attributions in understanding and predicting behaviors. Indeed, difficulties in ToM are suggested to be core deficits in autism and may underlie the social and communicational impairments characteristic to the disorder.

ToM abilities are described as rich and complex mentalistic conceptions of people that begin to develop between the ages of 3 and 5 (Flavell, 2000; Gopnik, 1990), and thus require an aggregated operationalization. Task batteries and broader ranges of tasks are used to assess different components of ToM across different levels of complexity (Baron-Cohen, 2000; Hughes et al., 2000; Tager-Flusberg, 2001; Wellman, Cross, & Watson, 2001). The classic procedure for evaluating ToM abilities is the well-known, standard "false-belief task." A child is told a story about an object that is moved from its original location to a new location, without the knowledge of the main protagonist. Thus the child must understand that a person's mental state may contradict reality; that is, a person may hold a false belief. Research has supported the notion that ToM abilities, as operationalized by the false-belief task, are associated with levels of skill in social behavior (Astington & Jenkins, 1995; Lalonde & Chandler, 1995; Watson, Nixon, Wilson, & Capage, 1999). However, this task has shown a ceiling effect for children with a mental age of 6 years; thus some children with autism, especially those with high functioning, pass these tasks even though they manifest mentalization difficulties in everyday-life situations (Klin, 2000; Tager-Flusberg, 2001). Therefore, other tests and procedures must be employed for high-functioning individuals, to increase task sensitivity and detect more subtle difficulties in ToM abilities. For example, the Strange Stories test (Happé, 1994) is considered a more advanced ToM measure, in that it consists of everyday interpersonal situations where people say things they do not literally mean (e.g., ironic or sarcastic statements). At the end of each story, participants are asked a comprehension question and a justification question to test their understanding of the mental state described. Individuals with autism fail to provide context-appropriate mental state explanations for the story characters' nonliteral utterances (Happé, 1994; Happé et al., 1996; Jolliffe & Baron-Cohen, 1999; Vogeley et al., 2001).

Furthermore, individuals with Asperger syndrome or high-functioning autism have difficulties on measures requiring the integration of cross-modal information from faces, voices, and context to understand the mental states and complex emotions of others. For example, Golan and Baron-Cohen (2006) demonstrated that the performance of adults with Asperger syndrome or high-functioning autism was lower than that of adults with typical development on such measures as the Cambridge Mindreading Face–Voice Battery (Golan, Baron-Cohen, & Hill, 2006). This instrument uses short silent clips of adult actors expressing emotions facially, as well as voice recordings of short sentences expressing various emotional intonations, to measure complex emotion and mental state recognition via more naturalistic methods. In a meta-analysis of ToM abilities in individuals with ASD, Yirmiya, Erel, Shaked, and Solomonica-Levi (1998) concluded that deficits in ToM are not unique to such individuals, but that they are more severe than those experienced by individuals with diagnoses other than autism.

CONCLUSIONS

In this chapter, we have described the assessment of social difficulties in individuals with ASD. We have first presented the screening and diagnostic instruments that are used to assess social deficits as one of the three domains of behaviors constituting the core symptoms of ASD. Next, we have discussed relationships that individuals with autism have with significant others—their attachment to their mothers, and their relationships with their agemates. We would like to end this chapter by returning to the diathesis–stress model with which we opened the chapter, emphasizing both genetic vulnerability and environmental factors.

A dysfunction of mirror neurons, which may underlie the ability to imitate, has recently been proposed as the biological explanation or "cause" of the social and some other difficulties of individuals with autism. Meltzoff and Prinz (2002) have suggested that the ability to understand another person's feelings, intentions, and actions, which is crucial for relationships with others and for ToM, is associated with the ability to imitate, which develops during the very first weeks and months of life. Impairment in imitation ability is indeed one of the core symptoms included in the domain of communication in the DSM-IV-TR criteria for autistic disorder (American Psychiatric Association, 2000). Thus being able to imitate may be a key to our human understanding of what it means "for others to be like us and for us to be like others" (Meltzoff & Decety, p. 491, 2003). These authors have suggested that behavioral imitation is innate, that it precedes ToM in development and evolution, and that behavioral imitation and its neural substrate provide the mechanism by which ToM and empathy develop in humans. It is not surprising, therefore, that imitation skills have attracted attention in the search for underlying causes of the social difficulties that characterizes autism.

A major step forward in understanding the brain mechanisms subserving imitation has been the discovery of the mirror neuron system in the macaque monkey. Mirror neurons are a particular class of visual–motor neurons that discharge both when a monkey performs a particular action and when it observes another individual (monkey or human) performing a similar action (Di Pellegrino, Fadiga, Fogassi, Gallese, & Rizzolatti, 1992; Gallese, Fadiga, Fogassi, & Rizzolatti, 1996; Rizzolatti, Fadiga, Gallese, & Fogassi, 1996; for a review, see Rizzolatti & Craighero, 2004). Such neurons were originally discovered in area F5 of the monkey premotor cortex, and later in the areas around the intraparietal sulcus (Fogassi et al., 2005). Interestingly, the parietal mirror neurons discharge differently in response to identical motor actions when they are embedded in different action contexts, presumably enabling the observer to understand the intention of the agent. Although, relative to humans, monkeys are not very good imitators (Tomasello & Call, 1997; Iriki, 2006), these neurophysiological properties have led investigators to suggest a connection between the mirror neuron system and imitation, at least in monkeys (for a review, see Rizzolatti, Fogassi, & Gallese, 2001).

The neural circuits connecting regions populated by mirror neurons in monkeys are anatomically interconnected and also connected with the superior temporal sulcus, where higher-order visual neurons respond to seeing the action of others (Jellema, Baker, Wicker, & Perrett, 2000). These circuits seem optimal as precursors of neural mechanisms of imitation in humans as well (Iacoboni, 2005). Indeed, functional imaging studies of imitative behavior in humans have identified similar circuitry in the human brain (Iacoboni et al., 1999; Koski, Iacoboni, Dubeau, Woods, & Mazziotta, 2003). This circuitry comprises the human superior temporal sulcus and the human mirror neuron system—namely, the inferior frontal cortex, which seems particularly important for coding the goal of the imitated action (Koski et al., 2002), and the rostral part of the inferior parietal lobule (Chaminade, Meltzoff, & Decety, 2005; Decety, Chaminade, Grèzes, & Meltzoff, 2002).

Corroborating the association of this cortical network with imitative behavior and ToM, recent functional magnetic resonance imaging data have shown that during observation and imitation of facial expressions, children with ASD show less activity in mirror neuron areas (particularly the inferior frontal gyrus—pars opercularis), as well as in the limbic system, than typically developing children do (Dapretto et al., 2006). More-over, this reduction is correlated with the independently evaluated severity of ASD, which suggests that the malfunctioning of this circuit during a task involving social mirroring may indeed be part of the clinical picture of ASD.

In summary, as reviewed in this chapter, our knowledge of the social deficits characterizing ASD is quite impressive. In addition, we now have more and more screening and diagnostic measures that are applicable across many developmental stages, from infancy to adulthood. Moreover, we are beginning to understand the neural circuitry that may be impaired in indi-viduals with ASD. Based on these data, our next goal should be devising and empirically testing more intensive early intervention programs during the time that the brain shows a high degree of plasticity.

REFERENCES

Adrien, J. L., Lenoir, P., Martineau, J., Perrot, A., Hameury, L., Larmande, C., et al. (1993). Blind ratings of early symptoms of autism based upon family home movies. *Journal of the American Academy of Child and Adolescent Psychiatry, 32,* 617–626.

Adrien, J. L., Perrot, A., Hameury, L., Martineau, J., Roux, S., & Sauvage, D. (1991). Family home movies: Identification of early autistic signs in infants later diagnosed as autistics. *Brain Dysfunction, 4,* 355–362.

Ainsworth, M. D. S. (1979). Infant–mother attachment. *American Psychologist, 34,* 932–937.

Ainsworth, M. D. S., Blehar, M. C., Waters, E., & Wall, S. (1978). *Patterns of attachment.* Hillsdale, NJ: Erlbaum.

Allison, C., Williams, J., Scott, F., Stott, C., Bolton, P., Baron-Cohen, S., et al. (2007). The Childhood Asperger Syndrome Test (CAST): Test–retest reliabil-ity in a high scoring sample. *Autism, 11,* 173–185.

American Psychiatric Association. (1994). *Diagnostic and statistical manual of mental disorders* (4th ed.). Washington, DC: Author.

American Psychiatric Association. (2000). *Diagnostic and statistical manual of mental disorders* (4th ed., text rev.). Washington, DC: Author.

Astington, J., & Jenkins, J. (1995). Theory of mind development and social under-standing. *Cognition and Emotion, 9,* 151–165.

Austin, E. J. (2005). Personality correlates of the broader autism phenotype as assessed by the Autism Spectrum Quotient (AQ). *Personality and Individual Differences, 38,* 451–460.

Baird, G., Charman, T., Baron-Cohen, S., Cox, A., Swettenham, J., Wheelwright, S., et al. (2000). A screening instrument for autism at 18 months of age: A 6-year follow-up study. *Journal of the American Academy of Child and Ado-lescent Psychiatry, 39,* 694–702.

Baird, G., Simonoff, E., Pickles, A., Chandler, S., Loucas, T., Meldrum, D., et al. (2006). Prevalence of disorders of the autism spectrum in a population cohort of children in South Thames: The Special Needs and Autism Project (SNAP). *Lancet, 368,* 210–215.

Baranek, G. T. (1999). Autism during infancy: A retrospective video analysis of sensory–motor and social behaviors at 9–12 months of age. *Journal of Autism and Developmental Disorders, 29,* 213–224.

Baron-Cohen, S. (2000). Theory of mind and autism: A fifteen year review. In S. Baron-Cohen, H. Tager-Flusberg, & D. J. Cohen (Eds.), *Understanding other minds: Perspectives from developmental cognitive neuroscience* (pp. 3–20). Oxford: Oxford University Press.

Baron-Cohen, S., Allen, J., & Gillberg, C. (1992). Can autism be detected at 18 months?: The needle, the haystack, and the CHAT. *British Journal of Psychiatry, 161,* 839–843.

Baron-Cohen, S., Cox, A., Baird, G., Swettenham, J., Nightingale, N., Morgan, K., et al. (1996). Psychological markers in the detection of autism in infancy in a large population. *British Journal of Psychiatry, 168,* 158–163.

Baron-Cohen, S., & Wheelwright, S. (2003). The Friendship Questionnaire: An investigation of adults with Asperger syndrome or high-functioning autism, and normal sex differences. *Journal of Autism and Developmental Disorders, 33,* 509–517.

Baron-Cohen, S., & Wheelwright, S. (2004). The Empathy Quotient: An investigation of adults with Asperger syndrome or high-functioning autism, and normal sex differences. *Journal of Autism and Developmental Disorders, 34,* 163–175.

Baron-Cohen, S., Wheelwright, S., Skinner, R., Martin, J., & Clubley, E. (2001). The Autism-Spectrum Quotient (AQ): Evidence from Asperger syndrome/ high functioning autism, males and females, scientists and mathematicians. *Journal of Autism and Developmental Disorders, 31,* 5–17.

Barrera, M. E., & Maurer, D. (1981). Recognition of mother's photographed face by the three-month-old. *Child Development, 52,* 558–563.

Bauminger, N., & Kasari, C. (2000). Loneliness and friendship in high-functioning children with autism. *Child Development, 71,* 447–456.

Bauminger, N., Shulman, C., & Agam, G. (2003). Peer interaction and loneliness in high-functioning children with autism. *Journal of Autism and Developmental Disorders, 33,* 489–507.

Bauminger, N., Shulman, C., & Agam, G. (2004). The link between perceptions of self and of social relationships in high-functioning children with autism. *Journal of Autism and Developmental Disorders, 16,* 193–214.

Berument, S. K., Rutter, M., Lord, C., Pickles, A., & Bailey, A. (1999). Autism Screening Questionnaire: Diagnostic validity. *British Journal of Psychiatry, 175,* 444–451.

Bowlby, J. (1969). *Attachment and loss: Vol. 1. Attachment.* New York: Basic Books.

Bryson, S. E., McDermott, C., Rombough, V., Brian, J., & Zwaigenbaum, L. (2000). *The Autism Observation Scale for Infants.* Unpublished manuscript.

Bryson, S. E., Zwaigenbaum, L., McDermott, C., Rombough, V., & Brian, J. (2008). The Autism Observation Scale for Infants: Scale development and reliability data. *Journal of Autism and Developmental Disorders, 38,* 731–738.

Campbell, J. M. (2005). Diagnostic assessment of Asperger's disorder: A review of five third-party rating scales. *Journal of Autism and Developmental Disorders, 35,* 25–35.

Chaminade, T., Meltzoff, A. N., & Decety, J. (2005). An fMRI study of imitation: Action representation and body schema. *Neuropsychologia, 43,* 115–127.

Channon, S., Charman, T., Heap, J., Crawford, S., & Rios, P. (2001). Real-life-type problem-solving in Asperger's syndrome. *Journal of Autism and Developmental Disorders, 31,* 461–469.

Clifford, S. M., & Dissanayake, C. (2008). The early development of joint attention in infants with autistic disorder using home video observations and parental interview. *Journal of Autism and Developmental Disorders, 38,* 791–805.

Clifford, S., Young, R., & Williamson, P. (2007). Assessing the early characteristics of autistic disorder using video analysis. *Journal of Autism and Developmental Disorders, 37,* 301–313.

Constantino, J. N., Gruber, C. P., Davis, S., Hayes, S., Passanante, N., & Przybeck, T. (2004). The factor structure of autistic traits. *Journal of Child Psychology and Psychiatry, 45,* 719–726.

Constantino, J. N., Lajonchere, C., Lutz, M., Gray, T., Abbacchi, A., McKenna, K., et al. (2006). Autistic social impairment in the siblings of children with pervasive developmental disorders. *American Journal of Psychiatry, 163,* 294–296.

Constantino, J. N., & Todd, R. D. (2005). Intergenerational transmission of sub-threshold autistic traits in the general population. *Biological Psychiatry, 57,* 655–660.

Corsello, C., Hus, V., Pickles, A., Risi, S., Cook, E. H., Leventhal, B. L., et al. (2007). Between a ROC and a hard place: Decision making and making decisions about using the SCQ. *Journal of Child Psychology and Psychiatry, 48,* 932–940.

Cox, A., Klein, K., Charman, T., Baird, G., Baron-Cohen, S., Swettenham, J., et al. (1999). Autism spectrum disorders at 20 and 42 months of age: Stability of clinical and ADI-R diagnosis. *Journal of Child Psychology and Psychiatry, 40,* 719–732.

Dapretto, M., Davies, M. S., Pfeifer, J. H., Scott, A. A., Sigman, M., Bookheimer, S. Y., et al. (2006). Understanding emotions in others: Mirror neuron dysfunction in children with autism spectrum disorders. *Nature Neuroscience, 9,* 28–30.

Dawson, G., Estes, A., Munson, J., Schellenberg, G., Bernier, R., & Abbott, R. (2007). Quantitative assessment of autism symptom-related traits in probands and parents: Broader Phenotype Autism Symptom Scale. *Journal of Autism and Developmental Disorders, 37,* 523–536.

Decety, J., Chaminade, T., Grèzes, J., & Meltzoff, A. N. (2002). A PET exploration of the neural mechanisms involved in reciprocal imitation. *NeuroImage, 15,* 265–272.

Dietz, C., Swinkels, S., van Daalen, E., van Engeland, H., & Buitelaar, J. K. (2006). Screening for autistic spectrum disorders in children aged 14–15 months: II. Population screening with the Early Screening of Autistic Traits Questionnaire (ESAT): Design and general findings. *Journal of Autism and Developmental Disorders, 36,* 713–722.

Di Pellegrino, G., Fadiga, L., Fogassi, L., Gallese, V., & Rizzolatti, G. (1992). Understanding motor events: A neurophysiological study. *Experimental Brain Research, 91,* 176–180.

Dissanayake, C., & Crossley, S. A. (1996). Proximity and sociable behaviors in autism: Evidence for attachment. *Journal of Child Psychology and Psychiatry, 37,* 149–156.

Dissanayake, C., & Crossley, S. A. (1997). Autistic children's responses to separation and reunion with their mothers. *Journal of Autism and Developmental Disorders, 27,* 295–312.

Downs, A., & Smith, T. (2004). Emotional understanding, cooperation, and social behavior in high-functioning children with autism. *Journal of Autism and Developmental Disorders, 24,* 625–635.

Duvall, J. A., Lu, A., Cantor, R. M., Todd, R. D., Constantino, J. N., & Geschwind, D. H. (2007). A quantitative trait locus analysis of social responsiveness in multiplex autism families. *American Journal of Psychiatry, 164,* 656–662.

Dworzynski, K., Ronald, A., Hayiou-Thomas, M., Rijsdijk, F., Happé, F., Bolton, P. F., et al. (2007). Aetiological relationship between language performance and autistic-like traits in childhood: A twin study. *International Journal of Language and Communication Disorders, 42,* 273–392.

Eaves, L. C., Wingert, H., & Ho, H. H. (2006a). Screening for autism: Agreement with diagnosis. *Autism, 10,* 229–242.

Eaves, L. C., Wingert, H. D., Ho, H. H., & Mickelson, E. C. R. (2006b). Screening for autism spectrum disorders with the Social Communication Questionnaire. *Journal of Developmental and Behavioral Pediatrics, 27,* S95–S103.

Ehlers, S., Gillberg, C., & Wing, L. (1999). A screening questionnaire for Asperger syndrome and other high-functioning autism spectrum disorders in school age children. *Journal of Autism and Developmental Disorders, 29,* 129–141.

Ehlers, S., Nydén, A., Gillberg, C., Sandberg, A. D., Dahlgren, S., Hjelmquist, E., et al. (1997). Asperger syndrome, autism and attention disorders: A comparative study of the cognitive profiles of 120 children. *Journal of Child Psychology and Psychiatry, 38,* 207–217.

Feldman, R. (2007). Parent–infant synchrony and the construction of shared timing: Physiological precursors, developmental outcomes, and risk conditions. *Journal of Child Psychology and Psychiatry, 48,* 329–354.

Fine, S. E., Weissman, A., Gerdes, M., Pinto-Martin, J., Zackai, E. H., McDonald-McGinn, D. M., et al. (2005). Autism spectrum disorders and symptoms in children with molecularly confirmed 22q11.2 deletion syndrome. *Journal of Autism and Developmental Disorders, 35,* 461–470.

Flavell, J. H. (2000). Development of children's knowledge about the mental world. *International Journal of Behavioral Development, 24,* 15–23.

Fogassi, L., Ferrari, P. F., Gesierich, B., Rozzi, S., Chersi, F., & Rizzolatti, G. (2005). Parietal lobe: From action organization to intention understanding. *Science, 308,* 662–667.

Gallese, V., Fadiga, L., Fogassi, L., & Rizzolatti, G. (1996). Action recognition in the premotor cortex. *Brain, 119*, 593–609.

Goddard, L., Howlin, P., Dritschel, B., & Patel, T. (2007). Autobiographical memory and social problem-solving in Asperger syndrome. *Journal of Autism and Developmental Disorders, 37*, 291–300.

Golan, O., & Baron-Cohen, S. (2006). Systemizing empathy: Teaching adults with Asperger syndrome or high-functioning autism to recognize complex emotions using interactive multimedia. *Development and Psychopathology, 18*, 591–617.

Golan, O., Baron-Cohen, S., & Hill, J. (2006). The Cambridge Mindreading (CAM) Face–Voice Battery: Testing complex emotion recognition in adults with and without Asperger syndrome. *Journal of Autism and Developmental Disorders, 36*, 169–183.

Gopnik, A. (1990). Developing the idea of intentionality: Children's theories of mind. *Canadian Journal of Philosophy, 20*, 89–114.

Happé, F. (1994). Wechsler IQ profile and theory of mind in autism: A research note. *Journal of Child Psychology and Psychiatry, 35*, 1461–1471.

Happé, F., Ehlers, S., Fletcher, P., Frith, U., Johansson, M., Gillberg, C., et al. (1996). "Theory of mind" in the brain: Evidence from a PET scan study of Asperger syndrome. *NeuroReport, 8*, 197–201.

Hauck, M., Fein, D., Waterhouse, L., & Feinstein, C. (1995). Social initiations by autistic children to adults and other children. *Journal of Autism and Developmental Disorders, 25*, 579–595.

Howes, C. (1980). Peer play scale as an index of complexity of peer interaction. *Developmental Psychology, 16*, 371–372.

Hughes, C., Adlam, A., Happé, F., Jackson, J., Taylor, A., & Caspi, A. (2000). Good test–retest reliability for standard and advanced false-belief tasks across a wide range of abilities. *Journal of Child Psychology and Psychiatry, 41*, 483–490.

Iacoboni, M. (2005). Neural mechanisms of imitation. *Current Opinion in Neurobiology, 15*, 632–637.

Iacoboni, M., Woods, R. P., Brass, M., Bekkering, H., Mazziotta, J. C., & Rizzolatti, G. (1999). Cortical mechanisms of human imitation. *Science, 286*, 2526–2528.

Iriki, A. (2006). The neural origins and implications of imitation, mirror neurons and tool use. *Current Opinion in Neurobiology, 16*, 660–667.

Jellema, T., Baker, C. I., Wicker, B., & Perrett, D. I. (2000). Neural representation for the perception of the intentionality of actions. *Brain and Cognition, 44*, 280–302.

Jolliffe, T., & Baron-Cohen, S. (1999). The Strange Stories Test: A replication with high-functioning adults with autism or Asperger syndrome. *Journal of Autism and Developmental Disorders, 29*, 395–406.

Kanner, L. (1943). Autistic disturbances of affective contact. *Nervous Child, 2*, 217–250.

Kanner, L. (1949). Nosology and psychodynamics in early childhood autism. *Journal of Orthopsychiatry, 19*, 416–426.

Ketelaars, C., Horwitz, E., Sytema, S., Bos, J., Wiersma, D., Minderaa, R., et al. (2008). Brief report: Adults with mild autism spectrum disorders (ASD): Scores on the Autism Spectrum Quotient (AQ) and comorbid psychopathology. *Journal of Autism and Developmental Disorders, 38,* 176–180.

Kleinman, J. M., Robins, D. L., Ventola, P. E., Pandey, J., Boorstein, H. C., Esser, E. L., et al. (2008). The Modified Checklist for Autism in Toddlers: A follow-up study investigating the early detection of autism spectrum disorders. *Journal of Autism and Developmental Disorders, 38,* 827–839.

Klin, A. (2000). Attributing social meaning to ambiguous visual stimuli in higher-functioning autism and Asperger syndrome: The Social Attribution Task. *Journal of Child Psychology and Psychiatry, 41,* 831–846.

Klin, A., Saulnier, C. A., Sparrow, S. S., Cicchetti, D. V., Volkmar, F. R., & Lord, C. (2007). Social and communication abilities and disabilities in higher functioning individuals with autism spectrum disorders: The Vineland and the ADOS. *Journal of Autism and Developmental Disorders, 37,* 748–759.

Koski, L., Iacoboni, M., Dubeau, M. C., Woods, R. P., & Mazziotta, J. C. (2003). Modulation of cortical activity during different imitative behaviors. *Journal of Neurophysiology, 89,* 460–471.

Koski, L., Wohlschläger, A., Bekkering, H., Woods, R. P., Dubeau, M. C., Mazziotta, J. C., et al. (2002). Modulation of motor and premotor activity during imitation of target-directed actions. *Cerebral Cortex, 12,* 847–855.

Kurita, H., Koyama, T., & Osada, H. (2005). Autism-Spectrum Quotient—Japanese version and its short forms for screening normally intelligent persons with pervasive developmental disorders. *Psychiatry and Clinical Neurosciences, 59,* 490–496.

Lalonde, C., & Chandler, M. (1995). False belief understanding goes to school: On the social-emotional consequences of coming early or late to a first theory of mind. *Cognition and Emotion, 9,* 167–185.

Landa, R. J., Holman, K. C., & Garrett-Mayer, E. (2007). Social and communication development in toddlers with early and later diagnosis of autism spectrum disorders. *Archives of General Psychiatry, 64,* 853–864.

Lawrence, E. J., Shaw, P., Baker, D., Baron-Cohen, S., & David, A. S. (2004). Measuring empathy: Reliability and validity of the Empathy Quotient. *Psychological Medicine, 34,* 911–924.

Lee, L., David, A. B., Rusyniak, J., Landa, R., & Newschaffer, C. J. (2007). Performance of the Social Communication Questionnaire in children receiving preschool special education services. *Research in Autism Spectrum Disorders, 1,* 126–138.

Lord, C., Rutter, M., DiLavore, P. C., & Risi, S. (2002). *Autism Diagnostic Observation Schedule.* Los Angeles: Western Psychological Services.

Losche, G. (1990). Sensorimotor and action development in autistic children from infancy to early childhood. *Journal of Child Psychology and Psychiatry, 31,* 749–761.

Maestro, S., Muratori, F., Cavallaro, M. C, Pei, F., Stern, D. D., Glose, B., et al. (2002). Attentional skills during the first 6 months of age in autism spectrum disorder. *Journal of the American Academy of Child and Adolescent Psychiatry, 41,* 1239–1245.

Maestro, S., Muratori, F., Cavallaro, M. C., Pecini, C., Cesari, A., Paziente, A., Stern, D., Golse, D., & Palacio-Espasa, F. (2005) How young children treat objects and people: An empirical study of the first year of life in autism. *Child Psychiatry and Human Development, 35,* 383–396.

Main, M., & Solomon, J. (1990). Procedures for identifying infants as disorganized/disoriented during the Ainsworth Strange Situation. In M. T. Greenberg, D. Cicchetti, & E. M. Cummings (Eds.), *Attachment in the preschool years* (pp. 121–160). Chicago: University of Chicago Press.

Mayes, S. D., & Calhoun, S. L. (2003). Analysis of WISC-III, Stanford–Binet:IV, and academic achievement test scores in children with autism. *Journal of Autism and Developmental Disorders, 33,* 329–341.

Mayes, S. D., & Calhoun, S. L. (2004). Similarities and differences in Wechsler Intelligence Scale for Children—Third Edition (WISC-III) profiles: Support for subtest analysis in clinical referrals. *Clinical Neurophysiology, 18,* 559–572.

McDuffie, A., Yoder, P., & Stone, W. (2005). Prelinguistic predictors of vocabulary in children with autism spectrum disorders. *Journal of Speech, Language, and Hearing Research, 48,* 1080–1097.

Meltzoff, A. N., & Decety, J. (2003). What imitation tells us about social cognition: A rapprochement between developmental psychology and cognitive neuroscience. *Philosophical Transactions of the Royal Society of London, Series B, 358,* 491–500.

Meltzoff, A. N., & Moore, M. K. (1977). Imitation of facial and manual gestures by human neonates. *Science, 198,* 75–78.

Meltzoff, A. N., & Moore, M. K. (1999). Persons and representations: Why infant imitation is important for theories of human development. In J. Nadel & G. Butterworth (Eds.), *Imitation in infancy* (pp. 9–35). Cambridge, UK: Cambridge University Press.

Meltzoff, A. N., & Prinz, W. (2002). *The imitative mind: Development, evolution and brain bases.* Cambridge, UK: Cambridge University Press.

Mundy, P., & Gomes, A. (1998). Individual differences in joint attention skill development in the second year. *Infant Behavior and Development, 21,* 469–482.

Mundy, P., Hogan, A., & Doehring, P. (1996). *A preliminary manual for the abridged Early Social-Communication Scales.* Coral Gables, FL: University of Miami. Retrieved from *www.psy.miami.edu/faculty/pmundy.*

Mundy, P., Sigman, M., & Kasari, C. (1990). A longitudinal study of joint attention and language development in autistic children. *Journal of Autism and Developmental Disorders, 20,* 115–128.

Mundy, P., Sigman, M., Ungerer, J., & Sherman, T. (1986). Defining the social deficits of autism: The contribution of non-verbal communication measures. *Journal of Child Psychology and Psychiatry, 27,* 657–669.

Oppenheim, D., Koren-Karie, N., Dolev, S., & Yirmiya, N. (in press). Maternal insightfulness and resolution of the diagnosis are related to secure attachment in preschoolers with autism spectrum disorders. *Child Development.*

Osterling, J. A., & Dawson, G. (1994). Early recognition of children with autism: A study of first birthday home videotapes. *Journal of Autism and Developmental Disorders, 24,* 247–257.

Osterling, J. A., Dawson, G., & Munson, J. A. (2002). Early recognition of 1-year-old infants with autism spectrum disorder versus mental retardation. *Development and Psychopathology, 14*, 239–251.

Pascalis, O., de Schonen, S., Morton, J., Deruelle, C., & Fabre-Grenet, M. (1995). Mothers' face recognition by neonates: A replication and an extension. *Infant Behavior and Development, 18*, 79–86.

Pine, E., Luby, J., Abbacchi, A., & Constantino, J. N. (2006). Quantitative assessment of autistic symptomatology in preschoolers. *Autism, 10*, 344–352.

Ponnet, K., Buysse, A., Roeyers, H., & De Corte, K. (2005). Empathic accuracy in adults with a pervasive developmental disorder during an unstructured conversation with a typically developing stranger. *Journal of Autism and Developmental Disorders, 35*, 585–600.

Reiersen, A. M., Constantino, J. N., Volk, H. E., & Todd, R. D. (2007). Autistic traits in a population-based ADHD twin sample. *Journal of Child Psychology and Psychiatry, 48*, 464–472.

Reznick, J. S., Baranek, G. T., Reavis, S., Watson, L. R., & Crais, E. R. (2007). A parent-report instrument for identifying one-year-olds at risk for an eventual diagnosis of autism: The First Year Inventory. *Journal of Autism and Developmental Disorders, 37*, 1691–1710.

Rizzolatti, G., & Craighero, L. (2004). The mirror-neuron system. *Annual Review of Neuroscience, 27*, 169–192.

Rizzolatti, G., Fadiga, L., Gallese, V., & Fogassi, L. (1996). Premotor cortex and the recognition of motor actions. *Cognitive Brain Research, 3*, 131–141.

Rizzolatti, G., Fogassi, L., & Gallese, V. (2001). Neurophysiological mechanisms underlying the understanding and imitation of action. *Nature Reviews Neuroscience, 2*, 661–670.

Robins, D. L., & Dumont-Mathieu, T. M. (2006). Early screening for autism spectrum disorders: Update on the Modified Checklist for Autism in Toddlers and other measures. *Journal of Developmental and Behavioral Pediatrics, 27*, S111–S119.

Robins, D. L., Fein, D., Barton, M. L., & Green, J. A. (2001). The Modified Checklist for Autism in Toddlers: An initial study investigating the early detection of autism and pervasive developmental disorders. *Journal of Autism and Developmental Disorders, 31*, 131–144.

Rodrigue, J. R., Morgan, S. B., & Geffken, G. R. (1991). A comparative evaluation of adaptive behavior in children and adolescents with autism, Down syndrome, and normal development. *Journal of Autism and Developmental Disorders, 21*, 187–196.

Rogers, S. J., Ozonoff, S., & Maslin-Cole, C. (1991). A comparative study of attachment behavior in young children with autism and other psychiatric disorders. *Journal of the American Academy of Child and Adolescent Psychiatry, 30*, 483–488.

Rogers, S. J., Ozonoff, S., & Maslin-Cole, C. (1993). Developmental aspects of attachment behavior in young children with developmental disorders. *Journal of the American Academy of Child and Adolescent Psychiatry, 32*, 1274–1282.

Ronald, A., Happé, F., Bolton, P., Butcher, L. M., Price, T. S., Wheelwright, S., et al. (2006a). Genetic heterogeneity between the three components of the autism spectrum: A twin study. *Journal of the American Academy of Child and Adolescent Psychiatry, 45,* 691–699.

Ronald, A., Happé, F., Price, T. S., Baron-Cohen, S., & Plomin, R. (2006b). Phenotypic and genetic overlap between autistic traits at the extremes of the general population. *Journal of the American Academy of Child and Adolescent Psychiatry, 45,* 1206–1214.

Rutgers, A. H., Bakermans-Kranenburg, M. J., van IJzendoorn, M. H., & van Berckelaer-Onnes, I. A. (2004). Autism and attachment: A meta-analytic review. *Journal of Child Psychology and Psychiatry, 45,* 1123–1134.

Rutter, M., Bailey, A., & Lord, C. (2003a). *Social Communication Questionnaire.* Los Angeles: Western Psychological Services.

Rutter, M., Le Couteur, A., & Lord, C. (2003b). Autism Diagnostic Interview—Revised (ADI-R). Los Angeles: Western Psychological Services.

Saemundsen, E., Magnusson, P., Smari, J., & Sigurdardottir, S. (2003). Autism Diagnostic Interview—Revised and the Childhood Autism Rating Scale: Convergence and discrepancy in diagnosing autism. *Journal of Autism and Developmental Disorders, 33,* 319–328.

Sally, D., & Hill, E. (2006). The development of interpersonal strategy: Autism, theory-of-mind, cooperation and fairness. *Journal of Economic Psychology, 27,* 73–97.

Sameroff, A. (2000). Developmental systems and psychopathology. In A. Sameroff, M. Lewis, & S. Miller (Eds.), *Handbook of developmental psychopathology* (2nd ed., pp. 23–40). New York: Kluwer Academic/Plenum.

Scheeren, A. M., & Stauder, J. E. A. (2008). Broader autism phenotype in parents of autistic children: Reality or myth? *Journal of Autism and Developmental Disorders, 38,* 276–287.

Schopler, E., Reichler, R. J., DeVellis, R. F., & Daly, K. (1980). Toward objective classification of childhood autism: Childhood Autism Rating Scale (CARS). *Journal of Autism and Developmental Disorders, 10,* 91–103.

Scott, F., Baron-Cohen, S., Bolton, P., & Brayne, C. (2002). The CAST (Childhood Asperger Syndrome Test): Preliminary development of a UK screen for mainstream primary-school age children. *Autism, 6,* 9–31.

Seibert, J. M., Hogan, A. E., & Mundy, P. C. (1982). Assessing interactional competencies: The Early Social-Communication Scales. *Infant Mental Health Journal, 3,* 244–245.

Seligman, M. E. P. (1970). On the generality of the laws of learning. *Psychological Review, 77,* 406–418.

Shapiro, T., Sherman, M., Calamari, G., & Koch, D. (1987). Attachment in autism and other developmental disorders. *Journal of the American Academy of Child and Adolescent Psychiatry, 26,* 480–484.

Siegel, D. J., Minshew, N. J., & Goldstein, G. (1996). Wechsler IQ profiles in diagnosing high-functioning autism. *Journal of Autism and Developmental Disorders, 26,* 389–406.

Sigman, M., & Mundy, P. (1989). Social attachment in autistic children. *Journal of the American Academy of Child and Adolescent Psychiatry, 28,* 74–81.

Sigman, M., & Ruskin, E. (1999). Continuity and change in the social competence of children with autism, Down syndrome, and developmental delays. *Monographs of the Society for Research in Child Development, 64*(1, Serial No. 256).

Sigman, M., & Ungerer, J. A. (1984). Attachment behaviors in autistic children. *Journal of Autism and Developmental Disorders, 14*, 231–244.

Sparrow, S. S., Cicchetti, D. V., & Balla, D. A. (2005). *Vineland Adaptive Behavior Scales, Second Edition (Vineland-II)*. Circle Pines, MN: American Guidance Service.

Stone, W. L., & Caro-Martinez, L. (1990). Naturalistic observations of spontaneous communication in autistic children. *Journal of Autism and Developmental Disorders, 20*, 437–453.

Stone, W. L., Coonrod, E. E., Turner, L. M., & Pozdol, S. L. (2004). Psychometric properties of the STAT for early autism screening. *Journal of Autism and Developmental Disorders, 34*, 691–701.

Stone, W. L., & Ousley, O. Y. (1997). *STAT manual: Screening Tool for Autism in Two-Year-Olds*. Unpublished manuscript, Vanderbilt University.

Swinkels, S., Dietz, C., van Daalen, E., Kerkhof, I. H. G. M., van Engeland, H., & Buitelaar, J. K. (2006). Screening for autistic spectrum disorders in children aged 14 to 15 months: I. The development of the Early Screening of Autistic Traits Questionnaire (ESAT). *Journal of Autism and Developmental Disorders, 36*, 723–732.

Tager-Flusberg, H. (2001). A reexamination of the theory of mind hypothesis of autism. In J. A. Burack, T. Charman, N. Yirmiya, & P. R. Zelazo (Eds.), *The development of autism: Perspectives from theory and research* (pp. 173–193). Mahwah, NJ: Erlbaum.

Tomanik, S. S., Pearson, D. A., Loveland, K. A., Lane, D. M., & Shaw, J. B. (2007). Improving the reliability of autism diagnoses: Examining the utility of adaptive behavior. *Journal of Autism and Developmental Disorders, 37*, 921–928.

Tomasello, M., & Call, J. (1997). *Primate cognition*. Oxford: Oxford University Press.

Travis, L. L., & Sigman, M. (1998). Social deficits and interpersonal relationships in autism. *Mental Retardation and Developmental Disabilities, 4*, 65–72.

van IJzendoorn, M. H., Rutgers, A. H., Bakermans-Kranenburg, M. J., Swinkels, S. H. N., van Daalen, E., Dietz, C., et al. (2007). Parental sensitivity and attachment in children with autism spectrum disorder: Comparison with children with mental retardation, with language delays, and with typical development. *Child Development, 78*, 597–608.

Ventola, P. E., Kleinman, J., Pandey, J., Barton, M., Allen, S., Green, J., et al. (2006). Agreement among four diagnostic instruments for autism spectrum disorders in toddlers. *Journal of Autism and Developmental Disorders, 36*, 839–847.

Vogeley, K., Bussfeld, P., Newen, A., Herrmann, S., Happé, F., Falkai, P., et al. (2001). Mind reading: Neural mechanisms of theory of mind and self-perspective. *NeuroImage, 14*, 170–181.

Volkmar, E. R., Sparrow, S. S., Gourgreau, D., Cicchetti, D. V, Paul, R., & Cohen, D. J. (1987). Social deficits in autism: An operational approach using the

Vineland Adaptive Behavior Scales. *Journal of the American Academy of Child and Adolescent Psychiatry, 26,* 156–161.

Wakabayashi, A., Baron-Cohen, S., Wheelwright, S., & Tojo, Y. (2006). The Autism-Spectrum Quotient (AQ) in Japan: A cross-cultural comparison. *Journal of Autism and Developmental Disorders, 36,* 263–270.

Watson, A. C., Nixon, C. L., Wilson, A., & Capage, L. (1999). Social interaction skills and the theory of mind in young children. *Developmental Psychology, 35,* 386–391.

Watson, L. R., Baranek, G. T., Crais, E. R., Reznick, J. S., Dykstra, J., & Perryman, T. (2007). The First Year Inventory: Retrospective parent responses to a questionnaire designed to identify one-year-olds at risk for autism. *Journal of Autism and Developmental Disorders, 37,* 49–61.

Wechsler, D. (1991). *Wechsler Intelligence Scale for Children—Third Edition (WISC-III).* San Antonio, TX: Psychological Corporation.

Weinfield, N.S., Sroufe, L.A., Egeland, B., & Carlson, E. (1999). The nature of individual differences in infant–caregiver attachment. In J. Cassidy & P. R. Shaver (Eds.), *Handbook of attachment: Theory, research, and clinical applications* (pp. 64–88). New York: Guilford Press.

Wellman, H. (1990). *The child's theory of mind.* Cambridge, MA: MIT Press.

Wellman, H., Cross, D., & Watson, J. (2001). Meta-analysis of theory-of-mind development: The truth about false belief. *Child Development, 72,* 655–684.

Werner, E., Dawson, G., Osterling, J., & Dinno, N. (2000). Brief report: Recognition of autism spectrum disorder before one year of age: A retrospective study based on home videotapes. *Journal of Autism and Developmental Disorders, 30,* 157–162.

Wetherby, A. M., Allen, L., Cleary, J., Kublin, K., & Goldstein, H. (2002). Validity and reliability of the Communication and Symbolic Behavior Scales Developmental Profile with very young children. *Journal of Speech, Language, and Hearing Research, 45,* 1202–1218.

Wetherby, A. M., Goldstein, H., Cleary, J., Allen, L., & Kublin, K. (2003). Early identification of children with communication disorders: Concurrent and predictive validity of the CSBS developmental profile. *Infants and Young Children, 16,* 161–174.

Wetherby, A. M., & Prizant, B. (1993). *Communication and Symbolic Behavior Scales—normed edition.* Baltimore: Brookes.

Wetherby, A. M., & Prizant, B. (2002). *Communication and Symbolic Behavior Scales Developmental Profile—first normed edition.* Baltimore: Brookes.

Wetherby, A. M., Watt, N., Morgan, L., & Shumway, S. (2007). Social communication profiles of children with autism spectrum disorders late in the second year of life. *Journal of Autism and Developmental Disorders, 37,* 960–975.

Wetherby, A. M., Woods, J., Allen, L., Cleary, J., Dickinson, H., & Lord, C. (2004). Early indicators of autism spectrum disorders in the second year of life. *Journal of Autism and Developmental Disorders, 34,* 473–493.

Williams, J., Allison, C., Scott, F., Stott, C., Bolton, P., Baron-Cohen, S., et al. (2006). The Childhood Asperger Syndrome Test (CAST): Test–retest reliability. *Autism, 10,* 415–427.

Williams, J., Scott, F., Stott, C., Allison, C., Bolton, P., Baron-Cohen, S., et al. (2005). The CAST (Childhood Asperger Syndrome Test): Test accuracy. *Autism, 9*, 45–68.

Woodbury-Smith, M. R., Robinson, J., Wheelwright, S., & Baron-Cohen, S. (2005). Screening adults for Asperger syndrome using the AQ: A preliminary study of its diagnostic validity in clinical practice. *Journal of Autism and Developmental Disorders, 35,* 331–335.

World Health Organization. (1992). *ICD-10 classification of mental and behavioral disorders: Clinical descriptions and diagnostic guidelines.* Geneva: Author.

Yirmiya, N., Erel, O., Shaked, M., & Solomonica-Levi, D. (1998). Meta-analyses comparing theory of mind abilities of individuals with autism, individuals with mental retardation, and normally developing individuals. *Psychological Bulletin, 124,* 283–307.

Yirmiya, N., & Ozonoff, S. (2007). The very early autism phenotype. *Journal of Autism and Developmental Disorders, 37,* 1–11.

Yirmiya, N., & Sigman, M. D. (2001). Attachment in autism. In J. Richter & S. Coates (Eds.), *Autism: Putting together the pieces* (pp. 53–63). London: Jessica Kingsley.

Yirmiya, N., Sigman, M. D., Kasari, C., & Mundy, P. (1992). Empathy and cognition in high-functioning children with autism. *Child Development, 63,* 150–160.

Zwaigenbaum, L., Bryson, S., Rogers, T., Roberts, W., Brian, J., & Szatmari, P. (2005). Behavioral manifestations of autism in the first year of life. *International Journal of Developmental Neuroscience, 23,* 143–152.

CHAPTER SEVEN

Assessing Speech, Language, and Communication in Autism Spectrum Disorders

Rhea Paul

Kaitlyn P. Wilson

In his initial descriptions of autism, Kanner (1943, 1946) highlighted atypical patterns of communication. Since then, autism and related disorders have been characterized as a spectrum of conditions; however, abnormal communication development remains central to the diagnostic criteria for these autism spectrum disorders (ASD). Whether verbal or nonverbal, communication deficits are a core symptom of ASD. Some people with ASD may begin talking at a later age than is typical, or they may remain nonverbal for life; others may gain minimally productive verbal skills, learning to produce words and sentences, but having difficulty using them effectively. This chapter explores how communication and its components (i.e., speech, language, pragmatics) are assessed for the dual purpose of establishing an ASD diagnosis and determining appropriate communication intervention goals for children with ASD. Before we begin this discussion, however, a group of key terms associated with this domain of functioning must be defined. These terms, and their relationships, are depicted graphically in Figure 7.1.

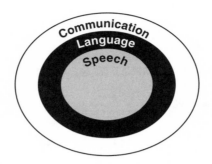

FIGURE 7.1. Domains of Communication.

"Communication" is an overarching term that refers to all forms of sending and receiving messages, whether through use of spoken language, gestures, body language, written language, or sign language. "Language" represents a specific type of communication involving the formulation of ideas and messages through rule-based combinations of words. "Speech" is the expression of language through the use of sounds produced by oral gestures. It is important to remember that other modes besides speech are used to express language-based ideas, such as writing or sign language. In the following discussion of communication and its assessment in children with ASD, these distinctions will be important to consider, as assessments of communication, of language, and of speech are distinct processes. In fact, ASD provide a useful model for understanding the difference between communication and language, as individuals with ASD may attain language skills, but be unable to use language for the purpose of communicating (Frith & Happe, 1994).

ASSESSING PRELINGUISTIC COMMUNICATION SKILLS

In the first years of life, children may show early signs of the communication deficits characteristic of ASD; however, ASD diagnoses are generally not made until the ages of 2–4 years (Chawarska, Klin, Paul, & Volkmar, 2007; Woods & Wetherby, 2003). Thus the assessment of communication skills in the first few years of life is based on the atypical development or presence of behaviors found in retrospective studies to be associated with a confirmed diagnosis of ASD later in early childhood (Klin et al., 1992; Volkmar, Stier, & Cohen, 1985; Baranek, 1999; Maestro et al., 2002; Osterling, Dawson,

& Munson, 2002); few studies have relied on direct observations (e.g., Charman et al., 2003; Lord & Risi, 2000; Wetherby et al., 2004). Research has suggested that atypical development of certain early communication skills is highly correlated with ASD risk. These include deficits in attention to people, social smiling, and sharing of affect, as well as in preverbal forms of social communication, including use of gaze and gestures for sharing attention to objects (joint attention) (e.g., Baron-Cohen et al., 1996; Charman et al., 1997; Lord, 1995; Mundy, Sigman, Ungerer, & Sherman, 1987; Swettenham et al., 1998; Wetherby et al., 2004). Communication impairments include limited responsiveness to speech, delayed development of language, and the use of others' bodies as tools (Lord, 1995; Wetherby et al., 2004). In one such study, Baron-Cohen et al. (1996) linked the absence of three key early communication skills (i.e., protodeclarative pointing, gaze monitoring, and pretend play) to a reliable risk of ASD at 18 months of age.

Assessing early communication skills can be difficult, as it requires analysis of many subtle behaviors and careful observation of the presence and nature (e.g., flexibility, appropriateness) of various aspects of communication. The communicative aspects assessed are typically considered within the following categories: the *frequency* of communicative attempts, the *functions* of these attempts, the *means* used to accomplish communicative goals, and the level of *responsiveness* to others' communicative attempts. These communicative aspects are discussed below, and within each discussion, the following considerations are outlined: signs of typical communication development, signs of possible ASD, and assessment methods.

Frequency of Communication

According to developmental benchmarks, typically developing children initiate communication at a rate of 2 acts/minute at 12 months, and 7 acts/minute at 24 months (Chapman, 2000). As these data illustrate, the second year of life is typically accompanied by a large increase in the number of communicative acts, whether preverbal gestures, vocalizations, or words. In children with ASD, a depressed rate of preverbal communicative acts (Wetherby, Prizant, & Hutchinson, 1998) is exhibited during this early developmental period. In addition, children with ASD often fail to engage others in communication surrounding interests or enjoyment, which results in a lower frequency of communicative attempts than that of typically developing children.

Assessing the frequency of communication involves recording the number of intentional communicative acts made by a child within a certain time period or communicative context. For example, if a child and caregiver are engaged in a caregiving routine (e.g., dressing, bathing, feeding) for a specified amount of time (generally 10–15 minutes for the purpose of assessment), the number of intentional communicative acts initiated by the child is recorded by an observer. During this observation, the observer should count only those acts initiated by the child, and only those that meet the criteria for intentional communication. That is, they must:

Consist of a gesture, vocalization, or verbal production.

Be directed toward another person, with gaze, touch, gesture, or movement toward the person.

Be interpretable as conveying a message or communicative function, such as a request, protest, or direction of attention of a person to create joint attention or engage in social interaction.

Several measures have been developed that provide specific opportunities, or temptations, for a child to communicate. For example, the Communication and Symbolic Behavior Scales (CSBS; Wetherby & Prizant, 2002) tempts the child to communicate a request for help (e.g., gesture, vocalization, gaze) when he or she is unable to open a container with a desired object inside. The number of times the child responds to such communicative opportunities is then observed and recorded. Additional examples of scales that make use of this format include the Early Social Communication Scales (ESCS; Mundy, Hogan, & Doehring, 1996) and the Prelinguistic Communication Assessment (PCA; Stone, Ousley, Yoder, Hogan, & Hebpurn, 1997).

Functions of Communication

Both "protoimperative" (acts intended to regulate others' actions) and "protodeclarative" (acts intended to create social interaction or joint attention) communicative functions are seen in typical children by 18 months of age. Bruner (1977) groups these intentions into three general functions:

1. *Regulatory*: Requests and protests.
2. *Comments*: Calling attention to objects and activities of interest, for the purpose of creating joint attention.
3. *Social interaction*: Showing off, calling attention to oneself, or seeking comfort or attention from others.

In children ages 18–24 months, more advanced communicative functions typically emerge, and an understanding of conversational structure becomes apparent. During this stage, typically developing children begin to attend more to others' speech and to acknowledge the back-and-forth nature of discourse. As such, the communicative functions acquired at this time are what Chapman (1981, 2000) called "discourse functions." These discourse functions include the following:

1. *Requests for information*: Using language to gain information about the world. At the earliest stages, this function may consist of requests for the names of things (i.e., labels: "Whazzat?"). At a later stage, these requests may begin to include "wh-" words, rising intonation contours, or both.
2. *Acknowledgments*: Confirming that the previous utterance was received, through such behaviors as verbal imitation, nonverbal mimicking of intonation pattern, or head nods.
3. *Answers*: Responding to another person's request for information with a semantically appropriate remark.

Compared to typically developing children, children with ASD exhibit a limited range of communicative behaviors. Children with ASD primarily use regulatory functions (i.e., requests or protests), with limited use of communication for the purposes of social interaction, commenting, or establishing joint attention (Mundy & Stella, 2000). This finding reflects Woods and Wetherby's (2003) similar conclusion that most children with ASD have early deficits in the use of joint attention.

The methods suggested for assessing the frequency of communicative acts may be applied similarly to the assessment of communicative functions. The purpose of assessing communicative functions is to determine the range of such functions being utilized by the child. This can be accomplished through observation of the child in various communicative contexts, whether caregiving activities or play situations. Data can be recorded by marking the frequency of each of the functions listed above, or by using one of the communication scales cited earlier.

Means of Communication

Early means of communication include gaze, "babbling" (i.e., speech-like vocalizations), and conventional gestures (such as pointing, showing, and waving). Infants generally begin using gestures such as pointing between the ages of 6 and 10 months (Zinober & Martlew, 1985). Use of babbling and "protowords" (i.e., consistent patterns of vocalization used to express meaning) are also expected before the onset of speech.

Research suggests that children with ASD use nonconventional communicative means as infants and toddlers. Instead of using a conventional gesture, such as pointing, to show or ask for an object, a child with an ASD may attempt to achieve the same communicative purpose through use of nonconventional gestures (Dawson, Meltzoff, Osterling, Rinaldi, & Brown, 1998; Stone et al., 1997). An example of this nonconventional means is a child who wants a pacifier and, instead of pointing to request the object, pulls the caregiver's hand to the pacifier. Children with ASD have been found to use atypical preverbal vocalizations as well (Sheinkopf, Mundy, Kimbrough-Oller, & Steffens, 2000).

Assessing a child's means of expressing communicative intent can be accomplished during structured observation of caregiver–child play, and can be evaluated concurrently with communicative frequency and function. Paul (2005, 2007) has provided a framework for structuring and compiling the observational data derived from this context (see Figure 7.2). This framework requires a record of each communicative act within the cell defined by its function and means. The frequency and range of both functions and means can be determined via this method when these data are compared to the frequency of communicative acts recorded. Measures such as the CSBS, ESCS, and PCA provide additional means for recording this type of observation, when structured communicative temptations are offered.

Responsiveness to Communication

By 12 months of age, typically developing children respond to their names by looking toward the speaker. By this time, children also have a receptive vocabulary of about 50 words (Chapman, 2000), and soon after, they produce their first word or approximation.

Nadig et al. (2007) found that a lack of response to hearing one's name is not necessarily universal among infants who are later diagnosed with ASD, but they suggest that a reduced response to name could be a characteristic of the broader autism phenotype during infancy. Osterling and Dawson (1994) agree that infants and toddlers with ASD exhibit reduced responsiveness to their names and to speech in general. Parents of children with this reduced responsiveness may suspect deafness at first; therefore, a hearing evaluation is often the first step to an ASD diagnosis in young children.

Responsiveness can be assessed by observing a caregiver–child play session, by using the communicative temptations listed below (see "Obtaining a Communication Profile"), or by using the CSBS or ESCS. During these structured opportunities, the observer will count the number of times the child shows a reaction to communications directed to him or her. This method results in a record of the child's response to gestural and verbal bids for attention and interaction.

	Request	Protest	Sharing enjoyment	Comment/ joint attention	Initiating social interaction	Responding to gesture	Responding to name	Responding to speech
				Function of communication				
Gaze to person								
Three-point gaze*								
Conventional gesture								
Unconventional gesture								
Typical vocalization								
Unusual vocalization								
Echo								
Spontaneous speech								

*Child looks at object, at person, then back at object; or at person, at object, then back at person.

FIGURE 7.2. Summary of communication assessment for prelinguistic children. (Adapted from Paul (2007). Copyright 2007 by C. V. Mosby, a division of Elsevier. Adapted by permission.

177

Spoken Language Assessment in Children with ASD

In 2001, the National Research Council reported that about 50% of children diagnosed with ASD would acquire functional speech. In 2005, Tager-Flusberg, Paul, and Lord estimated that more than 60% of children with ASD possessed spoken language. As an emphasis on early communication intervention continues for children diagnosed with ASD, the percentage of these children who will acquire speech is expected to increase as well. In general, when children with ASD acquire spoken language, they do so by the age of 6 (Paul & Cohen, 1984; Tager-Flusberg et al., 2005), although there have been reported cases of nonverbal children acquiring language during adolescence (Mirenda, 2003; Windsor, Doyle, & Siegel, 1994). Children with ASD tend to show more severe receptive language difficulties than do children with other language disorders (Paul, Chawarska, Klin, & Volkmar, 2007). These deficits are more difficult to target in an assessment than are expressive language deficits. A sampling of instruments that can be used at this level appears in Table 7.1.

Children with ASD generally acquire expressive language, or begin to use words as the primary form of communication, between 2 and 6 years of age. Below, we discuss communication assessment from this early stage of language use to the point at which a child produces more or less complete sentences. It is always important to remember that great variety exists in the language development of children with ASD. Some children may show delays in language development and be chronologically older than the typically expected age during this period of development. Others may show patterns of language acquisition similar to those seen in children with specific language disorders who are not on the autism spectrum (Tager-Flusberg & Joseph, 2003). Finally, some children with ASD may show normal or even precocious development of the forms of language (Landa, 2000; Tager-Flusberg et al., 2005); their deficits may be restricted to the pragmatic uses of communication.

Obtaining a Communication Profile

Following the identification of the presence or absence of basic language deficits through use of standardized tools, assessment efforts should focus on detailing a child's communication profile. The primary means for establishing a communication profile is collecting a sample of spontaneous speech during an interaction with the child. This interaction may consist of various play scenarios, a caregiving routine, or a shared book-reading activity. During these activities, language samples can be recorded on vid-

TABLE 7.1. Standardized Instruments for Assessing Early Language Development

Instrument	Areas assessed
Clinical Evaluation of Language Fundamentals—Preschool (Wiig, Semel, & Secord, 2004)	Concepts, syntax, semantics, morphology
Peabody Picture Vocabulary Test—Fourth Edition (Dunn & Dunn, 2007)	Receptive vocabulary/expressive vocabulary
MacArthur–Bates Communicative Development Inventories (3rd ed.) (Fenson et al., 2007)	Parent checklist that assesses receptive and expressive vocabulary, as well as use of play and gestures; later level assesses expressive vocabulary and early syntax
Preschool Language Scale—Fourth Edition (Zimmerman et al., 2002)	Receptive/expressive syntax, semantics, morphology
Reynell Developmental Language Scales–III (Edwards et al., 1999)	Receptive language/expressive language
Sequenced Inventory of Communicative Development—Revised (Hedrick et al., 1984)	Receptive language/expressive language
Test of Early Language Development (Hresko et al., 1999)	Receptive/expressive semantics and syntax
Test of Language Development—Primary: Third Edition (Newcomer & Hammill, 1997)	Receptive and expressive semantics and syntax
Vineland Adaptive Behavior Scales, Second Edition (Sparrow et al., 2005)	Receptive/expressive/written language

eotape or audiotape for later transcription and analysis. Increasingly, family members are being included in these processes, as they are asked to complete observation checklists, describe daily routines, interpret their child's actions, and/or validate assessment results (Crais, 1996).

As discussed above, young children with ASD often have a reduced frequency of communicative attempts; therefore, elicitation procedures may be necessary to gain an accurate picture of their communicative abilities. Communication elicitation generally involves tempting a child to communicate by setting up situations that produce desire for more or less of an action or object. Additional elicitation methods may strive to evoke confusion, surprise, or even disgust in the child. Here are some specific examples of temptations that can be used to elicit communication:

Keeping toys to oneself, so the child needs to request them.
Eating a snack without offering any to the child, to elicit requests.

Offering the child the chance to pull objects out of opaque containers, to elicit comments.

Engaging in a routine (such as rolling a ball back and forth), and then suddenly switching to another (such as pushing a truck).

Engaging in social routines, such as tickle games or finger plays, and interrupting the routine to get the child to request its continuation.

Offering the child an object or activity he or she does not like, to elicit a protest.

Offering parts of toys or puzzles, but withholding some, so the child needs to request them.

Pretending to misunderstand or not to hear a request or comment made by the child, in order to elicit a conversational repair.

Suddenly doing something silly or unexpected, such as putting on a funny hat or "Groucho" glasses, to elicit a comment.

Assessment of Language Forms and Meanings

Certain communicative patterns are typical of children with ASD, whether they involve restricted use of typical communicative behaviors or overuse of atypical behaviors. The kinds of communicative behaviors that can be observed and recorded in children with ASD, and methods of analysis for each behavior, are outlined below.

1a. *Responsiveness*: Compared to typically developing children, children with ASD do not respond as consistently to hearing their names called, and may show minimal understanding of the conversational responsibility to respond when spoken to.

1b. *Analysis methods*: The number of times a child responds to his or her name can be examined as a proportion of the number of times the name was called. Likewise, the number of adult utterances to which the child responds with speech or meaningful gestures can be compared to the total number of adult utterances offered.

2a. *Echolalia*: This behavior is common in children with ASD in the early stages of spoken language acquisition. It includes immediate or delayed imitation of what is heard, or the repetition of strings of memorized language (i.e., scripts).

2b. *Analysis methods*: The proportion of echoed to spontaneous utterances can be analyzed. Echoed utterances can be further separated into immediate and delayed echolalia. The function of the echoed language should be recorded, in order to design intervention to replace the echoed language with more conventional means of communication to achieve the given functions.

3a. *Pronoun use*: Children with ASD often use the pronoun "you" in place of "I" or "me" when referring to themselves. This is thought to reflect their tendency to echo what they hear others say. For example, when a caregiver asks a child with an ASD, "Are you hungry?", the child may respond with the phrase, "You hungry."

3b. *Analysis methods*: The number of inappropriate uses of pronouns in a speech sample can be calculated as a proportion of total pronoun use in the sample.

4a. *Vocabulary and syntax*: Children with ASD sometimes attach unusual or peculiar meanings to words or phrases. For example, a child with an ASD may say, "Go on red riding," to mean "I want to go in the wagon." However, whereas association of semantic meaning to words is a relative deficit, syntax is generally a relative strength in children with ASD. Therefore, syntactic level, often determined by mean length of utterance (MLU), can be a baseline measure against which other areas of language skill may be measured.

4b. *Analysis methods*: Vocabulary diversity can be analyzed simply by recording the number of different words in the speech sample, or more formally by calculating the "type–token" ratio (i.e. number of different words divided by total number of words spoken). Language analysis programs such as Miller and Chapman's (2000) Systematic Analysis of Language Transcripts (SALT) automatically compute both vocabulary and MLU measures from transcripts entered into their data systems. These values can be compared to those in the SALT's database of transcripts from typically developing children between the ages of 3 and 13 years. In addition, any idiosyncratic word use observed in children with ASD may be noted.

Assessing Pragmatics in Spoken Language

"Pragmatic" skills involve the *use* of language to communicate, as opposed to the content or form of language. Children with ASD may have above-average skills in language form (i.e., sound production, grammar) and/or content (i.e., vocabulary, semantic relations); yet they may struggle with pragmatic skills such as taking turns, offering greetings, and maintaining or changing a conversational topic. Pragmatic language deficits are readily apparent to others and are potentially stigmatizing to children with ASD. By understanding the domains of pragmatic language, clinicians, parents, and therapists of children with ASD can focus on goals that reflect the skills necessary for successful interaction with the social world. Chapman (1981) and Grice (1975) have outlined the domains of pragmatic language; these are described, along with corresponding assessment methods, below. Table 7.2 also lists some coding schemes for assessing pragmatics in conversation.

TABLE 7.2. Coding Schemes for Assessing Pragmatics in Conversation

Instrument	Description
Responsiveness/Assertiveness Rating Scale (Girolametto, 1997)	Parent rating, using a 5-point scale (never to always) to answer 25 questions about child's behaviors in conversation
Pragmatic Protocol (Prutting & Kirchner, 1983)	Checklist based on direct observation; global ratings of conversational skills in eight areas
Discourse Skills Checklist (Bedrosian, 1985)	Frequency analysis of 40 discourse behaviors
Functional Communication Scales—Revised (Kleiman, 2003)	Qualitative rating of 16 social uses of language

1a. *Communicative functions*: The intended purposes for which communication is used.

1b. *Assessment*: Through observation, parent checklist, or a structured play method, the range of functions expressed can be noted. The functions seen in typically-developing children between ages 5 and 7, as described by Tough (1977), appear in Figure 7.3. This form can be used as a recording device to assess the range of communicative functions expressed in free or structured play interactions between a child with an ASD and an adult or peer.

2a. *Discourse management*: The organization of turns and topics in conversation.

2b. *Assessment*: During observations of interactions with a variety of conversational partners (e.g. peers, adults, familiar, unfamiliar), a clinician may focus on and record the child's ability to:

- Take a conversational turn at the appropriate time.
- Give partners speaking turns at the appropriate time.
- Reduce perseveration on preferred topics.
- Switch topics when cues (e.g., facial expressions, body language) are offered.
- Use appropriate transition phrases or cues (e.g., "On another topic," "I was also thinking") when initiating topic change.
- Initiate and maintain conversation on topics of interest to conversational partners.

3a. *Register variation*: Flexible use of language forms in accordance with the specific context of an interaction.

Functions	Example from TD	Expressed by client: Frequency	Expressed by client: Example
Directing others	"You go there."		
Self-directing	"I'm gonna hide the ball."		
Reporting on past and ongoing events	"We played on the swings."		
Reasoning	"The gerbil ran away 'cause we forgot to lock the cage."		
Predicting	"Mom'll get mad if I play in the mud."		
Empathizing	"She's crying 'cause she fell down."		
Imagining	"I'm the mommy; I'll put the baby to bed."		
Negotiating	"If you give me the truck, I'll give you the ball."		

FIGURE 7.3. Chart for recording functions of communication expressed, with examples expressed by typically developing (TD) children at 4–7 Years. Based on Chapman (1981) and Tough (1977).

3b. *Assessment*: During interaction with the child and/or observation of the child interacting with a variety of other conversational partners, an evaluation is made of the the child's ability to:

- Use polite forms.
- Speak appropriately to people of various ages and social status, using different language and speaking tones (i.e., informal language with peers, more formal language with teachers and other adults).
- Ask in different ways, depending on whether request is a favor (to borrow something) or a right (to have a borrowed object returned).
- Use context-specific vocabulary, according to the topic, conversational partner, and situation.

4a. *Presupposition*: Assuming what information a conversational partner needs to be given and what the partner already knows.

4b. *Assessment*: Observing the child in conversation with a variety of conversational partners, the clinician can note whether the child:

- Gives the appropriate amount of information—that is, avoids excessively discussing a topic or sounding pedantic on the one hand, and being too vague or causing confusion on the other.
- Uses pronouns appropriately (e.g., "he" if the subject is known or has been stated previously).
- Uses ellipsis appropriately (e.g., answering "Yes, I did" instead of "Yes, I went to the store" when asked, "Did you go to the store?").
- Creating cohesive conversational flow by appropriately relating statements to ideas introduced earlier in the conversation.

5a. *Conversational manner*: According to Grice (1996), contributions to conversation should be "clear, brief, and orderly."

5b. *Assessment*: Assessment of this domain should involve observation of the ability to speak succinctly and fluidly. For example, the clinician may note use of overly long, complex utterances; blatantly sparse conversational contributions; and/or disorganized, tangential, cluttered, or repetitive styles of speech.

The skills described above may be probed most efficiently in semistructured interactions, during which communication may be elicited in response to various situations, such as the following:

- Asking the child to pretend to be the "mommy" or "daddy" to a doll or toy.
- Having the child ask for an object, then (if the original request is blunt or abrupt) telling him or her to "ask more nicely."
- Providing an opportunity for the child to use contrastive stress—for example, by giving him or her a choice of two objects and presenting the wrong one.
- Asking for clarification of something the child said.
- Asking the child to describe a sequence, such as a set of pictures depicting a child dressing, and noting whether the child changes appropriately from noun at first mention ("the boy") to pronoun ("he") in later references; changes appropriately from full sentence in the first description ("The boy puts his sock on his foot") to elliptical sentence ("He puts his shoe on" ["his foot" is ellipted because it is redundant the second time]); and relates the sequence in a logical, organized manner.

An example of a simple assessment form that might be used for this semistructured assessment activity appears in Figure 7.4.

	Yes	No	No opportunity
Communicative functions			
Directing others			
Self-directing			
Reporting			
Reasoning			
Predicting			
Empathizing			
Imagining			
Negotiating			
Discourse management			
Waits turn to speak			
Responds to speech w/speech consistently			
Responds to speech w/relevant remark			
Maintains other's topic for at least two turns			
Shifts topics appropriately			
Monitors interlocutor with gaze appropriately (looks at other when talking; looks at referents, then back at interlocutor)			
Register variation			
Talks appropriately to unfamiliar adult (clinician)			
Demonstrates at least one register shift (e.g., in talk to baby doll or stuffed animal)			
Uses politeness conventions in requests (e.g., "please")			
Can increase politeness when told to "ask nicer"			
Uses indirect requests spontaneously/ appropriately			
Presupposition			
Uses pronouns appropriately			
Uses ellipsis appropriately			
Uses stress appropriately for emphasis and contrast			
Gives enough background information			
Can provide additional information when requested ("A what?") for conversational repair			
Manner of communication			
Gives clear, relevant responses			
Talks appropriate amount			
Can relate sequence of actions clearly in organized fashion			

FIGURE 7.4. Example form for assessing pragmatics in semistructured conversation: Early language level. Adapted from Paul (2007). Copyright 2007 by C. V. Mosby, a division of Elsevier. Adapted by permission.

COMMUNICATION ASSESSMENT
IN HIGH-FUNCTIONING SPEAKERS WITH ASD

Establishing Eligibility for Speech–Language Services

In the context of ASD, the label "high-functioning" implies that an individual presents with a normal IQ (generally 70–80 or above) and can express ideas in a wide range of words and sentences. This label is sometimes also used to refer to individuals with Asperger syndrome, who are characterized by a significant discrepancy between their high intellectual abilities and their impaired social communication skills. As a group, high-functioning children with ASD tend to exhibit advanced vocabulary and sentence structures, but poor pragmatic and social interaction skills. This discrepancy in abilities presents a challenge to the practitioner who needs to represent such a child's complex communication needs and to provide justification for services for a child who presents with a relatively high verbal IQ and scores within or above the normal range on most standard language assessments. Despite these strengths in formal language, however, the high-functioning child with an ASD will experience pragmatic and higher-level language deficits, which will become more obvious and problematic as social and educational demands increase with age.

In such cases, when traditional assessment materials are not adequate measures of communicative need, less traditional assessment methods may be considered. However, some standardized tests have shown potential for documenting the pragmatic weaknesses of higher-functioning individuals with ASD, and may help to establish their eligibility for services from a speech–language pathologist to address their social communication deficits. Some of these tests are now described.

The Test of Pragmatic Language (TOPL; Phelps-Terasaki & Phelps-Gunn, 1992) was standardized with a sample of 1,016 students. The TOPL uses picture cues paired with verbal prompts to test social language skills in children ages 5–13 years. This test assesses six core components of pragmatic language (i.e., physical setting, abstraction, topic, purpose [speech acts], visual–gestural cues, and audience). Young, Diehl, Morris, Hyman, and Bennetto (2002) found the TOPL to be a viable tool in differentiating between children with and without ASD matched for verbal IQ and basic language skill, based on pragmatic language performance.

The Comprehensive Assessment of Spoken Language (CASL; Carrow-Woolfolk, 1999) has separate scales for both Pragmatic judgment and Supralinguistic forms (nonliteral uses of language, drawing inferences and understanding of idiomatic language), which can be contrasted with lexical and syntactic skills. Reichow, Salamack, Paul, Volkmar, and Klin (in press) showed that the Pragmatic and Inferences subtests of the CASL appeared to document the difficulties exhibited by speakers with ASD in adaptive use of language for communication.

The Test of Language Competence (TLC; Wiig & Secord, 1989) examines understanding of multiple meanings, figurative usage, and the ability to draw inferences and produce utterances appropriate for various contexts. Although the TLC and other tests aimed at assessing pragmatic skills can sometimes demonstrate significant discrepancies between language form and function in students with ASD at advanced language levels, even these measures occasionally fail to overcome the powerful cognitive strategies high-functioning individuals can marshal in the structured testing environment. For this reason, less formally structured, more naturalistic assessments are often necessary.

The Children's Communication Checklist–2 (CCC-2; Bishop, 2006) is a parent checklist that provides not only measures of basic language skills, but also a "communicative deviance" score that shows the discrepancy between language form and language use. The well-standardized CCC-2 can be used to document a significant discrepancy between semantic/syntactic and pragmatic skills that can be used to argue for the need for speech–language intervention, even in the presence of language test scores in the normal range.

The Autism Spectrum Screening Questionnaire (ASSQ; Ehlers, Gillberg, & Wing, 1999) is a checklist screener consisting of 27 items that can be completed by parents, teachers, or clinicians. Its aim is to identify symptoms characteristic of children and adolescents with high-functioning ASD, including Asperger syndrome. The ASSQ may indicate areas of specific weakness, including pragmatic deficits and language use difficulties, that may be contrasted with language test scores.

The Pragmatic Rating Scale (PRS; Landa et al., 1992) was designed for evaluating conversational skills in parents of individuals with ASD, to determine whether weaknesses in pragmatics are common across family members. This scale identifies 30 pragmatic behaviors that reflect abnormalities thought to be typical of autism, based on reports of major pragmatic behaviors in the literature. The rating involves analysis of a 30-minute conversational interview sample with topics based on the Autism Diagnostic Observation Scale (Lord et al., 2000). See Table 7.3 for an outline of these topics. Each behavior is rated on a 3-point scale (0 = "normal", 1 = "moderately inappropriate", 2 = "absent or highly inappropriate"). Paul et al. (2008) analyzed data comparing PRS scores from adolescents with typical development to those of high-functioning teens with ASD, and the data suggest that PRS scores above 6 are correlated with pragmatic deficits. The specific behaviors rated on the PRS appear in Figure 7.5.

TABLE 7.3. Topics of Discussion for Pragmatic Rating Scale (PRS) Interview

1. Greeting and small talk.
2. "Tell me about your school/job."
3. "Tell me about your friends."
4. "What makes you happy? Afraid? Angry? Annoyed? Proud?"
5. Ask individual to tell a story from a wordless picture book.
6. Ask individual to describe action in a comic strip; place strip out of reach to encourage use of gestures.
7. "What would you do if you won a million dollars?"

Assessing Pragmatics and Prosody

High-functioning children with ASD demonstrate a range of social communication deficits:

- An impaired "theory of mind," or a limited ability to draw appropriate conclusions about others' thoughts and feelings. These deficits affect their presuppositional ability.
- Difficulties in feeling empathy, expressing emotion appropriately, or understanding the emotions of others.
- Obsessive interest in unusual topics, ranging from newts to plumbing equipment. They often have difficulty discussing nonpreferred topics.
- A tendency to make blunt comments that may offend others, such as pointing out a person's weight or appearance inappropriately.
- A tendency to be overly friendly in inappropriate ways; this may sometimes include inappropriate touching or asking explicitly for things (like sex) usually only hinted at in polite conversation.
- Use of incessant, repetitive questions that others may find annoying.
- Difficulties in understanding irony and humor in peer conversations.
- Inability to negotiate entry into peer activities.

All the while, these children may be showing age-appropriate or superior performance on basic tests of verbal skills. As high-functioning children with ASD progress in their education, they may encounter difficulty when asked to make inferences about characters' feelings, write essays on nonpreferred topics, or work in peer groups to complete tasks. As such, their pragmatic deficits will affect not only their success with social interactions, but also their ability to achieve academic success and maintain self-confidence.

	0	1	2
Inappropriate or absent greeting	___	___	___
Strikingly candid	___	___	___
Overly direct or blunt	___	___	___
Inappropriately formal	___	___	___
Inappropriately informal	___	___	___
Overly talkative	___	___	___
Irrelevant or inappropriate detail	___	___	___
Content "out of sync" with interlocutor	___	___	___
Confusing accounts	___	___	___
Topic preoccupation/perseveration	___	___	___
Unresponsive to cues	___	___	___
Little reciprocal (to-and-fro) exchange	___	___	___
Terse	___	___	___
Odd humor	___	___	___
Insufficient background information	___	___	___
Failure to reference pronouns	___	___	___
Inadequate clarification	___	___	___
Vague accounts	___	___	___
Scripted, stereotyped discourse	___	___	___
Awkward expression of ideas	___	___	___
Indistinct or mispronounced speech	___	___	___
Inappropriate rate of speech	___	___	___
Inappropriate intonation	___	___	___
Inappropriate volume	___	___	___
Excessive pauses, reformulations	___	___	___
Unusual rhythm, fluency	___	___	___
Inappropriate physical distance	___	___	___
Inappropriate gestures	___	___	___
Inappropriate facial expression	___	___	___
Inappropriate use of gaze	___	___	___
Subject's total score:	___	___	___

FIGURE 7.5. Score form based on Landa et al.'s (1992) Pragmatic Rating Scale (PRS). Adapted from Paul (2005). Copyright 1992 by Wiley. Adapted by permission. Scoring: 0 = "normal," 1 = "moderately inappropriate," 2 = "absent or highly inappropriate." Total scores of 6 or above are typical or students with ASD and are indicative of pragmatic disorders.

Another area of notable disability in high-functioning people with ASD is "prosody," or the musical aspects of speech (i.e., rate, volume, melody, and rhythm patterns) that accompany the linguistic signal and modulate its meaning. Research suggests that prosodic problems commonly seen in this population include inappropriate use of stress, hypernasal speech, and decreased speech fluency (Shriberg et al., 2001). Anecdotal reports also suggest trouble with modulating volume in speech and unusual intonation patterns (Pronovost, Wakstein, & Wakstein, 1966). The unique prosodic patterns of these children may render them odd, unapproachable, or unpleasant to others. In addition, teachers may interpret prosodic difficulties as defiant or passive–aggressive behavior. Some formal and informal measures that may be used to assess prosody are outlined below.

1a. *Formal assessment*: One formal screening instrument is the Prosody–Voice Screening Profile (PVSP; Shriberg, Kwiatkowski, & Rasmussen, 1990). The PVSP can be used to examine prosodic variables (i.e., stress, rate, fluency, loudness, pitch, voice quality) in free speech samples. As a screening measure, the PVSP has a suggested cutoff score of 80% for identifying a prosodic deficit. That is, if more than 80% of the subject's utterances are rated as inappropriate in one of the six areas above, according to the PVSP scoring procedures, the speech sample is considered to be demonstrating prosodic difficulties in that area.

1b. *Benefits*: The PVSP has been used to study prosody in a variety of communication disorders, and has a database of typical speakers for comparison. It has undergone extensive interjudge agreement studies and demonstrates adequate reliability at the level of summative prosody–voice codes.

1c. *Drawbacks*: The PVSP is highly labor-intensive, requiring transcription and utterance-by-utterance judgements to be made for each prosody–voice code. It also requires intensive training and practice before raters can attain adequate skill levels.

2a. *Informal assessment*: Speech samples may be gathered as part of the pragmatic assessment and evaluated informally for their prosodic characteristics. A clinician can make a judgment ("appropriate," "inappropriate," "no opportunity to observe") on each of the relevant domains of prosody, with special attention paid to stress, fluency, volume, intonation, and nasality. A recording sheet like the one in Figure 7.6 can be used to summarize this assessment.

2b. *Benefits*: Informal assessment of a speech sample may allow for a more descriptive, qualitative analysis of prosody. This style of analysis and the impressions accompanying each judgment may be useful for describing

Prosodic Parameter	Clinical Judgment →		
	Appropriate	Inappropriate	No opportunity to observe
Rate			
Stress in words			
Stress in sentences			
Fluency, use of repetition, revision			
Phrasing, use of pauses			
Overall pitch level, relative to age/gender			
Intonation (melody, patterns of speech)			
Voice quality			
Voice resonance (nasality)			

FIGURE 7.6. Recording form for judging prosodic production in spontaneous speech. From Paul (2005). Copyright by Wiley. Adapted by permission.

prosodic traits in a school-based report, or for discussing these traits with a child's teacher or parent.

2c. *Drawbacks*: Although clinician judgments are often used to assess various aspects of communicative performance, prosody is an area in which few data exist to support the validity or reliability of these judgments. Clearly, the assessment of prosodic production is an area in which there is a great need for more research to establish boundaries of normality and develop more efficient methods of assessment.

Assessing Conversational and Narrative Skills

Speakers with high-functioning ASD are often most comfortable and successful when interacting with familiar, trusted adults (e.g., parents, teachers, therapists). The world of social interaction seems unregulated and unpredictable to these children, and responsive adults represent the safest, most predictable social partners. Interacting with peers, who are often unfamiliar and can seem fickle or intimidating, often evokes anxiety in these children, as peers generally will not understand or compensate for the interactive deficits these children display. During conversational interactions, children with ASD typically fail to take into account the interests of others, the need to share the conversational floor, and the necessity for reading nonverbal cues to gauge success of the conversation. Therefore, in order to assess their conversational skills and understand their difficulties in everyday social communication, it is important to observe them engaged in a variety of peer interactions.

Using a checklist or observational guide provides organization to a social communication observation. Larson and McKinley (2003) have provided several forms for guiding this type of assessment; a sample form appears in Figure 7.7. In the clinical setting, where it is usually not possible to observe a child in a natural interaction with a peer, social interaction skills may be assessed via a more structured method involving interaction with an adult. One such method is to use a seminaturalistic probe task, during which an adult conversational partner interjects specified questions into a conversation in order to assess the speaker's ability to provide appropriate responses. Examples of conversational probes useful for this purpose appear in Table 7.4.

An additional aspect of social communication that can be assessed in higher-functioning children with ASD is the ability to produce narratives. The pragmatic impairments that hinder these children during social interactions may affect their ability to create cohesive stories as well. That is, writing a narrative requires the ability to draw inferences and understand internal responses of characters, and these skills are often deficient in children with ASD. Asking a child to produce or interpret a narrative can be an efficient means of assessing their higher-level language abilities (e.g., use of inference, complex syntax, pronouns, sequential markers). Botting (2002) found narrative ability to have a direct correlation to pragmatic skill level. In another study, Norbury and Bishop (2003) reported on narratives from 8- to 10-year-old students with communication disorders, generated in response to the wordless picture book *Frog, Where Are You?* (Mayer, 1969). Their findings suggested a few key areas of higher-level language deficit that are common to children with ASD, including incorrect use of pronouns and nouns to refer to story characters, and reduced syntactic complexity and accuracy (compared to that of typical peers).

Several tools are commercially available for assessing narrative, including these:

The Bus Story Language Test (Renfrew, 1991)
The Strong Narrative Assessment Procedure (Strong, 1998)
Narrative Rubrics (McFadden & Gillam, 1996)
The Test of Narrative Language (Gillam & Pearson, 2004)

	Appropriate	Inappropriate	No opportunity to observe	Comments
Listener role				
Vocabulary				
Syntax				
Main ideas				
Cooperative manner				
Gives feedback				
Speaker role: Language features				
Syntax				
Questions				
Figurative language				
Nonspecific language				
Precise vocabulary				
Word retrieval				
Mazes and dysfluencies				
Speaker role: Paralinguistic features				
Suprasegmental features				
Fluency				
Intelligibility				
Speaker role: Communicative functions				
Give information				
Receive information				
Describe				
Persuade				
Express opinion/belief				
Indicate readiness				
Solve problems verbally				
Entertain				

(continued)

FIGURE 7.7. A form for assessing peer conversation in speakers with ASD. From Larson and McKinley (2003). Copyright 2003 by Thinking Publications. Reprinted by permission.

	Appropriate	Inappropriate	No opportunity to observe	Comments
Conversational rules				
Verbal turns/topics				
Initiation				
Topic choice				
Topic maintenance				
Topic switch				
Turn-taking				
Repair/revision				
Interruption				
Verbal politeness				
Quantity				
Sincerity				
Relevance				
Clarity				
Tact				
Nonverbal				
Gestures				
Facial expressions				
Eye contact				
Proxemics				

FIGURE 7.7. *(continued)*

COMMUNICATION ASSESSMENT IN NONVERBAL CHILDREN WITH ASD

Despite current efforts to increase the number of children with ASD who acquire spoken language (National Research Council, 2001), a substantial portion of the population with ASD will remain nonverbal. Many of these individuals will rely on modes of augmentative and alternative communication (AAC), such as signs, pictures, and speech-generating devices. This section outlines the AAC assessment considerations unique to this population, as well as specific tools designed for assessment of nonverbal children in order to determine the most appropriate communication system for each individual.

TABLE 7.4.   Probes for Eliciting Conversational Behavior in Speakers with ASD

Behavior Probed	Example	Target	Examples
Topic initiation	"By the way, I went camping over the weekend."	1. Responsiveness 2. Topic maintenance 3. Relevance	"I went canoeing." "My friend did that last month." "Weekends are the best!"
Questions	"So how was your vacation?"	1. Responsiveness 2. Topic maintenance 3. Relevance	"Not bad." "I met a guy from Canada." "I tried waterskiing." "Our hotel had dancing every night."
Requests for repair	"What kind of dancing?"	1. Responsiveness 2. Adjustment to listener 3. Repair strategy	"Samba." "Samba, it's a Latin dance." "Do you know any Latin dances?"
Sources of difficulty	"Can you get that pen for me? (no pen in sight)"	1. Assertiveness 2. Comprehension monitoring 3. Clarification requests	"I don't see any pen." "Did you say a pen?" "Do you mean a pencil?"

AAC Assessment Considerations

AAC systems take many forms and, according to Light (1988), may be used to communicate wants and needs, transfer information, create social closeness, and express social etiquette. Although this range of typical communicative functions is ultimately attainable through use of AAC systems, children with ASD must use AAC methods that match their current level of communicative functioning. An AAC assessment aims to determine this functioning level by assessing all of the communicative attributes discussed previously, including communicative frequency, functions, means, and responsiveness. However, there are additional domains of assessment to consider in planning an AAC system. The domains described by Beukelman and Mirenda (2005) that are particularly relevant in planning such a system for a child with an ASD are cognitive/linguistic capabilities and language capabilities.

Cognitive/Linguistic Capabilities

In order to choose the most appropriate AAC method, it is important to determine the child's level of cognitive/linguistic functioning. A basic question involves determining into which of the following four broad stages a child's cognition falls:

1. The *preintentional stage,* when few goals can be held in mind to be pursued through actions. This corresponds to a level below 8 months in typical development and may be manifested by difficulty in demonstrating an understanding of permanence of objects and cause–effect relationships.
2. The *presymbolic stage,* when a child may be able to develop goals and intentions, but has difficulty creating mental representations or using symbolic play and behavior. This stage occurs from 8 to 18 months in typical development and may be manifested in an inability to use pretend play schemes.
3. The *preliterate stage,* when a child can use pretend play and symbols, but has no phonological awareness or knowledge of letter names and sounds. This stage occurs between 2 and 5 years of age in typical development, and can be seen in an unfamiliarity with letters and difficulty in detecting rhymes.
4. The *literate stage,* when a child demonstrates knowledge of or interest in letter names and sounds, and can detect rhymes.

The level of cognitive development as indexed by these general stages can be used, along with other information gathered in the assessment, to select the most appropriate means of ACC for each child.

Language Capabilities

Nonverbal children with ASD may not attain speech as a means of communication, but it is important to determine their receptive language skills as part of the AAC assessment. Within this domain, considerations include single-word comprehension and understanding of grammar and morphological rules. When it is developmentally appropriate to do so, literacy skills may also be assessed, as many AAC methods utilize letters or the written word. These often represent areas of relative strength for children with ASD (Chawarska et al., 2007). Miller and Paul (1995) suggest methods for assessing comprehension in nonverbal children.

Following a comprehensive assessment of a child's communicative capabilities, a decision is made regarding the most appropriate AAC method for the child. In general, AAC methods are considered to fall into one of two categories: *unaided* systems, which involve only the communicator's own body as the means of communication (e.g., sign language or gesture systems); and *aided* systems, which make use of other tools, such as picture boards or computers. However, a combination of these methods may be deemed appropriate for some children. In addition, once a device has been selected, AAC assessment process should continue throughout the lifespan of the individual with an ASD as his or her communication environments, needs, and capabilities change.

Assessment Tools for Nonverbal Children with ASD

Formal, norm-referenced assessment tools often require verbal responses, motor movements, and/or timed performance. For nonverbal children with ASD, this type of assessment, which compares them to their age-matched peers, may serve little purpose. Instead, Beukelman and Mirenda (2005) suggest the use of criterion-referenced assessment tools, which establish a child's ability to use certain communication strategies or tools. In addition, communication assessment may involve interviews of caregivers and other team members, as well as observation of natural interactions between the child and his or her typical communication partners. Several structured methods have been developed for use with these types of assessment. Some examples of such tools are now described.

The Augmentative Communication Assessment Profile (Goldman, 2002) is intended for children with ASD between 3 and 11 years of age, and identifies skills related to use of unaided systems, including signing, pointing, and picture exchange.

The Matching Assistive Technology and Child (Scherer, 1997) tool is intended for an infant or young child and is used by the entire team to identify the family's goals and preferences for the child, to define the child's limitations, and to determine the most appropriate technologies and training methods for the child and family.

A Developmental Assessment for Individuals with Severe Disabilities— Second Edition (DASH-2; Dykes & Erin, 1999) assesses children who are functioning at an age level from birth to 6 years, 11 months. The DASH-2 identifies the level of assistance (if any) required by the child in completion of various tasks, and assesses the child's skill level in language, sensory–motor, daily living, academics, and social-emotional domains.

The Communication Supports Checklist (McCarthy et al., 1998) is for use by programs serving individuals with severe disabilities, and is intended as a tool for determining programs' strengths and weaknesses as these relate to the communication needs of the populations they serve. Once completed, this tool offers a program assistance in developing a communication supports action plan to better serve its clientele.

Checklists, such as the one provided in Figure 7.8, may be used to structure informal observations of the child's communication. During such observations, the clinician can note any maladaptive behaviors (such as head banging or rocking), record the situations during which these occur, and note the communicative functions they seem to serve. This information

Communicative function	Communicative means						
	Word	Vocal-ization	Point	Other gesture	Gaze direction	Body orientation/ movement	Mal-adaptive means
Request for objects							
Request for actions							
Request for information (question)							
Statement/comment							
Acknowledgment							
Response to yes–no question							
Response to "wh-" question							
Other response							

FIGURE 7.8. Checklist for communication needs assessment in nonverbal children with ASD. Adapted from Paul (2005). Copyright by Wiley. Adapted by permission.

will be important during intervention planning, as self-injurious and mal-adaptive communication must be replaced by safer, more functional means. Overall, the purpose of an AAC assessment is to collect information within the child's natural environments, both through observation and input from parents, caretakers, and educators, to establish the most functional, comfortable, user-friendly, and versatile communication system possible for the child and family.

MULTICULTURAL CONSIDERATIONS IN ASD ASSESSMENT

The diagnostic criteria for autism and related disorders, as outlined by the American Psychiatric Association (2000) and the World Health Organization (1992), have been accepted throughout the world. Thus we know that ASD are seen in every cultural, linguistic, and national group (Volkmar, 2005). Because, however, the core symptoms of ASD affect social and communicative skills, and because these skills are to some extent culturally determined, cultural sensitivity is necessary in assessing children with this condition. Within the United States, research has begun to explore the cultural differences, particularly those based on race and ethnicity, that affect diagnosis and treatment of ASD. For example, Mandell, Listerud, Levy, and Pinto-Martin (2002) studied Medicaid-eligible children to compare treatment time and age of diagnosis in African American and European American populations. They found that the European American children were typically diagnosed a year and a half earlier than their African American counterparts. In addition, it generally took more visits to the mental health office for African American children to receive a diagnosis of autism. The cultural differences that underlie this reality are important considerations for professionals interested in assessing, diagnosing, and treating ASD in the United States.

Differences between African American and European American parents in the management of their children with ASD may be affected by their previous clinical experiences, help-seeking behaviors, and support and advocacy networks. According to Diala et al. (2000), African Americans are less likely than their European American counterparts to seek mental health services, and are more likely to have negative experiences when they do seek help. Whaley (1998) explored the idea that attitudes of European American clinicians toward African American patients may be implicated in the observed racial differences in ASD treatment and outcomes. African Americans' negative experience of such attitudes may contribute to their reduced help-seeking behaviors. According to Kass, Weinick, and Monheit (1999), African Americans made 26% fewer visits to their regular medical care providers than did European Americans. Dyches et al. (2004) suggest that this relative reluctance to seek help from medical professionals may also be related to stronger support networks of families, friends, and churches in the African American culture. Whatever the underlying reason, it is increasingly clear that the cultural disparity regarding health care experiences in general is affecting the efficiency and quality of the ASD diagnostic process for people in the African American community.

Although the overall number of research studies on ASD is on the rise, racial and cultural differences as they relate to ASD in the United States have been generally overlooked in the literature. Even those studies that do investigate diagnosis and treatment of ASD in racially and culturally different groups often have limited validity, due to small sample sizes and other confounding factors (Dyches, Wilder, Sudweeks, Obiakor, & Algozzine, 2004). Dyches et al. (2004) cited recruiting strategies as a major factor in limiting the pool of potential subjects for ASD research, as minority groups in the United States may prefer not to participate in research efforts, due to language barriers, mistrust, or misunderstanding. The resulting paucity of research on American minority groups' use of health services and attitudes toward disorders such as ASD leaves clinicians ill equipped to address sociocultural issues in diagnosis and treatment. Beginning to consider the impact of cultural differences during assessment and treatment of ASD is a first step toward a more inclusive model. A few tools have already been developed to consider cultural differences in communication; these are now described.

The Diagnostic Evaluation of Language Variation (DELV; Seymour, Roeper, de Villiers, & de Villiers, 2005) comes in the form of a screening measure, a criterion-referenced test, and a norm-referenced test. The DELV is intended for children ages 4–12 years, and while it is sensitive to the linguistic and cultural characteristics of many African American children, it can be used for children of any race or ethnicity to identify the risk of a language disorder while considering the potential effects of variations from mainstream American English. It allows a culture-fair assessment of language form, and also contains a pragmatic section that can be useful for any client in documenting a discrepancy between skill levels in the formal and pragmatic domains of language.

Cultural Contexts for Early Intervention: Working with Families (Moore & Péréz-Méndez, 2003) is the title of both a video and a written manual designed for professionals who wish to become more skillful in assessment and intervention practices across cultures.

Multicultural Students with Special Language Needs: Practical Strategies for Assessment and Intervention (Roseberry-McKibbin, 2002) is a 364-page book that outlines key information about various cultural groups, including the groups' characteristics and traditions. In addition, this reference points out the variables that are most important to consider in assessing and planning intervention for children and families of various cultures.

In addition, the American Speech–Language–Hearing Association offers several manuals and compilations of articles to train clinicians to work with multicultural populations. These documents are available through its website (*www.asha.org*).

COMMUNICATION ASSESSMENT IN CONTEXT

The assessment of communication is, of course, part of the larger process of diagnostic evaluation and educational planning that goes into determining the strengths and needs of a child with an ASD. In conducting this process, professionals from various disciplines collaborate with family members and other caregivers to determine a child's diagnostic classification and eligibility for publicly funded services, to describe in detail the child's needs in all areas of functioning, to identify the most appropriate goals for an intervention program, and to monitor the program as it proceeds to ensure that it is efficient and effective.

Planning and Monitoring Communication Intervention

As we have seen, data from the communication assessment of a child with an ASD will be gathered through a range of methods, including standard testing, structured observations, and parental interviews/questionnaires, as well as input from others with knowledge of the child's history and current presentation, who collectively form the child's treatment team. The assessment data will then be used to do the following:

- Identify the frequency, range, and means of communicative acts expressed. This involves determining the degree to which language or some other means (such as gesture) is used to express communicative functions.
- Establish the degree of reciprocity or responsiveness to communication the child shows.
- Describe the pattern of formal language acquisition—whether it is delayed, absent, similar to that seen in specific language disorder, or a relative strength.
- Compare the use of words and sentences with pragmatic abilities.
- Identify language patterns characteristic of ASD, such as pronoun reversals, echolalia, or prosodic abnormalities.
- Determine the most accessible form of AAC if the child is nonverbal.

This information will be shared with members of the child's treatment or educational team, including parents, other caregivers, teachers, and therapists—both to ensure its congruence with their understanding of the child, and to increase understanding of the child's current strengths and needs. The data are then used by the team to identify a set of goals for the child's communication intervention program. These goals will be based both on the portrait drawn of the child's strengths and needs by the assessment data, and also on the particular areas identified by the team as being most important to address, in order to improve the child's functioning in day-to-day settings.

Once individualized goals for the child's communication program have been established collaboratively in this way, one additional form of assessment may be introduced to assist in planning the intervention program. "Dynamic assessment" is designed to take a closer look at what factors, supports, or modifications enhance the child's communication performance. In dynamic assessment, the communicative context is manipulated through the use of prompts, cues, or various scaffolds to determine which of these best support positive changes in communication. Thus dynamic assessment provides important initial information about what techniques or teaching styles may be appropriate to improve communication for a particular child. Dynamic assessment often takes place at the beginning of an intervention program, to identify the most effective ways to meet the aims identified by the assessment team.

SUMMARY

Communication assessment in individuals with ASD is a process that requires a broad understanding of both typical developmental patterns and those unique to ASD. Decisions regarding assessment methods will be made on the basis of each child's age, developmental level, verbal ability, and communication skills. Available and valid methods of assessing communication in children with ASD include formal evaluation of communication through standardized tools; informal evaluation through use of observations, checklists, and communication samples; and involvement of the family through interviews, questionnaires, and information sharing. A comprehensive assessment of communicative strengths and needs involves consideration of current performance, developmental history, cultural and linguistic factors, and the concerns expressed by caregivers and educators. It results in a family-centered plan to maximize the child's ability to communicate with the world.

Deficits in communication are core symptoms of ASD, and assessment of these skills is always a central part of the evaluation process. Children with ASD who are in the prelinguistic phase of communication may require assistance in establishing the communicative basis for a formal language system, while older nonverbal children may require assessment to identify the most appropriate AAC system. Assessment of communication for children in later stages of language use should consider the atypical communicative patterns that often accompany ASD, such as echolalia and pronoun errors, as well as the pragmatic and receptive language deficits that are common in this population. Although each communication assessment will be unique, due to the wide range of strengths and needs seen in this spectrum of disorders, the considerations discussed in this chapter offer a framework for thinking about the communication assessment process. A flexible, family-centered approach that includes everyone who cares for or provides treatment to a child will increase the validity of the information collected at each stage of the process, and will give the child the best possible chance to experience a communication intervention program that will open this vital channel between the child and his or her world.

REFERENCES

American Psychiatric Association. (2000). *Diagnostic and statistical manual of mental disorders* (4th ed., text rev.). Washington, DC: Author.

Baranek, G. T. (1999). Autism during infancy: A retrospective video analysis of sensory–motor and social behaviors at 9–12 months of age. *Journal of Autism and Developmental Disorders, 29,* 213–224.

Baron-Cohen, S., Cox, A., Baird, G., Swettenham, J., Nightingale, N., Morgan, K., et al. (1996). Psychological markers in the detection of autism in infancy in a large population. *British Journal of Psychiatry, 168,* 158–163.

Bedrosian, J. (1985). An approach to developing conversational competence. In D. Ripich & F. Spinelli (Eds.), *School discourse problems* (pp. 237–254). San Diego, CA: College-Hill Press.

Beukelman, D. R., & Mirenda, P. (2005). *Augmentative and alternative communication: Supporting children and adults with complex communication needs* (3rd ed.). Baltimore: Brookes.

Bishop, D. (2006). *Children's Communication Checklist–2 (American Standardization Version).* London: Harcourt Assessment.

Blischak, D., & Schlosser, R. (2003). Use of technology to support independent spelling by students with autism. *Topics in Language Disorders, 23,* 293–304.

Botting, N. (2002). Narrative as a tool for the assessment of linguistic and pragmatic impairments. *Child Language Teaching and Therapy, 18,* 1–22.

Brinton, B., & Fujiki, M. (1992). Setting the context for conversational language sampling. In W. Secord (Ed.), *Best practices in school speech–language pathology* (Vol. 2, pp. 9–19). San Antonio, TX: Psychological Corporation.

Bruner, J. (1977). Early social interaction and language acquisition. In R. Schaffer (Ed.), *Studies in mother–infant interaction* (pp. 155–177). New York: Academic Press.

Carrow-Woolfolk, E. (1999). *Comprehensive Assessment of Spoken Language.* Circle Pines, MN: American Guidance Service.

Chapman, R. (1981). Analyzing communicative intents. In J. Miller (Ed.), *Assessing language production in children: Experimental procedures* (pp. 111–138). Boston: Allyn & Bacon.

Chapman, R. (2000). Children's language learning: An interactionist perspective. *Journal of Child Psychology and Psychiatry, 41,* 33–54.

Charman, T., Baron-Cohen, S., Swettenham, J., Baird, G., Drew, A., & Cox, A. (2003). Predicting language outcome in infants with autism and pervasive developmental disorder. *International Journal of Language and Communication Disorders, 38,* 265–285.

Charman, T., Swettenham, J., Baron-Cohen, S., Cox, A., Baird, G., & Drew, A. (1997). Infants with autism: An investigation of empathy, pretend play, joint attention, and imitation. *Developmental Psychology, 33,* 781–789.

Chawarska, K., Klin, A., Paul, R., & Volkmar, F. (2007). Autism spectrum disorder in the second year: Stability and change in syndrome expression. *Journal of Child Psychology and Psychiatry, 48,* 128–138.

Crais, E. (1996). Applying family-centered principles to child assessment. In P. McWilliam, P. Winton, & E. Crais (Eds.), *Practical strategies for family-centered early intervention* (pp. 69–96). San Diego, CA: Singular.

Dawson, G., Meltzoff, A., Osterling, J., Rinaldi, J., & Brown, E. (1998). Children with autism fail to orient to naturally occurring social stimuli. *Journal of Autism and Developmental Disorders, 28,* 479–485.

Diala, C., Muntaner, C., Walrath, C., Nickerson, K., LaVest, T., & Leaf, P. (2000). Racial differences in attitudes toward professional mental health care in the use of services. *American Journal of Orthopsychiatry, 70,* 455–464.

Dunn, L., & Dunn, L. (1997). *Peabody Picture Vocabulary Test—Third Education.* Circle Pines, MN: American Guidance Service.

Dyches, T. T., Wilder, L. K., Sudweeks, R. R., Obiakor, F. E., & Algozzine, B. (2004). Multicultural issues in autism. *Journal of Autism and Developmental Disorders, 34,* 211–221.

Dykes, M., & Erin, J. (1999). *A Developmental Assessment for Students with Severe Disabilities—Second Edition.* Austin, TX: PRO-ED.

Edwards, S., Fletcher, P., Garman, M., Highes, A., Letts, C., & Sinka, I. (1999). *Reynell Developmental Language Scales–III.* Windsor, UK: NFER-Nelson.

Ehlers, S., Gillberg, C., & Wing, L. (1999). A screening questionnaire for Asperger syndrome and other high-functioning autism spectrum disorders in school age. *Journal of Autism and Developmental Disorders, 29,* 129–141.

Fensen, L., Dale, P., Reznick, S., Thal, D., Bates, E., Hartung, J., et al. (2007). *MacArthur–Bates Communicative Developmental Inventories (3rd Ed.).* Baltimore: Brookes.

Gillam, R., & Pearson, N. (2004). *Test of Narrative Language.* Greenville, SC: SuperDuper.

Girolametto, L. (1997). Development of a parent report measure for profiling the conversational skills of preschool children. *American Journal of Speech–Language Pathology, 6,* 25–33.

Goldman, H. (2002). *Augmentative Communication Assessment Profile.* London: Speechmark.

Grice, P. (1996). Logic and conversation. In H. Deirsson & M. Losonsky (Eds.). *Readings in language and mind* (pp. 121–133). New York: Wiley.

Hedrick, D., Prather, E., & Tobin, A. (1984). *Sequenced Inventory of Communication Development—Revised.* Austin, TX: PRO-ED.

Hresko, W., Reid, K., & Hamill, D. (1999). *Test of Early Language Development—Third Edition.* Austin, TX: PRO-ED.

Kanner, L. (1943). Autistic disturbances of affective contact. *Nervous Child, 2,* 217–250.

Kanner, L. (1946). Irrelevant and metaphorical language in early infantile autism. *American Journal of Psychiatry, 103,* 242–246.

Kass, B., Weinick, R., & Monheit, A. (1999). *Racial and ethnic differences in health* (MEPS Chartbook No. 2). Rockville, MD: U.S. Department of Health and Human Services.

Kleiman, K. (2003). *Functional Communication Scale—Revised.* East Moline, IL: LinguiSystems.

Klin, A., Volkmar, F., & Sparrow, S. (1992). Autistic social dysfunction: Some limitations of the theory of mind hypothesis. *Journal of Child Pschology and Psychiatry, 33,* 861–876.

Landa, R. (2000). Social language use in Asperger syndrome and high-functioning autism. In A. Klin, F. R. Volkmar, & S. S. Sparrow (Eds.), *Asperger syndrome* (pp. 125–155). New York: Guilford Press.

Landa, R., Piven, J., Wzorek, M., Gayle, J., Cloud, D., Chase, G., et al. (1992). Social language use in parents of autistic individuals. *Psychological Medicine, 22,* 245–254.

Larson, V., & McKinley, N. (2003). *Communication solutions for older students: Assessment and intervention strategies.* Eau Claire, WI: Thinking.

Light, J. (1988). Interaction involving individuals using augmentative and alternative communication systems: State of the art and future directions. *Augmentative and Alternative Communication, 4,* 66–82.

Lord, C. (1995). Follow-up of two-year-olds referred for possible autism. *Journal of Child Psychology and Psychiatry, 36,* 1365–1382.

Lord, C., & Risi, S. (2000). Diagnosis of autism spectrum disorders in young children. In A. M. Wetherby & B. M. Prizant (Eds.), *Autism spectrum disorders: A transactional developmental perspective* (pp. 11–30). Baltimore: Brookes.

Lord, C., Risi, S., Lambrecht, L., Cook, E. H., Jr., Leventhal, B. L., DiLavore, P. C., et al. (2000). The Autism Diagnostic Observation Schedule—Generic: A standard measure of social and communication deficits associated with the spectrum of autism. *Journal of Autism and Developmental Disorders, 30*(3), 205–223.

Maestro, S., Muratori, F., Cavallaro, M. C., Pei, F., Stern, D., Golse, B., et al. (2002). Attentional skills during the first 6 months of age in autism spectrum disorder. *Journal of the American Academy of Child and Adolescent Psychiatry, 41* 1239–1245.

Mandell, D. S., Listerud, J., Levy, S. E., & Pinto-Martin, J. A. (2002). Race differences in the age at diagnosis among Medicaid-eligible children with autism. *Journal of the American Academy of Child and Adolescent Psychiatry, 41,* 1447–1453.

McCarthy, C. F., Mclean, L. K., Miller, J. F., Brown, D. P., Romski, M. A., Rourk, J. D., et al. (1998). *Communication Supports Checklist for programs serving individuals with severe disabilities.* Baltimore: Brookes.

McFadden, T., & Gillam, R. (1996). An examination of the quality of narrative produced by children with language disorders. *Language, Speech and Hearing Services in Schools, 27,* 48–56.

Meyer, M. (1969). *Frog, where are you?* New York: Dial Books.

Miller, J., & Chapman, R. (2000). *Systematic Analysis of Language Transcripts.* Madison: University of Wisconsin.

Miller, J., & Paul, R. (1995). *The clinical assessment of language comprehension.* Baltimore: Brookes.

Mirenda, P. (2003). "He's not really a reader": Perspectives on supporting literacy development in individuals with autism. *Topics in Language Disorders, 23,* 271–282.

Moore, S. M., & Pérez-Méndez, C. (2003). *Cultural contexts for early interven-*

tion: Working with families. Rockville, MD: American Speech–Language–Hearing Association.

Mundy, P., Hogan, A., & Doehring, P. (1996). *Preliminary manual for the Abridged Early Social Communication Scales.* Retrieved from *www.psy.miami.edu/faculty/pmundy.*

Mundy, P., Sigman, M., Ungerer, J., & Sherman, T. (1987). Nonverbal communication and play correlates of language development in autistic children. *Journal of Autism and Developmental Disorders, 17,* 349–364.

Mundy, P., & Stella, J. (2000). Joint attention, social orienting, and nonverbal communication in autism. In A. M. Wetherby & B. M. Prizant (Eds.), *Autism spectrum disorders: A transactional developmental perspective* (pp. 55–77). Baltimore: Brookes.

Nadig, A. S., Ozonoff, S., Young, G. S., Rozga, A., Sigman, M., & Rogers, S. J. (2007). A prospective study of response to name in infants at risk for autism. *Archives of Pediatrics and Adolescent Medicine, 161,* 378–383.

National Research Council. (2001). *Educating children with autism.* Washington, DC: National Academy Press.

Newcomer, P. L., & Hammill, D. D. (1997). *Test of Language Development—Primary: Third Edition* (TOLD-P:4). Austin, TX: PRO-ED.

Norbury, C., & Bishop, D. V. M. (2003). Narrative skills of children with communication impairments. *International Journal of Language and Communication Disorders, 38,* 287–314.

Osterling, J., & Dawson, G. (1994). Early recognition of children with autism: A study of first birthday home videos. *Journal of Autism and Developmental Disorders, 24,* 247–258.

Osterling, J., Dawson, G., & Munson, J. A. (2002). Early recognition of 1-year-old infants with autism spectrum disorder versus mental retardation. *Developmental and Psychopathology, 14,* 239–251.

Paul, R. (2005). Assessing communication. In F. R. Volkmar, R. Paul, A. Klin, & D. Cohen (Eds.), *Handbook of autism and pervasive developmental disorders* (3rd ed, Vol. 2, pp. 799–816). Hoboken, NJ: Wiley.

Paul, R. (2007). *Language disorders from infancy through adolescence: Assessment and intervention* (3rd ed.). St. Louis, MO: Mosby.

Paul, R., Chawarska, K., Cicchetti, D., & Volkmar, F. R. (in press). Language outcomes in toddlers with ASD. Autism Research. *Journal of Speech, Language, and Hearing Research.*

Paul, R., Chawarska, K., Klin, A., & Volkmar, F. (2007) Dissociations in development of early communication in ASD. In R. Paul. (Ed.), *Language disorders from a developmental perspective: Essays in honor of Robin Chapman* (pp. 163–194). Hillsdale, NJ: Erlbaum.

Paul, R., & Cohen, D. (1984). Outcomes of severe disorders of language acquisition. *Journal of Autism and Developmental Disorders, 14,* 405–421.

Paul, R., Orlovski, S., Marchinko, H., & Volkmar, F. (in press). Conversational Behaviors In Youth With High-Functioning Autism and Asperger syndrome. *Journal of Autism and Developmental Disorders.*

Phelps-Terasaki, D., & Phelps-Gunn, T. (1992). *The Test of Pragmatic Language-2.* Austin, TX: PRO-ED.

Pronovost, W., Wakstein, M., & Wakstein, D. (1966). A longitudinal study of speech behavior and language comprehension in fourteen children diagnosed as atypical or autistic. *Exceptional Children, 33,* 19–26.

Prutting, C., & Kirchner, D. (1983). Applied pragmatics. In T. M. Gallager & C. A. Prutting (Eds.), *Pragmatic assessment and intervention issues in language* (pp. 29–64). San Diego, CA: College-Hill Press.

Reichow, B., Salamack, S., Paul, R., Volkmar, F. R., & Klin, A. (in press). Pragmatic assessment in speakers with autism spectrum disorders: A comparison of a standard measure with parent report. *Journal of Communication Disorders.*

Renfrew, C. (1991). *The bus story: A test of continuous speech* (22nd ed.). Old Headington, Oxford, UK: Author.

Roseberry-McKibbin, C. (2002). *Multicultural students with special language needs: Practical strategies for assessment and intervention* (2nd ed.). Oceanside, CA: Academic Communication Associates.

Scherer, M. (1997). *Matching Assistive Technology and Child.* Webster, NY: Institute for Matching Person and Technology.

Semel, E., Wiig, E. H., & Secord, W. (2004). *Clinical Evaluation of Language Fundamentals—Preschool, Second Edition.* (CELF-Preschool 2). San Antonio, TX: Harcourt Assessment.

Seymour, H. N., Roeper, T. W., de Villiers, J., & de Villiers, P. A. (2005). *Diagnostic Evaluation of Language Variation.* San Antonio, TX: Harcourt Assessment.

Sheinkopf, S. J., Mundy, P., Kimbrough-Oller, D., & Steffens, M. (2000). Vocal atypicalities of preverbal autistic children. *Journal of Autism and Developmental Disorders, 30*(4), 345–354.

Shriberg, L. D., Kwiatkowski, J., & Rasmussen, C. (1990). *The Prosody–Voice Screening Profile.* Tucson, AZ: Communication Skill Builders.

Shriberg, L., Paul, R., McSweeney, J., Klin, A., Cohen, D., & Volkmar, F. R. (2001). Speech and prosody characteristics of adolescents and adults with high functioning autism and Asperger syndrome. *Journal of Speech, Language, and Hearing Research, 44,* 1097–1115.

Sparrow, S. S., Cicchetti, D., & Balla, D. (2005). *Vineland Adaptive Behavioral Scales, Second Edition (Vineland-II).* Circle Pines, MN: American Guidance Service.

Stone, W. L., Ousley, O. Y., Yoder, P. J., Hogan, K. L., & Hepburn, S. L. (1997). Nonverbal communication in two- and three-year-old children with autism. *Journal of Autism and Developmental Disorders, 27,* 677–696.

Strong, C. (1998). *Strong Narrative Assessment Procedure (SNAP).* Eau Claire, WI: Thinking.

Swettenham, J., Baron-Cohen, S., Charman, T., Cox, A., Baird, G., Drew, A., et al. (1998). The frequency and distribution of spontaneous attention shifts between social and nonsocial stimuli in autistic, typically developing, and nonautistic developmentally delayed infants. *Journal of Child Psychology and Psychiatry, 39,* 747–753.

Tager-Flusberg, H., & Joseph, R. (2003). Identifying neurocognitive phenotypes in autism. *Philosophical Transactions of the Royal Society of London, Series B, 358,* 303–314.

Tager-Flusberg, H., Paul, R., & Lord, C. (2005). Language and communication in autism. In F. R. Volkmar, R. Paul, A. Klin, & D. Cohen (Eds.), *Handbook of autism and pervasive developmental disorders* (3rd ed., Vol. XX, pp. 335–364). Hoboken, NJ: Wiley.

Tough, J. (1977). *The development of meaning.* New York: Halsted Press.

Volkmar, F. R. (2005). International perspectives. In F. R. Volkmar, R. Paul, A. Klin, & D. Cohen (Eds.), *Handbook of autism and pervasive developmental disorders* (3rd ed., Vol. II, pp. 1193–1252). Hoboken, NJ: Wiley.

Volkmar, F. R., Stier, D. M., & Cohen, D. J. (1985). Age of recognition of pervasive developmental disorder. *American Journal of Psychiatry, 142,* 1450–1452.

Wetherby, A. M., & Prizant, B. M. (2002). *Communication and Symbolic Behavior Scales.* Baltimore: Brookes.

Wetherby, A. M., Prizant, B. M., & Hutchinson, T. (1998). Communicative, social-affective, and symbolic profiles of young children with autism and pervasive developmental disorder. *American Journal of Speech–Language Pathology, 7,* 79–91.

Wetherby, A. M., Woods, J., Allen, L., Cleary, J., Dickinson, H., & Lord, C. (2004). Early indicators of autism spectrum disorders in the second year of life. *Journal of Autism and Developmental Disorders, 34,* 473–493.

Whaley, A. L. (1998). Racism in the provision of mental health services: A social-cognitive analysis [Abstract]. *American Journal of Orthopsychiatry, 68,* 47–57.

Wiig, E. H., & Secord, W. (1989). *Test of Language Competence.* New York: Psychological Corporation.

Windsor, J., Doyle, S., & Siegel, G. (1994). Language acquisition after mutism: A longitudinal case study of autism. *Journal of Speech and Hearing Research, 37,* 96–105.

Woods, J., & Wetherby, A. M. (2003). Early identification of and intervention for infants and toddlers who are at risk for autism spectrum disorder. *Language, Speech and Hearing Services in Schools, 34,* 180–193.

World Health Organization. (1992). *International classification of diseases* (10th rev.). Geneva: Author.

Young, E. C., Diehl, J. J., Morris, D., Hyman, S. L., & Bennetto, L. (2005). The use of two language tests to identify pragmatic language problems in children with autism spectrum disorders. *Language, Speech, and Hearing Services in Schools, 36,* 62–72.

Zimmerman, I., Steiner, V., & Pond, R. (2002). *Preschool Language Scale, Fouth Edition (PLS-4).* San Antonio, TX: Psychological Corporation.

Zinober, B., & Martlew, M. (1985). Developmental changes in four types of gesture in relation to acts and vocalization from 10 to 21 months. *British Journal of Developmental Psychology, 3,* 293–306.

CHAPTER EIGHT

Assessment of Intellectual Functioning in Autism Spectrum Disorders

Laura Grofer Klinger
Sarah E. O'Kelley
Joanna L. Mussey

> Even though most of these children were at one time or another looked upon as feebleminded, they are all unquestionably endowed with good *cognitive potentialities*. . . . The astounding vocabulary of the speaking children, the excellent rote memory for events of several years before, the phenomenal rote memory for poems and names, and the precise recollection of complex patterns and sequences, bespeak good intelligence. . . .
> —Kanner (1943, p. 247: emphasis in original)

Kanner's (1943) original description of the intellectual abilities of children with autism spectrum disorders (ASD) highlights the juxtaposition of cognitive delays and cognitive strengths that characterizes these disorders. Although intellectual evaluations may suggest that a child with an ASD is developmentally delayed, children with ASD often have some peaks in their abilities. This combination of strengths and weaknesses creates an uneven profile of cognitive abilities in individuals with ASD (see Figure 8.1). This uneven cognitive profile presents a conundrum for psychologists trying to decide which IQ test to administer.

Consider the case example of Jason, an 8-year-old boy with a diagnosis of autistic disorder. Jason had an extensive vocabulary, although the majority of his speech consisted of delayed echolalia, and he was unable to participate in a lengthy reciprocal conversation. He loved puzzles and

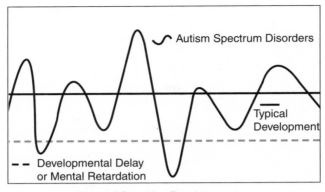

FIGURE 8.1. Uneven cognitive profile in ASD.

spent hours every day arranging objects into geometric patterns. Jason's mother referred him to our clinic for a psychological evaluation to assist in academic placement and accommodations for the third grade. If Jason were evaluated with an IQ test that required him to formulate answers to complex questions (e.g., the Wechsler Intelligence Scale for Children—Fourth Edition [WISC-IV]; Wechsler, 2003), he would be likely to show significant impairments and might receive a score in the range of mild mental retardation. However, in contrast, if Jason were administered a nonverbal test of intelligence measuring visual sequencing and pattern perception skills (e.g., the Leiter International Performance Scale—Revised [Leiter-R]; Roid & Miller, 1997), he would be likely to show average or above-average performance. Hence the conundrum faced by the psychologist: Which test would be most appropriate for Jason? Which would be the best measure of Jason's true abilities? Which would be the best measure of the "cognitive potentialities" that Kanner described?

The goal of this chapter is to provide a set of guidelines for deciding which intelligence test may be the most appropriate when evaluating a person with an ASD. There is no "best test" for measuring intellectual functioning in persons with ASD. Instead, the psychologist must consider the reasons why an intellectual evaluation is being requested for this particular individual; the literature on intellectual strengths and weaknesses in ASD; the unique social, communication, and behavioral symptoms of ASD that may interfere with intellectual testing; and the specific properties of the intellectual tests that are being considered. Thus, before we can provide a set of guidelines for choosing an intellectual assessment battery, each of these issues is discussed in detail.

OVERLAP BETWEEN ASD
AND MENTAL RETARDATION

Historically, it has been believed that the majority of children with autism have a dual diagnosis of mental retardation, although there has been little empirical evidence to support these claims (Edelson, 2006). In his review of 36 epidemiological studies published between 1966 and 2003, Fombonne (2005) reported that the median rate of mental retardation in individuals diagnosed with autistic disorder was 70.4% (range = 40–100%). Across these studies, 29.3% of individuals were reported to have mild to moderate mental retardation, and 38.5% were reported to have severe to profound mental retardation. More recent studies, however, suggest that the rate of mental retardation is considerably lower, with rates ranging from 40% to 71% for individuals diagnosed with autistic disorder and from 6% to 49% for individuals diagnosed with pervasive developmental disorder not otherwise specified (PDD-NOS) or Asperger's disorder (see Fombonne, 2005, for a review). A recent population-based epidemiological study showed a similar decrease in rates of mental retardation, with 55% of children with ASD receiving IQ scores within the range of mental retardation (Baird et al., 2006). These decreasing rates could be the results of a broadening of the ASD diagnostic criteria to include diagnoses such as Asperger's disorder (which by definition does not have a dual diagnosis of mental retardation), and/or they could be the results of more effective early intervention. Regardless of why the rates of comorbid diagnoses of ASD and mental retardation are decreasing, there is a growing need for intellectual assessments that are appropriate for both low- and high-functioning persons with ASD.

Lower IQ scores have been associated with both gender and the presence of comorbid medical conditions. Females with autism tend to receive lower scores on both verbal and nonverbal measures of intelligence (Volkmar, Szatmari, & Sparrow, 1993). Volkmar et al. (1993) also reported that proportionately more females with autism were in the range of severe mental retardation (IQ below 35), and that males with autism were 8.8 times more likely to have average intelligence. The prevalence rate of seizure disorders in persons with ASD ranges from 11% to 39% (see Ballaban-Gil & Tuchman, 2000, for a review). Individuals with ASD and a comorbid seizure disorder are more likely to have mental retardation.

REFERRAL QUESTIONS
FOR INTELLECTUAL TESTING IN ASD

When a clinician is choosing an appropriate instrument to assess developmental or intellectual functioning, it is important to consider the reason(s) why the testing is being conducted. There are several different reasons for evaluating developmental and intellectual abilities in individuals with ASD: (1) as part of a diagnostic battery to determine whether an ASD is present; (2) as part of an educational battery to evaluate the strengths and weaknesses that should be targeted by a child's individualized education program; (3) as a measure of treatment effectiveness; and (4) as an aid in estimating long-term prognosis.

Diagnostic Assessment

Intellectual testing is a recommended part of an interdisciplinary diagnostic evaluation (Filipek et al., 1999; Johnson, Myers, & the Council on Children with Disabilities, 2007). Klin, Saulnier, Tsatsanis, and Volkmar (2005) described developmental testing for infants and preschool-age children, and intellectual assessment for school-age children and older individuals, as a frame for interpreting the results of diagnostic testing. This "frame" can be used to evaluate whether a child's social and communication delays are greater than expected from the child's developmental level, or whether they are equivalent to the child's developmental level. In order for a child to receive an ASD diagnosis, social and communicative skills must be delayed below developmental level. For example, if a developmental evaluation indicates that a 4-year-old child has the cognitive development of a 2-year-old, then his or her social and communication skills (e.g., eye contact, pointing, symbolic play, reciprocal interactions, affect) should be compared to the skills expected of a 2-year-old. If a discrepancy between developmental level and social communication skills is not present, then diagnoses of other developmental delays or language disorder should be considered.

Intellectual assessment results can be used to assist in differentiating between autism and Asperger syndrome. According to *Diagnostic and Statistical Manual of Mental Disorders,* fourth edition, text revision (DSM-IV-TR) diagnostic criteria (American Psychiatric Association, 2000), a diagnosis of Asperger's disorder requires that no "clinically significant delay" in language, cognitive functioning, or adaptive behavior be present. The term "clinically significant delay" is not defined in the guidelines and has been interpreted as meaning that IQ scores must be more than one (i.e., 85) or two (i.e., 70) standard deviations below average. Thus the clinician has a wide range of interpretation in deciding whether a cognitive delay is present. However, the presence of mental retardation clearly rules out the presence of Asperger's disorder. It is important to note that IQ is not the sole factor in differentiating between these two disorders. Often a child meets the DSM-IV-TR criteria for Asperger's disorder, but also shows enough symptoms to meet diagnostic criteria for autistic disorder. In this case, a diagnosis of autistic disorder is required, although the term "high-functioning autism" may be more appropriate in describing this child's difficulties.

Assessment of Current Strengths and Weaknesses

Intellectual testing is often helpful in clarifying the specific strengths and weaknesses present in an individual child and highlighting the areas that need to be addressed by intervention. Klin et al. (2005) recommended that intellectual assessment should

> describe patterns of both verbal and nonverbal functioning across several domains: (1) problem solving (e.g., can the child generate strategies and integrate information?), (2) concept formation (e.g., can the child abstract rules from specific instances or understand principles of categorization, order, time, number, and causation, and generalize knowledge from one context to another?), (3) reasoning (e.g., can the child transform information to solve visual-perceptual and verbal problems?), (4) style of learning (e.g., can the child learn from modeling, imitation, using visual cues, or verbal prompts?), and (5) memory skills (e.g., how many items of information can the child retain; . . . are the child's memory skills in one modality better than in another such as visual or verbal?). (p. 777)

This assessment of strengths and weaknesses is especially important, given the uneven profile of cognitive skills that typically characterizes individuals with ASD.

Assessment of Intervention Effectiveness

Although IQ scores are commonly used as a measure of treatment effectiveness, there are many cautions involved in using IQ testing for this purpose. Importantly, the use of the same IQ test on multiple occasions raises concerns about possible practice effects and concerns about whether the testing is developmentally appropriate at both testing points. For example, a developmental test such as the Bayley Scales of Infant and Toddler Development, Third Edition (Bayley-III; Bayley, 2005) may be appropriate for a 2-year-old beginning intervention, but is no longer appropriate for a 4-year-old at the conclusion of intervention. However, if different tests are administered at pre- and posttreatment, it is unclear whether gains are due to testing error or to the different social and communication requirements of the test, or whether a true increase in developmental level or IQ has occurred. Even when the same test is administered at both time points, there are concerns that the items may measure different skills at different ages. For example, instruments may include measures of social skills (playing peek-a-boo, reading a book with the examiner) for infants and toddlers that may not be components of the same test at older ages. In this example, earlier scores could partially be attributed to a child's social rather than intellectual delays.

Despite these cautions, changes in cognitive abilities are considered a hallmark of effective interventions—especially early interventions, where the goal is often to facilitate inclusion in regular education kindergarten classrooms (e.g., Eikeseth, Smith, Jahr, & Eldevik, 2007; Lovaas, 1987; Smith, Groen, & Wynn, 2000). The National Research Council (2001) recommends that while intellectual testing provides useful information in measuring treatment effectiveness, this type of testing is not sufficient and should not be used as the sole measure of treatment outcome.

Predictions of Long-Term Outcome

IQ testing is often used as a prognostic indicator of long-term outcome for children and adolescents with ASD. Indeed, IQ scores in children with ASD are considered to be as stable as IQ scores in children with other forms of developmental disabilities (National Research Council, 2001). However, this does not mean that IQ scores are stable across the lifespan. Mayes and Calhoun (2003) found a significant correlation between age and full scale IQ in their sample of 164 children (ages 3–15 years) with autism. The average IQ score increased from 53 for children 3 years of age to 91 for children 8 years of age and older. For children with IQ scores below 80, both verbal and nonverbal IQ scores increased. For children with IQ scores greater than or equal to 80, only verbal IQ increased significantly with age. After 8 years of age, both verbal and nonverbal IQ scores were relatively stable. Because this was a cross-sectional study, it is possible that the increase in IQ can be attributed to the fact that more severely disordered children are generally evaluated at a younger age, while more high-functioning children are usually not seen until school age. However, longitudinal studies have also reported some significant improvement in IQ, particularly when comparing preschool performance to school-age performance (Mayes & Calhoun, 2003; Sigman & McGovern, 2005) and when focusing on children with high-functioning autism (Freeman, Ritvo, Needleman, & Yokota, 1985). Less improvement has been observed in children with a dual diagnosis of autism and mental retardation (Lord & Schopler, 1989). This significant change in IQ scores from early to middle childhood suggests that low IQ scores in early childhood do not necessarily predict later outcome.

However, more stability in IQ scores has been reported from middle childhood to adolescence and adulthood (Beadle-Brown, Murphy, & Wing, 2006; Howlin, Goode, Hutton, & Rutter, 2004; Seltzer, Shattuck, Abbeduto, & Greenberg, 2004; Sigman & McGovern, 2005). In Sigman and McGovern's (2005) longitudinal study of IQ in a sample of 48 individuals with autism, 74% of participants showed stable IQ between middle childhood and adolescence/early adulthood. Notably, 21% of their sample reported a significant decrease in IQ scores (i.e., a loss of 10 or more points); this decrease during adolescence may have been due to a failure to make gains rather than a regression in skills. This stability in IQ scores from middle childhood to adolescence and early adulthood suggests that IQ scores may assist in predicting long-term cognitive ability and outcome.

Howlin et al. (2004) conducted a long-term follow-up study on 68 individuals who were seen initially at an average age of 7 years and followed until the average age of 29 years. All participants were required to have an initial IQ score of 50 or greater, to ensure that long-term outcome was not confounded with severe mental retardation. Among the 45 children receiving initial IQ scores greater than or equal to 70 at the initial assessment, 78% remained in this range of intellectual functioning during adulthood. This higher-functioning group was also more likely to live independently, although outcome varied considerably in this group. Those with initial IQ scores between 50 and 69 appeared to have a much poorer prognosis in terms of independent living, education attainment, employment, and friendships. Howlin et al. (2004) concluded that "only individuals with an IQ in the normal range (70+) have a real chance of living independently as they reach adulthood" (p. 225). Other follow-up studies from middle childhood to adulthood (Beadle-Brown et al., 2006; see Seltzer et al., 2004, for a review) have reported similar findings indicating that IQ is a good predictor of long-term educational attainment, communication skills, and independent living skills.

Taken together, these studies suggest that IQ scores may be an important predictor of long-term outcome in terms of cognitive functioning and independent living skills once a child reaches middle childhood. Thus an IQ test is an important component of an assessment battery designed to estimate long-term prognosis.

PROFILE OF STRENGTHS AND WEAKNESSES IN ASD

Approximately 10% of children with ASD show unusual islets of ability or "splinter skills" that represent relative strengths in comparison to other skills, or absolute strengths in comparison to the skills of same-age peers (National Research Council, 2001). These splinter skills have been reported in drawing, block design, musical skills, memory for specific facts, and calendar calculation. Individuals with ASD who do not have these isolated splinter skills still tend to display uneven cognitive abilities (see Figure 8.1).

Because of this characteristically uneven cognitive profile, a child's overall IQ scores may be an average of widely discrepant scores and thus may not meaningfully describe the child's true ability (Klin et al., 2005). An average IQ score may overestimate ability in a child's weakest skills and underestimate ability in the child's strongest skills. Isolated peaks in performance on some tasks are not necessarily indicative of skills in other areas, or even in related areas. For example, an 8-year-old child may be able to decode written material at the level of a 10-year-old, but may have the reading comprehension ability of a 6-year-old. Klin et al. (2005) note that it is critical for the evaluator to have knowledge of the varying cognitive profiles that occur in ASD, in order to avoid erroneous conclusions by focusing on islets of strengths when interpreting testing results.

Traditionally, it has been believed that individuals with ASD have a specific profile of intellectual ability characterized by a higher nonverbal IQ than verbal IQ (Lincoln, Allen, & Kilman, 1995; see Lincoln, Hansel, & Quirmbach, 2007, for a review). For example, individuals with ASD have frequently shown relative and absolute strengths on nonverbal visual–spatial tasks involving puzzles and arranging patterns or blocks into designs (e.g., Ghaziuddin & Mountain-Kimchi, 2004; Lincoln et al., 1995; Ozonoff, South, & Miller, 2000). However, this profile has not received uniform support in the literature (Ehlers et al., 1997; Siegel, Minshew, & Goldstein, 1996; Venter, Lord, & Schopler, 1992). Mayes and Calhoun (2003) examined the intellectual profiles of 164 children with autism across a wide range of chronological ages (3–15 years) and intellectual functioning (IQs of 14–143). In their sample, the profile of greater nonverbal than verbal IQ was present in preschool children, but gradually disappeared during the school-age years. Children with IQ scores above 80 displayed an even pattern of verbal and nonverbal abilities by 6–7 years of age. Children with IQ scores below 80 maintained a higher nonverbal than verbal IQ through the preschool years and did not show similar verbal and nonverbal scores until they were 9–10 years of age. Thus discrepancies between verbal and nonverbal IQ scores are related to both age and IQ, and, contrary to prevailing beliefs, no single pattern is indicative of an ASD diagnosis.

Several studies have compared the intellectual profile of individuals with high-functioning autism and individuals with Asperger syndrome. By definition, individuals with Asperger syndrome must have language skills in the average range or higher. Not surprisingly, such individuals have higher verbal IQ scores than individuals with high-functioning autism (Ghaziuddin & Mountain-Kimchi, 2004). There has been some evidence that individuals with Asperger syndrome display an intellectual profile characterized by higher verbal IQ than nonverbal IQ (Ehlers et al., 1997; Ghaziuddin & Mountain-Kimchi, 2004; Joseph, Tager-Flusberg, & Lord, 2002; Ozonoff et al., 2000). For example, Ghaziuddin and Mountain-Kimchi (2004) reported that 82% of individuals with Asperger syndrome in their study showed a higher verbal IQ than nonverbal IQ, with 45% of these participants showing a discrepancy of 10 or more points. However, this profile was not unique to individuals with Asperger syndrome. Fifty percent of individuals with high-functioning autism also showed a higher verbal than nonverbal IQ, although only 25% of these participants had a discrepancy of 10 or more points. Although a profile of greater verbal than nonverbal IQ is present in many individuals with Asperger syndrome, it is not ubiquitous and cannot be used to make a differential diagnosis between Asperger sydrome and high-functioning autism.

Rather than focusing on specific strengths and weaknesses across broad categories of verbal and nonverbal abilities assessed by IQ tests, investigators have begun to identify specific cognitive skills that are impaired and specific skills that are intact in persons with ASD. Cognitive impairments are thought to have a significant impact on daily life, particularly with regard to social interactions. There are several theories regarding early-developing cognitive impairments; specifically, researchers have proposed that ASD are characterized by atypical perception, attention, intuitive learning, flexible thinking, and perspective taking.

Perceptual theories suggest that individuals with ASD tend to focus on the details rather than the bigger picture, which may account for their success on nonverbal perceptual tasks such as block designs (i.e., weak central coherence; Happé & Frith, 2006). Furthermore, Mottron, Dawson, Soulieres, Hubert, and Burack (2006) have suggested that this type of enhanced perceptual processing is present not only in visual perception, but across a wide range of perceptual domains. Attention theories have highlighted difficulties in disengaging and shifting attention, with sustained attention relatively intact in persons with ASD (Courchesne et al., 1994; Renner, Klinger, & Klinger, 2006). Difficulties in shifting focus have been described as part of an overall impaired learning style characterized by rigid, inflexible thinking (i.e., impaired executive functioning; Ozonoff & Jenson, 1999). Difficulties in taking into account both one's own perspective and the perspective of another person (i.e., impaired theory of mind; Baron-Cohen, 2001) are considered hallmark cognitive problems experienced by individuals with ASD. Other learning theories have highlighted difficulties in integration of information due to impaired complex information processing (Minshew, Goldstein, & Siegel, 1997; Williams, Goldstein, & Minshew, 2006) and impaired implicit or intuitive learning (Klinger, Klinger, & Pohlig, 2007). For example, Minshew and colleagues (Minshew et al., 1997; Williams et al., 2006) have hypothesized that individuals with ASD have a cognitive profile characterized by impaired complex information processing requiring integration of information (e.g., memory for large amounts of complex material on a reading comprehension test), with

relatively intact skills in the same domains on tasks requiring simple information processing (e.g., associative learning, vocabulary, and spelling). In
summary, this pattern of strengths (i.e., perceptual processing, sustained
attention, and simple information processing) and weaknesses (i.e., shifting
attention, flexible thinking, perspective taking, implicit learning, and complex information processing) may explain the uneven profile of cognitive
ability that characterizes individuals with ASD.

DEVELOPMENTAL AND BEHAVIORAL ISSUES IN ASSESSING PERSONS WITH ASD

Successful performance on an IQ test requires the ability to sit and attend
to another person's instructions. However, as discussed above, the characteristics of ASD include difficulties with attention, social interaction, and
language understanding. Thus the traditional standardized assessment paradigm is often a challenge for individuals with ASD (and for the examiners
trying to administer the tests). At a minimum, an examiner should have
experience administering intellectual assessments, as well as some knowledge about how the symptoms of ASD may interfere with test administration and performance. Ideally, the examiner will have experience interacting with individuals with ASD. An understanding of the symptoms and
treatment approaches for ASD will assist the examiner in choosing an
appropriate test and structuring the testing session to ensure that an individual's performance is representative of his or her true abilities.

Developmental Issues in IQ Assessment

It is important for an examiner to consider chronological and mental
ages when choosing and administering an IQ test. This is particularly
important in testing children with significant developmental delays, who
demonstrate a wide discrepancy between chronological and mental age.
Such a child is likely to receive the lowest standard score provided by
an assessment instrument. When this happens, it is difficult to translate
the score into a meaningful description of the child's current ability. For
example, if an IQ score of 50 is the lowest standard score provided by the
assessment instrument, it is impossible to know whether the child's IQ
is truly in this moderate range of mental retardation, or whether a test
with a wider range of standard scores would indicate severe or profound
mental retardation.

For older individuals with significant developmental delays, it would
be more appropriate to administer a test with a wider age range that will
accommodate their level of delay. For example, a 12-year-old who is functioning at a 4-year-old level will probably be unable to complete any items

on a test designed for elementary-school-age children, but may be able to perform some of the simpler tasks on a test designed for ages that span the preschool and elementary school years. For a young child, it may be more useful to consider the child's mental age (by calculating age equivalent scores) than to focus on a standard score (Akshoomoff, 2006). A focus on mental age equivalent scores in young children has several advantages. First, it highlights a focus on current developmental level rather than IQ. This is particularly important for young children with ASD, as the research discussed above on the stability of IQ in children with ASD suggests that children can show large improvements in IQ scores from the preschool to elementary school years. Thus the use of mental age scores provides information about current ability without implying permanent intellectual disability. Second, the use of mental age equivalents may be more meaningful to caregivers or teachers, as they provide estimates of developmentally appropriate academic, behavioral, and adaptive expectations. For example, it would be developmentally inappropriate to expect a 3½-year-old child who is functioning at the 15-month level to learn to write his or her name, be toilet-trained, or understand the link between his or her actions and time out as a discipline technique.

Finally, when an examiner is testing a child with significant developmental delay, Akshoomoff (2006) recommends allowing parents to observe developmental testing and asking the parents for feedback about whether the child seemed to be performing to the best of his or her abilities. Indeed, this is the approach we use in our ASD clinic. We have found that this extra information is useful in helping the examiner consider how to interpret the current results. For example, when an examiner is trying to decide whether a child's refusal behavior occurred because the task demands were too complicated for the child or because the child was simply not interested in trying the task, a parent's view is often helpful, particularly when the parent indicates that the child has never been able to complete similar tasks at home or school. Allowing parents to observe and provide their opinions is also helpful in preparing the parents for the feedback meeting. Parents who feel that their child showed his or her best skills during tests are more likely to accept estimates of developmental level or IQ as accurate representations of their child's current abilities.

Interference of ASD Symptoms

Individuals with ASD have the most difficulty on tests involving the use of social and language skills, and the least difficulty on nonverbal tasks that do not require speed or motor skills (National Research Council, 2001). More specifically, tests requiring skills that are specifically impaired in ASD—including attending to social information (Dawson et al., 2004), imitation (Rogers, Hepburn, Stackhouse, & Wehner, 2003), joint attention (Sigman, Mundy, Sherman, & Ungerer, 1986), and understanding of personal pronouns—are likely to produce lower scores than tests requiring skills that are often strengths in individuals with ASD (e.g., perception, rote memory). This is particularly evident in testing very young children with ASD (e.g., 2- to 4-year-old children). For example, such children may have difficulty completing tasks that assess the ability to play reciprocal social games (e.g., peek-a-boo), the ability to use an index finger to point to objects, the ability to imitate the examiner's actions, and the ability to understand directions that use the pronouns "I" and "you."

Akshoomoff (2006) reported that young children with ASD spent significantly less time attending to tasks as they were being presented, and significantly more time in off-task behaviors (e.g., leaving their seats, whining, or crying). Furthermore, she observed that performance on the Mullen Scales of Early Learning (usually referred to simply as the Mullen; Mullen, 1995) was positively correlated with engagement and negatively correlated with off-task behavior. Akshoomoff hypothesized that this relationship reflected poor cooperation and attention to the tasks (i.e., behavioral regulation problems), as well as task demands that were related to the core symptoms of ASD. For example, she noted that both imitation and pointing skills are required for several of the Mullen subtests. Similarly, other tests designed for this age group, such as the Bayley-III and the Stanford–Binet Intelligence Scales, Fifth Edition (SB5; Roid, 2003), include items that involve these types of skills. Although it may be impossible to find a test that does not involve these social and communication skills, an examiner should be aware of which tasks are likely to be particularly difficult for a child with ASD.

Ideas for Structuring the Testing Session

In order for an assessment to be considered valid, it must be administered in a standardized fashion, involving correct object placement and verbal and nonverbal directions. However, an experienced clinician can combine standardized administration with behavior management techniques that increase cooperation and motivation, and thus lead to a more valid estimate of the individual's ability. If a child spends the entire testing session screaming or running in circles in the testing room, the results are unlikely to be a true estimate of the child's abilities, no matter how standardized the administration of materials may be.

Lincoln et al. (2007) offer several ideas for how to encourage cooperation and reduce a child's attempts to leave the testing situation. For example, they suggest that it is often helpful for the examiner to position the side of the testing table against a wall, to have an assistant or parent sit next to the child, to position him- or herself behind the child (although this requires the examiner to be flexible enough to administer items from a different perspective than is typically used), or to conduct the testing while sitting on the floor. In our clinical experiences, we have successfully used each of these strategies. For graduate students learning test administration, it is often helpful to have an assistant in the room who can manage the child's behavior (e.g., by providing rewards, encouraging the child to stay seated) while the examiner focuses on administering test items. This not only provides the examiner an opportunity to display testing materials correctly, but reduces the overall test-taking time.

Individuals with ASD often become quite anxious when aspects of their routine are changed. For instance, parents of very young children with ASD frequently report that their children become upset when they take a different route to school or home. IQ testing is clearly not part of a regular daily routine; thus, being brought to a new place, meeting a new person, and being asked to do new tasks can be extremely stressful for a child with ASD. The use of a visual schedule can significantly reduce the child's anxiety about the testing session. Pictures depicting the various subtests (e.g., blocks, puzzles, book, and a question mark) can be put in vertical order on a piece of paper, with a check box next to each picture. As the child moves through each task, he or she can check each box (or put a sticker in each box) as a task is completed. Ideally, the examiner will know that this type of structure is needed ahead of time. However, if necessary, a quickly written column of numbers with boxes associated with each number will work. With higher-functioning children and adolescents, a written list will suffice (e.g., a simple list of words associated with each task—"Blocks," "Questions," "Find the same," etc.).

Typically, we vary our social interaction style with young children by using facial expressions, eye contact, and different words of praise throughout the testing session. However, given that difficulties with social skills are the hallmark deficits of ASD, it is often helpful to minimize the social component of the testing by developing a social routine. This is particularly important for young children with ASD, who may not understand a visual schedule (unless they are in an intervention program that uses this technique). For example, the examiner can establish a routine of saying, "Time to work. Look," presenting the test item, waiting for a response, and then saying, "Good working." This type of routine not only minimizes the child's anxiety about being in a new place, but also makes the examiner more predictable.

Individuals with ASD often have intense interests that interfere with their performance on standardized testing. For example, a young boy obsessed with trains may bring trains to the testing room, insist on holding a train during testing, and talk repetitively about the train that he saw on the way to the clinic. In this example, IQ scores will certainly be affected by his obsession; timed motor tasks will be hindered by the fact that the child is clutching a train, and verbal items will be hindered by the fact that he answers every question by talking about the train he saw. Koegel, Koe-gel, and Smith (1997) have suggested that such children can be motivated to complete assessment tasks if they are rewarded with breaks to play with objects related to their interests or to talk about their interests. Thus, in this example, the child may be given the opportunity to play with trains as a reward for completing a task. For instance, the examiner can build a train station (e.g., a tissue box) and tell the child that the trains need to stay in the station until the puzzles are done: "After we finish the puzzles, we can play with the trains. The trains need to stay in the station until the puzzles are finished." The examiner can further structure the environment by adding train play to the schedule (i.e., a picture of a train or the word "train" after every subtest) and by using a timer to tell the child how long he has to play with the train before returning to the IQ test. This level of structure helps to improve the child's understanding of when he will be allowed to play with the trains, and thus to improve the child's motiva-tion to complete the IQ subtests. As a result, the child is eminently more "testable" and is likely to receive higher IQ scores than would have been obtained by allowing the child to clutch a train and talk about it inces-santly during testing.

Overall, if an examiner has experience and an understanding of ASD symptoms and intervention approaches, few children with ASD should truly be "untestable" (Ozonoff, Goodlin-Jones, & Solomon, 2007). Koegel et al. (1997) found significant improvements in IQ when the testing ses-sion was modified to increase attention and motivation (e.g., by providing predictable breaks contingent upon on-task performance, allowing a child's mother to be present in the testing room, permitting the child to sit on the floor). However, unless the structure of the assessment session is adapted to fit the specific needs of the child with ASD, the "test session becomes one of assessing motivation, attention, or compliance more than of assessing language or intelligence" (Koegel et al., 1997, p. 241).

MEASURES OF INTELLECTUAL FUNCTIONING

Clinicians and researchers have a number of tools available to them for assessing the developmental level and intellectual ability of individu-als with ASD. Some of these measures were standardized on individuals with ASD, although inclusion criteria for each measure may have differed. However, other measures did not specifically include individuals with ASD during standardization, although individuals with ASD were not explicitly excluded according to the norming criteria provided in the technical manu-als. Table 8.1 briefly summarizes of the characteristics of the instruments reviewed below.

TABLE 8.1. Features of Available Cognitive and Adaptive Measures for Individuals with ASD

Measure	Age range	Administration time (minutes)	Required level of verbal ability[a]/Administration format[b]	Individuals with ASD included in standardization
		Cognitive measures		
Preschool age				
Bayley-III	1 to 42 m	30–90	V & NV	All five PDD diagnoses
DAS-II (Early Years battery)	2 y, 6 m to 3 y, 5 m	20	V & NV	None
WPPSI-III (young level)	2 y, 6 m to 3 y, 11 m	25–35	V	AD
Mullen	Birth to 5 y, 8 m	15–60	V	None
School age				
DAS-II (School-Age battery)	3 y, 6 m to 17 y, 11 m	30	V & NV	None
WPPSI-III (older level)	4 y, 0 m to 7 y, 3 m	40–50	V	AD
WISC-IV	6 y, 0 m to 16 y, 11 m	65–80	V	AD & AS
Leiter-R	2 y, 0 m to 20 y, 11 m	25–40	NV	None
Adult				
WAIS-III	16 to 89 y	65–95	V	None
Lifespan				
SB5	2 to 85 y	45–75	V & NV	AD
WASI	6 to 89 y	15–30	V	None
KBIT-2	4 to 90 y	15–30	V & NV	None
		Adaptive measures		
Vineland-II	Birth to 90 y	20–60	Interview or checklist	AD (V & NV)
ABAS-II	Birth to 89 y	20	Checklist	AD & AS
SIB-R	Infancy to over 80 y	15–60	Interview or checklist	None

Note: Bayley-III, Bayley Scales of Infant and Toddler Development, Third Edition; DAS-II, Differential Ability Scales—Second Edition; WPPSI-III, Wechsler Preschool and Primary Scale of Intelligence—Third Edition; Mullen, Mullen Scales of Early Learning; WISC-IV, Wechsler Intelligence Scale for Children—Fourth Edition; Leiter-R, Leiter International Performance Scale—Revised; WAIS-III, Wechsler Adult Intelligence Scale—Third Edition; SB5, Stanford–Binet Intelligence Scales, Fifth Edition; WASI, Wechsler Abbreviated Scale of Intelligence; KBIT-2, Kaufman Brief Intelligence Test, Second Edition; Vineland-II, Vineland Adaptive Behavior Scales, Second Edition; ABAS-II, Adaptive Behavior Assessment System—Second Edition; SIB-R, Scales of Independent Behavior—Revised; m, months; y, years; NV, nonverbal; V, verbal; PDD, pervasive developmental disorder; AD, autistic disorder; AS, Asperger syndrome; ASD, Autism spectrum disorders. [a]For cognitive measures. [b] For adaptive measures.

Bayley Scales of Infant and Toddler Development, Third Edition

The Bayley-III (Bayley, 2005) measures the strengths and abilities of children from 1 month to 42 months of age in the areas of cognitive, motor, language, social-emotional, and adaptive behaviors. Composite scores are available for each area assessed. Depending on a child's age, the Bayley-III can be administered in approximately 30–90 minutes. Administration time for the entire battery is approximately 50 minutes for children ages 12 months and younger, and approximately 90 minutes for children ages 13 months and older.

During standardization, data were collected on a group of 70 children between the ages of 16 months to 42 months who met DSM-IV criteria for a pervasive developmental disorder (PDD), including autistic disorder, Asperger's disorder, Rett's disorder, childhood disintegrative disorder, and PDD-NOS. On the Bayley-III, these children obtained significantly lower scores on all subtest scales (Cognitive, Receptive Communication, Expressive Communication, Fine Motor, Gross Motor, and Social-Emotional) and composite measures (Language and Motor) than did children in the matched control group.

The Bayley-III is one of the few standardized instruments that are available to evaluate young children with significant developmental delays who would not meet basal requirements on most preschool instruments, resulting in an inability to calculate meaningful standard scores. The most recent version of the Bayley was extended upward to include 3½-year-old children; thus the Bayley-III is a good choice for testing a 2- or 3-year-old who is functioning below the 24-month level of development. However, a standard score of 50 is the lowest score provided by the Bayley-III, making it impossible to get a specific standard score for extremely delayed children and necessitating the use of age equivalent scores. The Bayley-III can also be administered to a child older than 42 months to estimate the child's developmental level, if other measures are inappropriate due to a low mental age. However, these results must be interpreted cautiously, as a standard score cannot be computed.

Mullen Scales of Early Learning

The Mullen (Mullen, 1995) is designed to measure cognitive functioning in children from birth through 68 months of age. This instrument assesses a child's gross motor, fine motor, visual reception, receptive language, and expressive language abilities. Each of the individual scales yields T scores (mean = 50) and age equivalents. The Mullen also provides an overall Early Learning Composite standard score, which is based on the standardized T scores from the four cognitive scales (Visual Reception, Fine Motor, Receptive Language, and Expressive Language). The amount of time necessary to administer the Mullen varies between approximately 15 and 60 minutes, depending on a child's age, with older children requiring more time. During standardization of the Mullen, children with known physical or mental disabilities (including ASD) were not included in the sample.

Several recent studies have used the Mullen in young children with ASD (Akshoomoff, 2006; Landa & Garrett-Mayer, 2006). The Mullen was used to examine the early development of children at high risk for ASD at 6, 14, and 24 months of age in a prospective study conducted by Landa and Garrett-Mayer (2006). They separated children into three subgroups: children with ASD (showing clinical symptoms of autism), with language delay, or with no impairment. By 14 months of age, the children with ASD were delayed in all areas except the Visual Reception domain, compared to children in the no impairment group. In addition, the children with ASD showed higher Visual Reception scores than Receptive Language scores. This is consistent with the profile research described earlier in this chapter, indicating that preschool children with ASD show a strength in visual–spatial processing and a weakness in verbal processing. Nearly half of the group with ASD showed decreasing composite scores between 14 and 24 months, suggesting that this is a particularly vulnerable developmental period for children with ASD. It is difficult to know whether this indicates a true decline, whether children were experiencing a plateau in skill development leading to lower standard scores, or whether task demands at 24 months involved skills that are more specifically impaired in children with ASD.

Akshoomoff (2006) compared Mullen scores in children with ASD (16–43 months old) and an age-matched group of children with typical development. The children with ASD had significantly lower standard scores on every scale. In addition, the children with ASD performed relatively better on the Fine Motor scale and relatively worse on the Receptive Language scale, again supporting a specific weakness in verbal processing in young children with ASD.

Like the Bayley-III, the Mullen is one of the few standardized instruments that are available to evaluate young children with significant developmental delays who would not meet basal requirements on most preschool assessment instruments. The Mullen is appropriate for children up to 5½ years of age, and thus is a good choice for testing preschool-age children with significant delays. Because the Mullen covers the entire preschool-age range, it is also a good choice for early intervention studies examining change across the preschool years. However, even with this range, 73% of children with ASD in Akshoomoff's (2006) study received the lowest standard score (a T score of 20) provided by the Mullen on one or more scales. A T score of 20 is more than three standard deviations below average and represents an overall standard score of 55 or below. In this situation, age equivalent scores may be a more appropriate way to interpret test performance (Akshoomoff, 2006).

Differential Ability Scales—Second Edition

The Differential Ability Scales—Second Edition (DAS-II; Elliott, 2007) is a brief but comprehensive measure of ability, which makes it attractive for use with individuals with ASD. The DAS-II is designed to measure cognitive strengths and weaknesses in individuals between the ages of 2 years, 6 months and 17 years, 11 months. The Early Years battery, which was labeled the Preschool level in the original DAS (Elliott, 1990), consists of a lower level (four subtests for ages 2 years, 6 months to 3 years, 5 months, which take approximately 20 minutes to administer) and an upper level (six subtests for ages 3 years, 6 months to 6 years, 11 months, which take approximately 30 minutes to administer). The School-Age battery consists of six subtests for individuals ages 7 years, 0 months to 17 years, 11 months, which take approximately 40 minutes to administer. Testing at each level of the DAS-II yields a General Conceptual Ability (GCA) composite score. For the lower-level Early Years battery, cluster scores for Verbal Ability and Nonverbal Ability are also calculated. For both the upper-level Early Years and the School-Age batteries, cluster scores for Verbal Ability, Nonverbal Reasoning Ability, and Spatial Ability are calculated. In addition, for children 3 years, 6 months of age or older, a Special Nonverbal Composite may be derived from the appropriate nonverbal core subtests from each battery, which may be a useful measure of cognitive ability for nonverbal individuals with ASD. For individuals between the ages of 5 years, 0 months and 8 years, 11 months, examiners have the option of administering either the Early Years battery or the School-Age battery "out of level" to either lower- or higher-functioning individuals. The DAS-II provides norms for this full age range across the tasks contributing to these batteries; this is particularly useful for assessing an individual with ASD, as it allows for more accurate assessment based on the individual's mental rather than chronological age. Additional diagnostic subtests that measure working memory, processing speed, and school readiness are available for individuals of different ages in the DAS-II.

Unlike most other cognitive assessment instruments, the DAS-II does not require a strict administration order for its subtests, which allows the testing session to be individualized for each examinee. For example, it may be beneficial to begin with a nonverbal task for an individual with ASD, to build rapport and familiarity with the testing environment. An examiner may also choose to begin with a subtest that overlaps batteries, such as the Pattern Construction subtest, in order to observe and estimate informally the examinee's level of functioning (e.g., receptive and expressive language, cognitive flexibility) as a guide in selecting the most appropriate test battery (i.e., choosing either the Early Years or School-Age level, or only administering tasks that yield the Special Nonverbal Composite).

Because individuals with ASD were not included in the standardization samples, no information is available regarding specific profiles of individuals with ASD. Furthermore, given the newness of the DAS-II, no research studies are yet available regarding its utility with individuals with ASD. Joseph et al. (2002) administered the original version of the DAS (Elliott, 1990) to 120 individuals with autism who were considered high-functioning (i.e., mean GCA was 76.7 and 84.5 for the Preschool and School-Age levels of the DAS, respectively) in an exploration of cognitive profiles and symptomatology in ASD. A profile of higher nonverbal than verbal abilities was observed in 48% of the preschool-age group and 34% of the school-age group of children; this is consistent with research showing nonverbal–verbal discrepancies in preschool children with ASD. In comparison, a profile of higher verbal than nonverbal abilities was observed in 8% of preschool-age children and 28% of school-age children.

Overall, the DAS-II offers the opportunity to identify a child's specific strengths and weaknesses; is appropriate across a wide chronological and mental age range; and has some flexibility in test administration, which is helpful when testing children with ASD. Because of the large age range, the DAS-II may be a good choice for intervention studies that will use IQ testing as one measure of outcome across an extended period of time. However, the DAS-II is less useful in testing young children with ASD who are performing below the 2½-year level, as they are unlikely to meet basal requirements on most subtests, resulting in an inability to calculate meaningful standard scores.

Stanford–Binet Intelligence Scales, Fifth Edition

The SB5 (Roid, 2003) assesses intelligence and cognitive abilities in individuals from 2 to 85+ years of age. To obtain a Full Scale IQ, the SB5 requires an average of 45–75 minutes of testing time. In addition, the SB5 contains separate sections for Nonverbal IQ (based on five nonverbal subtests) and Verbal IQ (based on five verbal subtests), which can be useful for testing individuals with ASD who are nonverbal or have limited language abilities. Each of these sections requires approximately 30 minutes. In addition, five factor scores can be computed (Fluid Reasoning, Knowledge, Quantitative Reasoning, Visual–Spatial Processing, and Working Memory); these can be used to identify a pattern of strengths and weaknesses in performance. Each factor score includes a verbal and a nonverbal subtest. Moreover, an Abbreviated Battery IQ can be calculated from two subtests if necessary. This is often helpful when the child is displaying difficulty attending to task demands and the examiner is concerned about being able to complete the lengthier full battery of tests. The SB5 revision was designed to make the test more sensitive to assessing younger children with developmental delays than the previous version.

The SB5 standardization sample included 83 children and adolescents with diagnoses of autistic disorder between the ages of 2 and 17 years. This sample included 79% males and was predominantly European American. Individuals with autistic disorder performed similarly to those in the developmental delay group, but had slightly lower means on all subtest and composite scales. Although no studies to date have looked for a specific pattern of subtest performance on the SB5 in children with ASD, several studies have examined the performance of children with ASD on the fourth edition of this test (SB-IV; Carpentieri & Morgan, 1994; Harris, Handleman, & Burton, 1990; Mayes & Calhoun, 2003). Overall, children with ASD were found to be more impaired on verbal reasoning tasks (especially the Absurdities task, which requires social comprehension and reasoning) than on nonverbal reasoning tasks (such as Pattern Analysis, Bead Memory, or Quantitative Reasoning, which involve visual-perceptual skills). The children with ASD obtained verbal reasoning scores that were significantly lower than those of chronological-age-matched children with mental retardation (Carpentieri & Morgan, 1994). Further research is needed to identify the profile of SB5 scores in children with ASD.

Because of its wide age range, the SB5 may be an appropriate measure for testing a child with significant developmental delays (e.g., a 10-year-old child with the mental age of a preschool child) who might not meet basal requirements on tests that are solely developed for school-age children. In addition, the SB5 may be a good choice for intervention studies that will use IQ testing as one measure of outcome across an extended period of time. Although the SB5 provides a Nonverbal IQ score that may be appropriate for children with limited language, some of the nonverbal tasks require imitation and receptive language skills, which are both areas of weakness in children with ASD. For example, the Nonverbal Working Memory task requires the child to imitate the examiner's motor movements by tapping a series of blocks. At a more sophisticated level, children are asked to imitate the examiner's movements in reverse order, requiring that the child understand the verbal directions to do so. Thus the nonverbal measures on the SB5 are not completely independent of language understanding and can be negatively affected by symptoms of ASD.

Wechsler Preschool and Primary Scale of Intelligence—Third Edition

The Wechsler Preschool and Primary Scale of Intelligence—Third Edition (WPPSI-III; Wechsler, 2002) is designed to assess intelligence in children ages 2 years, 6 months through 7 years, 3 months. For younger children (2 years, 6 months to 3 years, 11 months), the WPPSI-III yields a Verbal IQ, a Performance IQ, an overall Full Scale IQ, and an optional supplemental General Language Composite. The core subtests can be completed in 25–35 minutes for this age group. For older children (4 years, 0 months to 7 years, 3 months), the WPPSI-III yields a Verbal IQ, a Performance IQ, a Full Scale IQ, and an optional supplemental Processing Speed Quotient. For older children, the core subtests can be completed in approximately 40–50 minutes.

To determine the clinical utility of the WPPSI-III, a group of 21 children between the ages of 3 years, 0 months and 6 years, 11 months who met DSM-IV criteria for autistic disorder were included in the standardization sample. This group of children contained more males than females, to reflect the higher prevalence rate of autistic disorder in males. Children were excluded from this group if they had existing overall cognitive ability scores more than 2.67 standard deviations below the mean. On all composites, children in the autistic disorder group scored significantly lower than the matched control group. As expected from research on intellectual profiles in children with ASD, they obtained higher mean Performance IQ scores than Verbal IQ scores. Scaled scores on all subtests, except for the Block Design and Object Assembly subtests, were lower for the children in the autistic disorder group than for the control group.

Because the WPPSI-III provides both Verbal and Performance IQ scores, it offers an opportunity to identify a pattern of strengths and weaknesses in children with ASD. However, some of the Performance IQ tasks require language understanding; thus the Performance IQ score is not completely independent of a child's language delays. The WPPSI-III was extended to include both younger preschool-age children and older children entering elementary school, making it appropriate for beginning school-age children who have significant developmental delays. However, the WPPSI-III is less useful for testing 2- and 3-year-old children with ASD who are performing below the 2½-year level, as they are unlikely to meet basal requirements on most subtests, resulting in an inability to calculate meaningful standard scores.

Wechsler Intelligence Scale for Children—Fourth Edition

The WISC-IV (Wechsler, 2003) is designed to assess intelligence in children ages 6 years, 0 months to 16 years, 11 months. It yields scores in the cognitive domains of Verbal Comprehension, Perceptual Reasoning, Working Memory, and Processing Speed, as well as providing a composite Full Scale IQ score. The amount of time required to administer the WISC-IV varies, depending on the number of subtests administered to the child, but administration of the 10 core subtests can be completed within approximately 65–80 minutes. During standardization testing, 182 children ages 6–7 years were given both the WISC-IV and the WPPSI-III. There was less than a 1-point difference between the two tests on the corresponding Index and Full Scale IQ scores (Wechsler, 2003). Thus the WISC-IV may be a good choice for reevaluating a child who has previously been given the WPPSI-III.

A sample of 19 children between the ages of 7 and 16 years who met DSM-IV criteria for autistic disorder were included in the standardization sample. This sample included 89% males, and all children received an IQ score above 60. Compared to a matched control group of children, the children with autistic disorder scored significantly lower on all composites. There were also significant group differences on all subtests except Block Design and Arithmetic. For children with autistic disorder, there was some support for a higher Perceptual Reasoning Index score than a Verbal Comprehension Index score, although the difference was relatively small (5.5 points).

Lincoln et al. (2007) administered the WISC-IV to a sample of 41 children between the ages of 6 and 14 years who met DSM-IV criteria for autistic disorder. These children showed the strongest performance on the Block Design subtest and the weakest performance on the Comprehension subtest. In comparison to the standardization sample, the children in Lincoln and colleagues' younger sample showed a much larger discrepancy (18.5 points) between the Perceptual Reasoning Index and Verbal Comprehension Index scores. When children with IQ scores below 60 were excluded, the large discrepancy remained (16.7 points). More research is needed to confirm whether the profile of scores on the WISC-IV will parallel research on the WISC-III suggesting that visual–verbal processing differences are most pronounced in younger and more intellectually delayed individuals with ASD (Lincoln et al., 1995; Manjiviona & Prior, 1999; Mayes & Calhoun, 2003).

In the standardization testing, an additional group of 27 children between the ages of 9 and 15 years who met DSM-IV criteria for Asperger's disorder were administered the WISC-IV. This group consisted of 93% males, and children were excluded if they had existing overall cognitive ability scores lower than 70. In this sample, the individuals in the Asperger's disorder group exhibited significantly lower performance on the Processing Speed Index, Working Memory Index, and Full Scale IQ when compared to a matched control group. These results are consistent with previous research on the WISC-III showing difficulties on timed motor tests such as the Coding and Symbol Search subtests, as well as with reported motor awkwardness and clumsiness in children with Asperger syndrome (Mayes & Calhoun, 2003, 2004).

Because the WISC-IV provides separate measures of verbal and non-verbal reasoning, working memory, and processing speed, it provides an opportunity to identify a pattern of strengths and weaknesses in children with ASD. The addition of the Working Memory Index and Processing Speed Index to the WISC-IV provides measurement of the poor motor skills and attention difficulties experienced by individuals with ASD. However, the use of timed tests and the need for verbal understanding even on measures of perceptual reasoning may lead examiners to underestimate the nonverbal abilities of some individuals with ASD (Klin et al., 2005). Furthermore, younger school-age children with significant delays are unlikely to meet basal requirements on most subtests, resulting in an inability to calculate meaningful standard scores.

Wechsler Adult Intelligence Scale—Third Edition

The Wechsler Adult Intelligence Scale—Third Edition (WAIS-III; Wechsler, 1997) is designed to assess intelligence in individuals between the ages of 16 and 89 years. Based on the 11 core subtests, Verbal IQ, Performance IQ, and Full Scale IQ scores are computed. An additional two subtests can be administered to compute Index scores for Verbal Comprehension, Perceptual Organization, Working Memory, and Processing Speed abilities. The standardization data indicate that administration of the 11 subtests required to calculate IQ scores can be completed in approximately 75 minutes (range = 60–90 minutes). Administration of the 13 subtests required to calculate IQ and Index scores can be completed in approximately 80 minutes (range = 65–95 minutes). During the standardization process of the WAIS-III, individuals with ASD were not excluded from the sample, but this group was not included during the validation process. However, individuals with other psychoeducational and developmental disorders, such as mental retardation, attention-deficit/hyperactivity disorder (ADHD), deafness/hearing impairment, or learning disabilities in reading and math were included in the clinical group.

Because ASD was not specifically examined in the standardization sample, no information is available regarding specific profiles of individuals with ASD. Furthermore, few publications have examined the WAIS-III in this population. Previous studies examining profiles on the previous version of the WAIS (WAIS-R) reported the typical pattern of a strength on the Block Design subtest and a weakness on the Comprehension subtest (Goldstein, Beers, Siegel, & Minshew, 2001). More research is needed to examine the profile associated with ASD on the WAIS-III. The fact that the WAIS-III provides separate measures of verbal and nonverbal reasoning, along with the more specific Index scores measuring Verbal Comprehension, Perceptual Organization, Working Memory, and Processing Speed, suggests that the WAIS-III may be a good choice for identifying a profile of strengths and weaknesses in adults with ASD. However, as with the WISC-IV, the use of timed tests and the need for verbal understanding even on measures included in the Performance IQ score may lead examiners to underestimate the nonverbal abilities of some individuals with ASD.

Leiter International Performance Scale—Revised

The Leiter-R (Roid & Miller, 1997) is designed to assess nonverbal intellectual ability, memory, and attention in children and adolescents between the ages of 2 years, 0 months and 20 years, 11 months. Administration requires no verbal instructions from the examiner or verbal responses from the child. This instrument contains 20 subtests, which are equally divided between a Visualization and Reasoning Battery and an Attention and Memory Battery. Although the number of subtests administered varies according to the child's age, the two batteries combined can generally be completed within 90 minutes. In addition to a Full Scale IQ score, a Brief IQ screener can be computed based on four subtests. The Brief IQ screener can be completed in approximately 25 minutes, while the Full Scale IQ measure requires approximately 40 minutes to administer. In a comparison of the Leiter-R Brief and Full Scale IQ scores in a group of children with autism and language limitations, Tsatsanis et al. (2003) found a very strong relationship ($r = .97$) between these two measures of intelligence. Thus the Leiter-R Brief IQ is particularly useful when a child is unable to complete the full battery of tests.

Although children with ASD were not among the special groups included in the Leiter-R standardization sample, the test was administered to 634 individuals with other developmental, sensory, or learning difficulties. These included children diagnosed with severe speech/language impairment; severe hearing impairment; severe motor delay or deviation; traumatic brain injury; significant cognitive delay (mild, moderate, or severe mental retardation); ADHD with and without hyperactivity; learning disability—nonverbal type; and learning disability—verbal type.

When investigating the profile of scores obtained on the Leiter-R in a group of children with autism who had limited language abilities and low nonverbal IQ (average Leiter-R Brief IQ of 68), Tsatsanis et al. (2003) found that in three out of four cases, these children performed significantly better on the Fundamental Visualization composite than on Fluid Reasoning. These findings are consistent with research findings of higher perceptual and visual–spatial reasoning skills in children with ASD. Kuschner, Bennetto, and Yost (2007) used the Leiter-R Brief IQ to examine the cognitive profile of preschool-age children with high-functioning ASD (average Leiter-R Brief IQ of 80). They found that, compared with children of similar chronological and nonverbal mental age with developmental delays, the children with ASD showed specific strengths in tasks measuring the ability to focus on specific visual details (Figure Ground subtest) and to mentally manipulate and synthesize visual information (Form Completion subtest). The children with ASD were specifically impaired on a subtest measuring abstract reasoning and concept formation (Repeated Patterns subtest). These results suggest that children with ASD do not have overall strengths in nonverbal processing, and instead have strengths in visual perception. This is consistent with cognitive theories of ASD, including the theories of weak central coherence (Happé & Frith, 2006) and enhanced perceptual processing (Mottron et al., 2006).

The Leiter-R is an excellent choice for testing either a nonverbal child with ASD or a child with significantly impaired receptive and expressive language. This is one of the few tests that would be appropriate for an older child with a very small vocabulary (e.g., a 15-year-old who is able to speak in single words only). An additional strength of the Leiter-R is the presence of teaching trials, including demonstrating and even taking the child's hand to teach task demands. However, a great many instructions are provided via gestures and facial expressions—both social stimuli that are very difficult for children with ASD to understand. Furthermore, this test is not appropriate for young delayed children. As on other tests that begin at the 2½-year range, preschool children with ASD who have developmental delays are unlikely to understand task demands and achieve a basal score on the Leiter-R.

Brief IQ Measures

Brief IQ measures are frequently used when time constraints do not allow administration of an entire battery. When a full battery of tests is desired, but the examiner is unsure whether a child will be able to maintain attention and motivation, it is often helpful to administer a measure with a short form that allows IQ to be calculated from performance on a few subtests. Both the SB5 and the Leiter-R have these types of brief IQ measures, which provide standardized scores based on their respective standardization samples. However, when the original purpose is to use a brief IQ measure—as is often the case when a lengthy research battery is being administered—the examiner can choose a stand-alone brief measure of intelligence.

Wechsler Abbreviated Scale of Intelligence

The Wechsler Abbreviated Scale of Intelligence (WASI; Wechsler, 1999) was developed to be a short measure of intelligence that can be used in clinical, psychoeducational, and research settings for individuals between the ages of 6 and 89 years. The two-subtest form of the WASI requires approximately 15 minutes to complete, and the four-subtest form can be completed in approximately 30 minutes. The profile of scores available from the WASI includes Verbal IQ, Performance IQ, and Full Scale IQ. Although individuals with ASD were not excluded from the WASI standardization sample, they were also not included as a special group while the clinical validity of this measure was being established. The clinical populations assessed with the WASI included individuals with mental retardation, ADHD, learning disabilities in reading and math, and traumatic brain injury.

Kaufman Brief Intelligence Test, Second Edition

The Kaufman Brief Intelligence Test, Second Edition (KBIT-2; Kaufman & Kaufman, 2004) is designed to be a brief measure of verbal and nonverbal intelligence for individuals ages 4 through 90 years. The KBIT-2 requires approximately 15–30 minutes to administer and yields a Verbal domain score, a Nonverbal domain score, and an IQ Composite score. During the standardization process, ASD was not included as an exclusionary condition, but it was also not included within the sample of conditions or diagnoses for validity purposes. The special populations included in the standardization sample were individuals with learning disability, speech–language disorders, ADHD, mental retardation, traumatic brain injury, and dementia.

MEASURES OF ADAPTIVE BEHAVIOR

Assessments of individuals with any suspected developmental disability, including ASD, should include a measure of adaptive functioning in addition to cognitive functioning. This is necessary for classification and diagnostic purposes (e.g., ascertaining whether an individual meets criteria for mental retardation), as well as in determining an individual's personal strengths and weaknesses beyond cognitive ability. Measures of adaptive functioning are also useful in planning interventions and for measuring response to intervention, as they do not necessarily involve the risk of practice effects from repeated administration.

A survey by Luiselli et al. (2001) of assessment practices of national service centers for individuals with autism in 30 states in the United States reported that 60.6% of centers reported using the original version of the Vineland Adaptive Behavior Scales (Sparrow, Balla, & Cicchetti, 1984) as their primary measure of adaptive behavior, and a review of available research in the area of ASD would certainly support similar popularity in research protocols as well. In addition to the recent revision of this instrument—the Vineland Adaptive Behavior Scales, Second Edition (Vineland-II; Sparrow, Cicchetti, & Balla, 2005)—there are several other measures of adaptive behavior, including the Adaptive Behavior Assessment System—Second Edition (ABAS-II; Harrison & Oakland, 2003) and the Scales of Independent Behavior—Revised (SIB-R; Bruininks, Woodcock, Weatherman, & Hill, 1996). All three of these measures offer potential benefits for clinicians and researchers working with individuals with ASD that warrant discussion. Each of these measures is reviewed below and is also summarized in Table 8.1.

Vineland Adaptive Behavior Scales, Second Edition

As noted above, the Vineland-II (Sparrow et al., 2005) is a recent revision of the widely popular Vineland Adaptive Behavior Scales (Sparrow et al., 1984). Although it is very similar in format to the former version, the Vineland-II represents efforts to obtain a more sensitive measure of developmental change in the early childhood years and throughout the lifespan. There are several versions of administration: two survey forms (a 383-item Survey Interview Form, which is administered by an examiner, and a Parent/Caregiver Rating Form, which is a checklist); an Expanded Interview Form, which permits more comprehensive assessment for use in planning interventions; and a Teacher Rating Form, which is based on classroom observation and focuses on academic functioning. The Survey Interview Form may be completed in 20–60 minutes, and the Parent/Caregiver Rating Form generally takes between 30 and 60 minutes to complete. The Vineland-II may be used with individuals from birth to age 90 to assess functioning in four domains and 11 subdomains. Individuals 7 years, 0 months and older are assessed in the domains of Communication (Receptive, Expressive, and Written); Daily Living Skills (Personal, Domestic, and Community); and Socialization (Interpersonal Relationships, Play and Leisure Time, and Coping Skills). Children 6 years, 11 months of age and younger are assessed on an additional Motor Skills domain (Gross and Fine). An optional Maladaptive Behavior Index consisting of three subscales (Internalizing, Externalizing, and Other), and a group of Maladaptive Critical Items, are available for individuals older than 3 years and provide additional measures of how an individual's adaptive functioning may be limited by difficult behaviors. Standard scores with a mean of 100 (standard deviation = 15) are calculated for each of the four domains and for an overall Adaptive Behavior Composite. Age equivalents are available for subdomains, but not for summary domains.

The Vineland-II manual provides data regarding 77 individuals with autism that were obtained during standardization. This sample included 31 children between the ages of 2 and 10 who were considered nonverbal (i.e., using five or fewer words) and 46 individuals between the ages of 3 and 19 who were considered verbal. Significant differences ($p < .01$) were obtained for both groups in comparison to an age-matched nonclinical reference group for the domain, subdomain, and Adaptive Behavior Composite scores. Adaptive Behavior Composite means were 50.7 for the nonverbal group and 65.7 for the verbal group. For the verbal group, the lowest domain score was found in Socialization. In both groups, the largest adaptive functioning deficits were found in the Interpersonal Relationships, Play and Leisure Time, and Expressive Language subdomains. Within the Maladaptive domain, both groups obtained significantly higher mean scores on the Internalizing subscale than the nonclinical sample did, but their Externalizing subscale scores were within the average range. The nonverbal group was rated overall as having more maladaptive behaviors than the verbal group, with scores in the elevated range.

Although the Vineland-II is too recent to have been widely studied for individuals with ASD, a wealth of literature is available regarding how individuals with ASD typically score on the original measure. Vineland profiles have been studied in individuals with varying levels of ASD and cognitive ability across the age span, with overall patterns of results indicating that individuals with ASD show the greatest deficits in the area of Socialization, moderate impairments in Communication, and relative strengths in Daily Living Skills and Motor Skills (Bölte & Poustka, 2002; Loveland & Kelley, 1991; Rodrigue, Morgan, & Geffken, 1991; Volkmar et al., 1987). Others have replicated the finding of lower Socialization skills, but have also found relative deficits in Daily Living Skills and Communication (Gillham, Carter, Volkmar, & Sparrow, 2000; Stone, Ousley, Hepburn, Hogan, & Brown, 1999; Szatmari, Archer, Fisman, & Streiner, 1994). A number of researchers have also found evidence that Vineland score profiles may be useful in distinguishing individuals with ASD from those with mental retardation, other developmental delay, or other clinical disorders (Gillham et al., 2000; Paul et al., 2004; Stone et al., 1999).

Adaptive Behavior Assessment System—Second Edition

The ABAS-II (Harrison & Oakland, 2003) provides five different forms to be used across the age range of birth to 89 years, each of which takes about 20 minutes to complete. Each form is completed by the relevant rater. A Parent/Primary Caregiver Form and a Teacher/Day Care Form are available for children. The Adult Form can be self-rated or completed by a family member, or by a supervisor or other respondent familiar with the individual. In addition to rating the frequency of behaviors, raters are asked to check a box for each item indicating whether they guessed about the individual's performance for that item, which allows for interpreting whether the respondent is an appropriate rater for the individual being assessed. The ABAS-II describes the level of an individual's functional skills that are required for daily living (i.e., self-care and interactions with others) without the assistance of others. Specific skill areas assessed by the ABAS-II include Communication, Community Use (depending on the individual's age), Functional (Pre-)Academics, Home/School Living (depending on the rater), Motor (depending on the individual's age), Health and Safety, Leisure, Self-Care, Self-Direction, Social, and Work (depending on whether the individual is employed). Scores for each skill area are combined into three separate Adaptive Domain composite scores: Conceptual (communication and academic skills), Social (interpersonal and social competence skills), and Practical (independent living and daily living skills). The sum of scaled scores for each skill area is also used to calculate a General Adaptive Composite (GAC). Each composite score has a mean of 100 and standard deviation of 15. The Vineland-II (Sparrow et al., 2005) reports moderate to high correlations with scores from the ABAS-II.

The authors of the ABAS-II made efforts to include individuals with a representative range of clinical diagnoses in the standardization sample, including individuals with diagnoses of PDD-NOS and autistic disorder. These diagnoses were represented in development of the Parent/Primary Caregiver and Teacher/Day Care Forms specifically. Reliability coefficients for individuals within these groups were high ($r \geq .92$ for composites). In a comparison of the children with autistic disorder to age-matched controls, the clinical group showed significant deficits in each skill area, adaptive domain, and the GAC (e.g., mean GAC between 64 and 67), with the largest skill deficits in the areas of Communication, Health and Safety, Leisure, and Social. Functional Pre-Academics emerged as a strength for the children below the age of 6 years, but their scaled score mean was still below one standard deviation below the mean for the measure. To date, there are no published studies using the ABAS-II with individuals with ASD.

Scales of Independent Behavior—Revised

The SIB-R (Bruininks et al., 1996) measures both adaptive and problem behaviors in individuals from infancy to over 80 years of age. The SIB-R is available in three separate forms, any of which may be administered as a structured interview or as a checklist completed directly by the respondent. The Full Scale form takes less than an hour to complete, addressing a range of adaptive skills in four clusters consisting of 14 subscales. Specific areas assessed include Motor Skills (Gross and Fine Motor subscales); Social and Communication Skills (Social Interaction, Language Comprehension, and Language Expression subscales); Personal Living Skills (Eating and Meal

Preparation, Toileting, Dressing, Personal Self-Care, and Domestic Skills subscales); and Community Living Skills (Time and Punctuality, Money and Value, Work Skills, and Home/Community Orientation subscales). The two additional forms of the SIB-R are the Short Form (a screening measure consisting of items selected from all 14 subscales of the Full Scale form) and an Early Development form (for use with children from early infancy through 6 years, or with older individuals whose developmental levels are below 8 years of age). The Early Development form includes items sampled from the Full Scale form that are useful in assessing development of an individual. Each of the short forms takes between 15 and 20 minutes to complete. All three SIB-R forms also include questions to address Maladaptive Behavior. Moreover, the SIB-R includes Individual Plan Recommendations forms designed to aid in planning and monitoring interventions for individuals based on the obtained SIB-R scores.

As with other measures, a Broad Independence score is calculated with a mean of 100 and a standard deviation of 15 that summarizes overall adaptive skill. A unique feature of the SIB-R, however, is the calculation of a Support Score, which combines the individual's adaptive level (70% of the Support Score) and the presence, frequency, and severity of maladaptive behaviors (30% of the Support Score). The Support Score is intended to describe an individual's overall functional independence and level of need for support and supervision.

Children and adults with mild, moderate, and severe mental retardation as well as high ability, and children from special education classes or programs described as exhibiting chronic aggression, behavior disorders, learning disabilities, or hearing impairments, were included in standardization procedures. However, there was no specific inclusion or description of individuals with ASD in the SIB-R development. Furthermore, no published studies of using the SIB-R with individuals with ASD are available.

GUIDELINES FOR CHOOSING ASSESSMENT INSTRUMENTS

As is clear from this review, there are multiple options for assessment of cognitive and adaptive functioning in individuals with ASD. Unlike some other aspects of assessment, such as determining appropriate diagnosis, there is no clear "gold standard" for assessing either area of functioning in children, adolescents, or adults with ASD. Instead, the flexibility of available instruments allows researchers and clinicians to adopt an *individualized* assessment approach rather than a static ASD cognitive and adaptive battery. The present review of existing measures and assessment issues indicates that examiners should take the following considerations into account when choosing the appropriate tools for a cognitive and/or adaptive assessment.

Considerations in Choosing a Measure of Cognitive Ability

Language Ability

One of the most limiting factors in cognitive assessment of an individual with ASD is often the verbal ability of the examinee. Some of the available measures permit separate assessment of nonverbal and verbal ability in producing qualitatively and quantitatively useful scores. However, some assessments, including the Wechsler intelligence tests and the SB5, require a certain level of receptive language for the examinee to understand nonverbal task directions. As a result, determining both the individual's level of language use and his or her level of understanding of verbal directions is essential in choosing an appropriate measure. Even when the nonverbal tasks are appropriate, individuals with limited language may not receive any credit on the language measures, resulting in an invalid assessment.

For older children who have no or limited language, the Leiter-R is an appropriate choice, as no language use on the part of the examiner or examinee is required. Although the Leiter-R is normed for children from 2 years of age onward, young nonverbal children with ASD may not understand task directions and may not be able to complete enough items to obtain a valid score. For these children, instruments that are appropriate from birth onward (i.e., the Bayley-III or the Mullen) may be the most beneficial.

Chronological Age and Developmental Level

With measures available spanning the age range from birth to 90 years, there is no age level at which an individual's ability may not be assessed. In measuring cognitive skills, it is best to choose a measure for which population norms are available for the individual's chronological age. Choosing an age-appropriate measure will add to the reliability and validity of the scores yielded by a cognitive measure, and will aid in greater understanding regarding the individual's abilities. When several measures are appropriate, the examiner should consider choosing an instrument that is appropriate for children several years younger than the examinee. For example, when deciding which developmental test to administer to a 3-year-old with ASD, the examiner has a wide range of tests that are appropriate for the child's chronological age, including the Bayley-III, the Mullen, DAS-II, SB5, and WPPSI-III. However, if the child is delayed, he may have difficulty completing tests that are designed for children 2½ years of age or older, and floor effects are likely. Thus the examiner might consider a developmental test that is appropriate for children several years younger, such as the Bayley-III or the Mullen. In the case that the age-appropriate measure is too diffi-cult (e.g., requires too much receptive or expressive language) and no other instruments are available, it is reasonable to choose an alternative measure that may provide age equivalents rather than standard scores. For example, if an individual is 5½ years through adulthood in chronological age, but below 2½ years in mental age, there is no appropriate instrument. In this case, either the Bayley-III or Mullen may be administered, and age equiva-lent scores should be calculated.

Behavioral Difficulties

Even when the testing session is structured as described earlier in this chap-ter, some examinees may exhibit behavioral difficulties that make it diffi-cult to complete a lengthy evaluation or raise concerns about the validity of the results. Behavioral difficulties are often a sign of frustration and fatigue in individuals with ASD. Examiners are therefore encouraged to choose the most succinct measure that will yield informative data for the purpose of the assessment when individuals have short attention spans or low toler-ance of seated, formalized testing. This approach will prove much more satisfying for both examiners and examinees than choosing a standard test or group of tests for every individual will. The DAS-II was designed to be a relatively quick assessment instrument and is a good choice when time is a concern; in addition, for children older than 2½ years of age, a brief IQ can be obtained after the first few subtests are completed. The KBIT-2 is also appropriate for children at least 4 years of age, and the WASI is appropriate for children at least 6 years of age.

The Purpose of the Assessment

Determining the need for an assessment and the value of its results for the individual with ASD is of ultimate importance in choosing a measure of cognitive ability. The underlying need for the assessment is typically for a comprehensive measure of a range of cognitive abilities, but in other situa-tions a screener of general cognitive ability will suffice. Examiners should keep in mind what will happen to the scores after the assessment is com-pleted as well. For example, certain agencies (e.g., school systems) may only accept comprehensive measures and full scale IQs or composite scores when making eligibility decisions. If an assessment is intended to be part of a series of administrations to track an individual's development over time, one of the instruments that covers a wider age range may be of preference (e.g., the SB5 for the entire lifespan, the Mullen for measurements across the preschool years, or the Leiter-R or DAS-II for multiple assessments throughout childhood and adolescence).

Because of the uneven profile of strengths and weaknesses character-izing individuals with ASD, an examiner is often faced with the decision to choose an instrument that highlights an examinee's strengths or weak-nesses. For example, a child with limited language but good nonverbal per-ception abilities may receive higher scores on a nonverbal IQ test such as the Leiter-R, but perform much more poorly on a test with receptive and expressive language demands such as the WISC-IV. This choice between these measures depends on the purpose of the evaluation. If the goal of the evaluation is to highlight the fact that the child is not developmentally delayed in all areas, and in fact has some age-level skills, the Leiter-R may be a good choice. However, if the purpose of the assessment is to identify strengths and weaknesses that may have an impact on school performance, a test that includes verbal ability is important for providing a good predic-tor of the child's performance in a classroom that requires verbal compre-hension and expression. Identifying the child's verbal weaknesses is likely to result in additional school accommodations; this may not occur if only a nonverbal IQ test is administered.

Considerations in Choosing an Adaptive Behavior Measure

With several available measures of adaptive functioning that are gener-ally similar in underlying concepts, type of information obtained, and age ranges of the standardization, the main decision for an examiner lies in whether detailed, qualitative information or simply a quick measure of an individual's adaptive level is needed. Test format is another consideration. Both the Vineland-II and the SIB-R are available in both interview and checklist forms, while the ABAS-II is exclusively a checklist. Still another aspect to consider in choosing an adaptive measure is the desired respon-dent (i.e., parent/caregiver, teacher, employer, or the examinee him- or her-self). The ABAS-II provides forms for the largest range of respondents, including a self-report, but the Vineland-II and the SIB-R also both allow data from caregivers and teachers to be obtained. Examiners are encour-aged to obtain data regarding adaptive functioning from multiple respon-dents when possible, particularly in clinical assessments, because research has found that parents and other raters tend to provide qualitatively differ-ent data from their different perspectives on an individual. For example, Szatmari et al. (1994) reported that while overall correlations of parent and teacher reports were good, teachers rated individuals with PDD as having higher adaptive skills on the Vineland than their parents did. Furthermore, parental reports on the Vineland yielded greater distinction at the subdo-main level between individuals with high-functioning autism and Asperger syndrome than were apparent from teacher reports (Szatmari et al., 1994); this suggests that researchers interested in distinguishing among ASD subtypes should carefully consider the feasibility of multiple respondents as well.

Given that the newest versions of the available adaptive measures have taken efforts to expand the available variability of scores for very young children with ASD, it may also be possible to choose any of these measures to assess response to intervention. For example, a screener form of the Vineland showed promise in detecting progress in preschool-age children over an 11-month period, with gains in the Vineland domain scores reported after a year of schooling was received (Charman, Howlin, Berry, & Prince, 2004).

SUMMARY

In this chapter, we have asserted that there is no "best test" for measuring intellectual functioning in persons with ASD. Because of the uneven profiles that characterize individuals with ASD and the behavioral difficulties that often occur during standardized testing, the examiner needs to have experience administering and interpreting standardized assessments and an understanding of how the symptoms of ASD may interfere with test performance. The examiner is encouraged to provide additional structure to increase the examinee's attention and motivation to complete the assessment, while still maintaining a standardized test administration. In addition, it is important to choose the right instrument in order to ensure that an accurate estimate of developmental ability is obtained. The examiner is encouraged to consider the following sequence of questions when deciding which test is most appropriate:

1. Which instruments are appropriate for the examinee's chronological age?
2. Is the child nonverbal, necessitating a nonverbal IQ test?
3. Given the examinee's estimated mental age, is it appropriate to choose a test that extends several years below the examinee's chronological age? If there are no appropriate measures that include both the examinee's chronological age and expected mental age, is a test that provides age equivalents available?
4. Is a full battery or a brief IQ score more appropriate? The answer to this question depends on whether the referral agency would prefer one type of measure and whether behavioral difficulties may interfere with testing success.

5. If the assessment is being conducted to measure whether the examinee is showing an increase or decrease in skills across time, which measure is most appropriate, given the proposed range of assessments? For example, if the child was previously evaluated with a Wechsler scale, it may be most appropriate to administer another Wechsler scale. If the child is participating in a longitudinal research project, which measure is most appropriate, given the proposed age range of the study?

6. Is the assessment being conducted to highlight the individual's strengths or to highlight areas of weakness that may need additional intervention? This is particularly important if the examinee has discrepant verbal and nonverbal abilities.

CASE STUDY

At the beginning of this chapter, we introduced Jason, a young boy with a diagnosis of autistic disorder, and raised a question about which IQ test would be the most appropriate for him. After interviewing his mother to obtain his developmental and social history, we used the questions above to choose an appropriate test. Below is a summary of the developmental history that we obtained, a discussion of our decision-making process in choosing IQ and adaptive behavior instruments, a condensed version of the test results, and a discussion of the appropriateness of these results in addressing the referral questions.

Developmental and Social History

Jason, age 8 years, 6 months, was referred to the autism clinic by his school system. An updated evaluation was requested to provide additional recommendations for school accommodations. Jason was currently in the third grade. He received resource room services daily for reading and math, and spent the remainder of his day in a regular education classroom. He also received speech therapy services two times per week for 30 minutes each time.

Jason's mother reported that she first became concerned about Jason's development when he was 12 months old, because he was not responding to his name and had not yet begun to speak. Although his motor milestones developed within normal limits (e.g., he walked at 11 months), Jason's language was delayed. He spoke his first words at 2½ years and did not combine words into short sentences until he was 3½ years old. His mother reported that Jason did not use gestures, eye contact, or facial expressions to help compensate for his language difficulties. He was diagnosed with autistic disorder at the age of 3 years.

In the area of language and communication skills, Jason's mother reported that he had an extensive vocabulary, although the majority of his speech consisted of delayed echolalia, in which he repeated lines from his favorite movies. She noted that it was difficult to hold a conversation with Jason because he did not comment on remarks made by others, responded only when asked a direct question, and tended to initiate only conversations that were related to his own interests. He occasionally mixed up his pronouns, referring to himself as "you" and other people as "I," although this was much improved from when he was a preschooler. He had learned to use gestures such as nodding his head "yes" or "no," but did not use descriptive gestures.

In the area of social development, Jason's mother reported that he referred to his classmates as his "friends," but that these friendships were not reciprocated and he did not see these children outside of school. His mother commented that Jason often watched other children and seemed to want to join in their games. However, he rarely approached other children, and she thought that he didn't know how to join their activities. When other children approached Jason, he was beginning to respond to them, but typically insisted that they play games according to his own rules. His eye contact had improved from his preschool years, especially with familiar people, although it was mostly fleeting.

In the area of repetitive behavior and play, Jason's mother reported that he was "obsessed" with stuffed animals (Beanie Babies) and has collected hundreds of them. She noted that he had memorized the names and "birthdates" of every animal in his collection. He spent his free time either reading the guide that described the characteristics of each of the stuffed animals in his collection or arranging his animals into geometric shapes and patterns. His mother noted that Jason was excellent at completing puzzles and could even complete them "upside down" (i.e., when he was only looking at the blank cardboard on the back of the pieces).

Choosing an Appropriate IQ Test and Structuring the Environment

We used the sequence of questions recommended earlier to identify the appropriate IQ test for Jason. Because his mother wanted a comprehensive evaluation to identify his strengths and weaknesses, including appropriate academic accommodations, we chose to administer a full IQ battery. Jason's mother was concerned about how his IQ might change across time; thus we wanted to choose an instrument that could be given again in the future to track any changes. Although we considered the Leiter-R because

of Jason's poor use of language for communicative purposes, we decided
that a measure of his verbal skills was necessary to provide a realistic estimate of the difficulties he was likely to encounter in the third grade. However, we wanted to choose an instrument that would show the discrepancy
between his verbal and nonverbal skills, so that his strengths would also
be identified. Given his chronological age and these other considerations,
we identified the WISC-IV, SB5, and DAS-II as being appropriate measures
for Jason's evaluation. We chose the WISC-IV because we suspected that
Jason's autism might interfere with some of the imitation demands on the
Nonverbal Working Memory subtest of the SB5, and we were concerned
that he might perform at the floor level of the DAS-II School-Age battery
because it begins at 7 years. Jason was given a picture schedule showing a
picture denoting each of the 10 subtests on the WISC-IV. For every subtest
that he completed, he earned a sticker of an animal. In addition, Jason
brought several of his stuffed animals with him to the testing session and
was allowed several minutes to play with the animals after he completed
two subtests. Following the WISC-IV, Jason's mother was interviewed with
the Vineland-II to assess Jason's adaptive behavior.

WISC-IV Results

Jason obtained a Verbal Comprehension Index of 75 (5th percentile), a Perceptual Reasoning Index of 92 (30th percentile), a Working Memory Index
of 71 (3rd percentile), and a Processing Speed Index of 53 (below the 1st
percentile). Jason's Full Scale IQ was 69 and was at the 2nd percentile compared to other children his age. This score was classified by the WISC-IV
as Extremely Low. There was a 95% chance that his true IQ score was
within the range of 65–75. The Full Scale IQ is an aggregate of the four
Index scores and is usually considered the best measure of global intellectual functioning. However, Jason showed significant differences across
Index scores, suggesting that the Full Scale IQ might not be an accurate
representation of his overall ability. Specifically, Jason's Perceptual Reasoning Index was significantly higher than all of his other Index scores. It was
17 points higher than his Verbal Comprehension Index; this discrepancy is
only seen in 12% of children Jason's age. Furthermore, Jason's Processing
Speed Index was significantly lower than all of his other Index scores. It
was 39 points lower than his Perceptual Reasoning Index; this discrepancy
is seen in 0.4% of children Jason's age.

The Verbal Comprehension Index is a measure of verbal concept formation, verbal reasoning, and knowledge acquired from one's environment. Jason's Verbal Comprehension Index was classified as Borderline;
his subtest scores ranged from 2 to 8 (8–12 is average). Jason scored in the
average range on a task requiring him to say how two things were alike

(Similarities subtest), but received a very low score on a task requiring him to verbalize solutions to everyday problems and social concerns (Comprehension subtest).

The Perceptual Reasoning Index assesses skills such as the ability to think in terms of visual images and manipulate objects or images. Jason's Perceptual Reasoning Index was in the average range; his subtest scores ranged from 6 to 11 (8–12 is average). His highest score was on a task requiring him to use objects to recreate a visual pattern (Block Design).

The Working Memory Index is a measure of an individual's ability to attend to verbally presented information, to process information in memory, and then to formulate a response. Jason's Working Memory Index was classified as Borderline; his subtest scores ranged from 7 to 8 (8–12 is average). Jason could remember small amounts of information, but seemed to have more difficulty as the subtests increased the amount of information he had to remember and manipulate.

The Processing Speed Index is a measure of an individual's ability to process simple or routine visual information efficiently, and to perform tasks quickly based on that information. Jason's Processing Speed Index was in the Extremely Low Range; his subtest scores ranged from 1 to 9 (8–12 is average). It should be noted that Jason had particular difficulty on the Symbol Search subtest, because he became anxious and upset when he made a mistake and could not correct his work. He began to repeat lines from a movie rather than complete the task. His level of anxiety and frustration probably interfered with his ability to complete this task within the time constraints, resulting in a Processing Speed Index that might be an underestimate of his true abilities in this area.

Vineland-II Results

Jason's mother was the respondent for the Vineland-II. Based on the information gathered from the interview, Jason obtained an Adaptive Behavior Composite of 71, which falls in the Moderately Low range of adaptive functioning. Jason's mother reported moderately low levels of skills in all areas assessed. In the area of Communication, Jason obtained a score of 79 (8th percentile). His mother reported that he could follow simple and complex instructions, speak in full sentences, and print simple words from memory. However, he had not yet learned to follow three-step commands or engage in back-and-forth conversation. In the area of Daily Living Skills, Jason obtained a score of 74 (4th percentile). His mother reported that he could brush his teeth and dress independently, but had not yet learned to use simple appliances. In the Socialization domain, Jason obtained a score of 64 (1st percentile). His mother described him as showing interest in same-age peers and answering questions when familiar adults made small talk;

however, he had not yet learned to talk about shared interests with others, play with other children his own age, or share his toys. In the Motor Skills domain, Jason obtained a score of 78 (7th percentile) and was described as being able to draw shapes and run easily. He had difficulty using a keyboard to type short words, catching a ball, tying knots, and using a bicycle without training wheels.

Discussion of Case Study Information

Jason's performance on the WISC-IV was consistent with previous research reviewed in this chapter, indicating that individuals with ASD often display an uneven profile of performance. Jason's WISC-IV profile was characterized by some skills that were significantly below his chronological age and other skills that were equivalent to his chronological age. He also showed the commonly observed pattern of significantly greater visual–spatial perception skills than verbal reasoning skills. Fitting this pattern, his lowest subtest score was on the Comprehension subtest (which measures verbal reasoning about social situations) and his highest subtest score was on the Block Design subtest (which measures visual–spatial perception). The WISC-IV highlighted Jason's strengths and weaknesses, providing an opportunity to recommend additional school assistance when receptive or expressive language was required by building on his strengths (e.g., increased used of written or picture directions rather than verbal directions, and use of manipulatives when solving math problems).

Similarly, the Vineland-II provided a profile that was consistent with previous research showing overall delays with specific deficits in social skills. Specific ideas for adaptive behavior goals could be developed from the Vineland-II (e.g., use of social scripts to teach him how to interact with peers, use of visual schedules to teach the steps involved in such daily living skills as using a microwave). Thus a consideration of the recommended questions for choosing an appropriate IQ and adaptive behavior assessment provided the desired information for making suggestions for school and home accommodations to help Jason reach his full potential.

REFERENCES

Akshoomoff, N. (2006). Use of the Mullen Scales of Early Learning for the assessment of young children with autism spectrum disorders, *Child Neuropsychology, 12,* 269–277.

American Psychiatric Association (2000). *Diagnostic and statistical manual of mental disorders* (4th ed., text rev.). Washington, DC: Author.

Baird, G., Simonoff, E., Pickles, A., Chandler, S., Loucas, T., Meldrum, D., & Charman, T. (2006). Prevalence of disorders of the autism spectrum in a population cohort of children in South Thames: The Special Needs and Autism Project (SNAP). *Lancet, 368,* 210–215.

Ballaban-Gil, K., & Tuchman, R. (2000). Epilepsy and epileptiform EEG: Association with autism and language disorders. *Mental Retardation and Developmental Disabilities Research Reviews, 6,* 300–308.

Baron-Cohen, S. (2001). Theory of mind and autism: A review. *International Review of Research in Mental Retardation, 23,* 169–184.

Bayley, N. (2005). *Manual for the Bayley Scales of Infant and Toddler Development, Third Edition (Bayley-III).* San Antonio, TX: Harcourt Assessment.

Beadle-Brown, J., Murphy, G., & Wing, L. (2006). The Camberwell cohort 25 years on: Characteristics and changes in skills over time. *Journal of Applied Research in Intellectual Disabilities, 19,* 317–329.

Bölte, S., & Poustka, F. (2002). The relation between general cognitive level and adaptive behavior domains in individuals with autism with and without co-morbid mental retardation. *Child Psychiatry and Human Development, 33,* 165–172.

Bruininks, R. H., Woodcock, R. W., Weatherman, R. F., & Hill, B. K. (1996). *Scales of Independent Behavior—Revised.* Chicago: Riverside.

Carpentieri, S. C., & Morgan, S. B. (1994). Brief report: A comparison of patterns of cognitive functioning of autistic and nonautistic retarded children on the Stanford–Binet—Fourth Edition. *Journal of Autism and Developmental Disorders, 24,* 215–223.

Charman, T., Howlin, P., Berry, B., & Prince, E. (2004). Measuring developmental progress of children with autism spectrum disorder on school entry using parent report. *Autism, 8,* 89–100.

Courchesne, E., Townsend, J.P., Akshoomoff, N.A., Yeung-Courchesne, R., Press, G.A., Murakami, J.W., et al. (1994). A new finding: Impairment in shifting attention in autistic and cerebellar patients. In H. Broman & J. Grafman (Eds.), *Atypical cognitive deficits in developmental disorders: Implications for brain function.* (pp. 101–137) Hillsdale, NJ: Erlbaum.

Dawson, G., Toth, K., Abbott, R., Osterling, J., Munson, J., Estes, A., et al. (2004). Early social attention impairments in autism: Social orienting, joint attention, and attention to distress. *Developmental Psychology, 40,* 271–283.

Edelson, M. G. (2006). Are the majority of children with autism mentally retarded? *Focus on Autism and Other Developmental Disabilities, 21,* 66–83.

Ehlers, S., Nyden, A., Gillberg, C., Sandberg, A. D., Dahlgren, S., Hjelmquist, E., et al. (1997). Asperger syndrome, autism, and attention disorders: A comparative study of the cognitive profiles of 120 children. *Journal of Child Psychology and Psychiatry, 38,* 207–217.

Eikeseth, S., Smith, T., Jahr, E., & Eldevik, S. (2007). Outcomes for children with autism who began intensive behavioral treatment between ages 4 and 7: A comparison controlled study. *Behavior Modifications, 31,* 264–278.

Elliott, C. D. (1990). *Differential Ability Scales.* San Antonio, TX: Psychological Corporation.

Elliott, C. D. (2007). *Differential Ability Scales—Second Edition.* San Antonio, TX: Harcourt Assessment.

Filipek, P. A., Accardo, P. J., Baranek, G. T., Cook, E. H., Jr., Dawson, G., Gordon,

B., et al. (1999). The screening and diagnosis of autistic spectrum disorders. *Journal of Autism and Developmental Disorders, 29,* 439–484.

Fombonne, E. (2005). Epidemiological studies of pervasive developmental disorders. In F.R. Volkmar, R. Paul, A. Klin, & D. Cohen (Eds.), *Handbook of autism and pervasive developmental disorders: Vol. 1. Diagnosis, development, neurobiology, and behavior* (3rd ed., pp. 42–69). Hoboken, NJ: Wiley.

Freeman, B. J., Ritvo, E. R., Needleman, R., & Yokota, A. (1985). The stability of cognitive and linguistic parameters in autism: A five-year prospective study. *Journal of the American Academy of Psychiatry, 24,* 459–464.

Ghaziuddin, M., & Mountain-Kimchi, K. (2004). Defining the intellectual profile of Asperger syndrome: Comparison with high-functioning autism. *Journal of Autism and Developmental Disorders, 34,* 279–284.

Gillham, J. E., Carter, A. S., Volkmar, F. R., & Sparrow, S. S. (2000). Toward a developmental operational definition of autism. *Journal of Autism and Developmental Disorders, 30,* 269–278.

Goldstein, G., Beers, S.R., Siegel, D. J., & Minshew, N. J. (2001). A comparison of WAIS-R profiles in adults with high-functioning autism or differing subtypes of learning disability. *Applied Neuropsychology, 8,* 148–154.

Happé, F., & Frith, U. (2006). The weak coherence account: Detail-focused cognitive style in autism spectrum disorders. *Journal of Autism and Developmental Disorders, 36,* 5–25.

Harris, S. L., Handleman, J. S., & Burton, J. L. (1990). The Stanford Binet profiles of young children with autism. *Special Services in the Schools, 6,* 135–143.

Harrison, P. L., & Oakland, T. (2003). *Adaptive Behavior Assessment System— Second Edition.* San Antonio, TX: Psychological Corporation.

Howlin, P., Goode, S., Hutton, J., & Rutter, M. (2004). Adult outcomes for children with autism. *Journal of Child Psychology and Psychiatry, 45,* 212–229.

Johnson, C. P., Myers, S. M., & the Council on Children with Disabilities. (2007). Identification of and evaluation of children with autism spectrum disorders. *Pediatrics, 120,* 1183–1215.

Joseph, R. M., Tager-Flusberg, H., & Lord, C. (2002). Cognitive profiles and social-communicative functioning in children with autism spectrum disorder. *Journal of Child Psychology and Psychiatry, 43,* 807–821.

Kanner, L. (1943). Autistic disturbances of affective contact. *Nervous Child, 2,* 217–250.

Kaufman, A. S., & Kaufman, N. L. (2004). *Kaufman Brief Intelligence Test— Second Edition (KBIT-2).* Circle Pines, MN: American Guidance Service.

Klin, A., Saulnier, C., Tsatsanis, K., & Volkmar, F. R. (2005). Clinical evaluation in autism spectrum disorders: Psychological assessment within a transdisciplinary framework. In F. R. Volkmar, R. Paul, A. Klin, & D. J. Cohen (Eds.), *Handbook of autism and pervasive developmental disorders: Vol. 2. Assessment, interventions, and policy* (3rd ed., pp. 772–798). Hoboken, NJ: Wiley.

Klinger, L.G., Klinger, M.R., & Pohlig, R.L. (2007). Implicit learning impairments in autism spectrum disorders: Implications for treatment. In J.M. Perez, P. M. Gonzalez, M.L. Comi, & C. Nieto (Eds.), *New developments in autism: The future is today* (pp. 76–103). London: Jessica Kingsley.

Koegel, L. K., Koegel, R. L., & Smith, A. (1997). Variables related to differences in standardized test outcome for children with autism. *Journal of Autism and Developmental Disorders, 27,* 233–243.

Kuschner, E. S., Bennetto, L., & Yost, K. (2007). Patterns of nonverbal cognitive functioning in young children with autism spectrum disorders. *Journal of Autism and Developmental Disorders, 37,* 795–807.

Landa, R., & Garrett-Mayer, E. (2006). Development in infants with autism spectrum disorders: A prospective study, *Journal of Child Psychology and Psychiatry, 47,* 629–638.

Lincoln, A. J., Allen, M. H., & Kilman, A. (1995). The assessment and interpretation of intellectual abilities in people with autism. In E. Schopler & G. B. Mesibov (Eds.), *Learning and cognition in autism* (pp. 89–117). New York: Plenum Press.

Lincoln, A. J., Hansel, E., & Quirmbach, L. (2007). Assessing intellectual abilities of children and adolescents with autism and related disorders. In S. R. Smith & L. Handler (Eds.), *The clinical assessment of children and adolescents: A practitioner's handbook* (pp. 527–544). Mahwah, NJ: Erlbaum.

Lord, C., & Schopler, E. (1989). The role of age at assessment, developmental level, and test in the stability of intelligence scores in young autistic children. *Journal of Autism and Developmental Disorders, 19,* 483–499.

Lovaas, I. (1987). Behavioral treatment and normal educational and intellectual functioning in young autistic children. *Journal of Consulting and Clinical Psychology, 55,* 3–9.

Loveland, K. A., & Kelley, M. L. (1991). Development of adaptive behavior in adolescents and young adults with autism and Down syndrome. *American Journal of Mental Retardation, 93,* 84–92.

Luiselli, J. K., Campbell, S., Cannon, B., DiPietro, E., Ellis, J.T., Taras, M., et al. (2001). Assessment instruments used in the education and treatment of persons with autism: Brief report of a survey of national service centers. *Research in Developmental Disabilities, 22,* 389–398.

Manjiviona, J., & Prior, M. (1999). Neuropsychological profiles of children with Asperger syndrome and autism. *Autism, 3,* 327–356.

Mayes, S. D., & Calhoun, S. L. (2003). Analysis of the WISC-III, Stanford-Binet: IV, and academic achievement test scores in children with autism, *Journal of Autism and Developmental Disorders, 33,* 329–341.

Mayes, S. D., & Calhoun, S. L. (2004). Similarities and differences in Wechsler Intelligence Scale for Children—Third Edition (WISC-III) profiles: Support for subtest analysis in clinical referrals. *The Clinical Neuropsychologist, 18,* 559–572.

Minshew, N. J., Goldstein, G., & Siegel, D. J. (1997). Neuropsychologic functioning in autism: Profile of a complex information processing disorder. *Journal of the International Neuropsychological Society, 3,* 303–316.

Mottron, L., Dawson, M., Soulieres, I., Hubert, B., & Burack J. (2006). Enhanced perceptual functioning in autism: An update, and eight principles of autistic perceptions. *Journal of Autism and Developmental Disorders, 36,* 27–43.

Mullen, E. M. (1995). *The Mullen Scales of Early Learning.* Circle Pines, MN: American Guidance Service.

National Research Council. (2001). *Educating children with autism.* Committee on Educational Interventions for Children with Autism, C. Lord & J.P. McGee (Eds.). Division of Behavioral and Social Sciences and Education. Washington, DC: National Academy Press.

Ozonoff, S., Goodlin-Jones, B. L., & Solomon, M. (2007). Assessment of autism spectrum disorders. In E. J. Mash & R. A. Barkley (Eds.), *Assessment of childhood disorders* (4th ed., pp. 487–525). New York: Guilford Press.

Ozonoff, S., & Jensen, J. (1999). Brief report: Specific executive function profiles in three neurodevelopmental disorders. *Journal of Autism and Developmental Disorders, 29,* 171–177.

Ozonoff, S., South, M., & Miller, J. N. (2000). DSM-IV defined Asperger syndrome: Cognitive, behavioral and early history differentiation from high-functioning autism. *Autism, 4,* 29–46.

Paul, R., Miles, S., Cicchetti, D., Sparrow, S., Klin, A., Volkmar, F., et al. (2004). Adaptive behavior in autism and pervasive developmental disorder not otherwise specified: Microanalysis of scores on the Vineland Adaptive Behavior Scales. *Journal of Autism and Developmental Disorders, 34,* 223–228.

Renner, P., Klinger, L.G., & Klinger, M.R. (2006). Exogenous and endogenous attention orienting in autism spectrum disorders. *Child Neuropsychology, 12,* 361–382.

Rodrigue, J. R., Morgan, S. B., & Geffken, G. R. (1991). A comparative evaluation of adaptive behavior in children and adolescents with autism, Down syndrome, and normal development. *Journal of Autism and Developmental Disorders, 21,* 187–196.

Rogers, S. J., Hepburn, S., Stackhouse, T., & Wehner, E. (2003). Imitation performance in toddlers with autism and those with other developmental disorders. *Journal of Child Psychology and Psychiatry, 44,* 763–781.

Roid, G. H. (2003). *Stanford–Binet Intelligence Scales, Fifth Edition.* Itasca, IL: Riverside.

Roid, G. H., & Miller, L. J. (1997). *Leiter International Performance Scale— Revised: Examiner's manual.* Wood Dale, IL: Stoelting.

Seltzer, M. M., Shattuck, P., Abbeduto, L., & Greenberg, J. (2004). Trajectory of development in adolescents and adults with autism. *Mental Retardation and Developmental Disabilities Research Reviews, 10,* 234–247.

Siegel, D. J., Minshew, N. J., & Goldstein, G. (1996). Wechsler IQ profiles in diagnosis of high-functioning autism. *Journal of Autism and Developmental Disorders, 26,* 389–406.

Sigman, M., & McGovern, C. W. (2005). Improvement in cognitive and language skills from preschool to adolescence in autism. *Journal of Autism and Developmental Disorders, 35,* 15–23.

Sigman, M., Mundy, P., Sherman, T., & Ungerer, J. (1986). Social interactions of autistic, mentally retarded, and normal children with their caregivers. *Journal of Child Psychology and Psychiatry, 27,* 647–656.

Smith, T., Groen, A. D., & Wynn, J. W. (2000). A randomized trial of intensive early intervention for children with pervasive developmental disorder. *American Journal on Mental Retardation, 105,* 269–285.

Sparrow, S. S., Balla, D. A., & Cicchetti, D. V. (1984). *Vineland Adaptive Behavior Scales.* Circle Pines, MN: American Guidance Service.

Sparrow, S. S., Cicchetti, D. V., & Balla, D. A. (2005). *Vineland Adaptive Behavior Scales, Second Edition*. Circle Pines, MN: American Guidance Service.

Stone, W. L., Ousley, O. Y., Hepburn, S. L., Hogan, K. L., & Brown, S. (1999). Patterns of adaptive behavior in very young children with autism. *American Journal on Mental Retardation, 104*, 187–199.

Szatmari, P., Archer, L., Fisman, S., & Streiner, D. L. (1994). Parent and teacher agreement in the assessment of pervasive developmental disorders. *Journal of Autism and Developmental Disorders, 24*, 703–717.

Tsatsanis, K. D., Dartnall, N., Cicchetti, D., Sparrow, S. S., Klin, A., & Volkmar, F. R. (2003). Concurrent validity and classification accuracy of the Leiter and Leiter-R in low-functioning children with autism. *Journal of Autism and Developmental Disorders, 33*, 23–30.

Venter, A., Lord, C., & Schopler, E. (1992). A follow-up study of high-functioning autistic children. *Journal of Child Psychology and Psychiatry, 33*, 489–507.

Volkmar, F. R., Sparrow, S. S., Goudreau, D., Cicchetti, D. V., Paul, R., & Cohen, D. J. (1987). Social deficits in autism: An operational approach using the Vineland Adaptive Behavior Scales. *Journal of the American Academy of Child and Adolescent Psychiatry, 26*, 156–161.

Volkmar, F. R., Szatmari, P., & Sparrow, S. S. (1993). Sex difference in pervasive developmental disorders. *Journal of Autism and Developmental Disorders, 23*, 579–591.

Wechsler, D. (1997). *Wechsler Adult Intelligence Scale—Third Edition (WAIS-III)*. San Antonio, TX: Psychological Corporation.

Wechsler, D. (1999). *Wechsler Abbreviated Scale of Intelligence (WASI)*. San Antonio, TX: Psychological Corporation.

Wechsler, D. (2002). *Wechsler Preschool and Primary Scale of Intelligence—Third Edition (WPPSI-III)*. San Antonio, TX: Psychological Corporation.

Wechsler, D. (2003). *Wechsler Intelligence Scale for Children—Fourth Edition (WISC-IV)*. San Antonio, TX: Psychological Corporation.

Williams, D. L., Goldstein, G., & Minshew, N. J. (2006). Neuropsychologic functioning in children with autism: Further evidence for disordered complex information processing. *Child Neuropsychology, 12*, 279–298.

CHAPTER NINE

Assessment of Neuropsychological Functioning in Autism Spectrum Disorders

Blythe A. Corbett
Vanessa Carmean
Deborah Fein

Neuropsychology can be defined as a bridge between neurology and psychology; it examines the relationship between the brain and behavior. It has emerged as a clinical and research discipline in the last 50 years. The field has progressed from the administration of basic paper-and-pencil tasks to elaborate, comprehensive batteries evaluating many domains of functioning. The goals can include integrating the factors of development, brain function, behavior, and social context to inform clinical judgments and research.

The purposes of a neuropsychological evaluation can be to identify strengths and weaknesses, establish a baseline of functioning, document performance status and changes in performance, and guide treatment. In addition, it can assist with differential diagnosis and the identification of between- and within-group differences. In research, the use of neuropsychological instruments permits the exploration of theoretical frameworks and provides useful dependent measures for comparison across groups or conditions. The field of pediatric neuropsychology has evolved as a specialized division within neuropsychology to emphasize child development, and to clarify how such factors as learning and behavior are related to the development of brain systems and structures. In addition, pediatric neu-ropsychology provides a model for the understanding of neuroplasticity in development.

A comprehensive neuropsychological assessment includes information from a variety of sources, in addition to the standardized tests described in this chapter. These sources can include medical and educational records, clinical observation, parent and teacher reports and ratings, and diagnostic interviews. This chapter is intended to provide an overview of the neu-ropsychological assessment process in relation to autism spectrum disor-ders (ASD) as well as a brief review of research findings. However, it is not intended to provide the necessary training and extensive knowledge required of a pediatric neuropsychologist—knowledge that includes a deep appreciation of child development, the central nervous system, and the emergence of cognitive processes across the lifespan (Batchelor & Dean, 1995). In addition, it is not possible within the scope of this chapter to pres-ent an exhaustive list of measures that can be used within each domain of functioning. Rather, the ones described below are examples of tools within each domain, and we have tried to include those that we have found helpful and that have good reported reliability and validity.

Neuropsychological assessment utilizes quantitative approaches that involve standardized behavior ratings and norm-referenced test data. Qualitative data, such as patient history, observations of behavior during testing, observations of social interaction, play, and communication, and neurological signs, are also very important; however, the interpretation of these data ultimately relies on the expertise of the examiner (Turkheimer, 1989).

Neuropsychological measures provide standardized scores based on normative data, which are derived (ideally) from a large sample of children representing the population of interest. Although various scores may be generated, the majority provide metrics that are derived by subtracting the population mean from an individual's raw score and then divided by the population standard deviation. A standardized score allows us to deter-mine how close the child's performance is to that of a comparison group. Psychological measures usually provide standardized scores with a mean of 100 and a standard deviation of 15, or scaled scores with a mean of 10 and a standard deviation of 3, or T scores with a mean of 50 and a standard deviation of 10.

DOMAINS OF FUNCTIONING

A neuropsychological assessment typically involves the assessment of many areas of functioning, including overarching cognitive or intellectual ability, adaptive skills, attention, sensory processing, motor ability, language, executive functioning, visual–spatial and visual–motor ability, memory, academic skills, and social-emotional functioning. The neuropsychological assessment can assist in corroborating diagnostic procedures, contribute to defining a unique profile of abilities and deficits, and assist in formulating appropriate treatments and interventions (Lezak, 1995).

In the following discussion, we address assessment of the primary domains of functioning; we focus on describing standardized measures of these various areas of ability. Several neuropathological models have been proposed over the years in an attempt to explain the core or related symptoms in ASD. When these core or "primacy" models are applicable, we present summaries of them within the relevant domains.

Cognitive Functioning

At the foundation of a neuropsychological assessment is intellectual testing, which provides the framework for the interpretation of other quantitative and qualitative measures and observations. In ASD, children's level of measured intelligence is affected by some factors that are either not relevant or not as important in typical development; these include the severity of autistic symptoms, level of adaptive functioning, motivation to participate in testing, and treatment provided (Filipek et al., 1999). It has been estimated that 50–70% of children with autism have intelligence quotients (IQs) falling in the impaired range (an IQ below 70 on most standardized measures) (American Psychiatric Association, 1994; Stevens et al., 2000; Waterhouse et al., 1996). Since intellectual ability is dependent on many factors (and influences many cognitive skills in turn), cognitive impairment may be due to difficulties in a number of contributing areas, including language, processing speed, broad knowledge, and social comprehension. It is important to note that although impairments in social behavior are usually considered the hallmark deficits in ASD, it is cognitive ability that serves as a better predictor of outcome (Filipek et al., 1999; Stevens et al., 2000). In addition, cognitive level influences the expression of autistic symptoms, including social behavior and repetitive interests. For example, for children with low IQ, social disability may manifest itself as a lack of interest in peers; for higher-IQ (and older) children, social disability may be manifested in social awkwardness, immaturity, and rigidity, which prevent actual mutual friendships from developing even when these children want to have friends. In the repetitive behavior domain, the low-IQ child may present with multiple motor stereotypes and unusual visual behaviors, whereas the higher-IQ child may manifest this characteristic more in resistance to changes in routines and preoccupations with unusual topics. As with any child, when the profile of cognitive subtests is uneven (as is the rule rather than the exception in ASD), the overall IQ score must be interpreted with caution and used more as a rough index of overall current functioning than as a real measure of cognitive ability.

Measures

A brief overview of several of the overall cognitive measures is now provided. (The reader is directed to Klinger, O'Kelley, & Mussey, Chapter 8, this volume, for a more comprehensive overview of assessing intelligence.)

The Wechsler Intelligence Scale for Children—Fourth Edition (WISC-IV; Wechsler, 2003) is considered one of the gold standards for measuring intellectual functioning. It provides separate scores based on verbal and nonverbal problem-solving skills, short-term memory, and processing speed. The WISC-IV is used to measure cognitive functioning in children from 6 years, 0 months to 16 years, 11 months of age. It is an improvement over previous Wechsler scales, but the instrument is not a stand-alone neuropsychological test (for a review, see Baron, 2005). The normative sample for the WISC-IV consisted of 2,200 English-speaking U.S. children stratified according to U.S. Bureau of the Census data; it included specialized populations, such as children with ASD. The WISC-IV is conormed with the Wechsler Individual Achievement Test—Second Edition, making it useful in assessing learning disability.

The Wechsler Preschool and Primary Scale of Intelligence—Third Edition (WPPSI-III; Wechsler, 2002) is a measure of general intellectual abilities that provides separate scores based on verbal and nonverbal problem-solving skills. It is intended for use with young children from 2 years, 6 months to 7 years, 3 months of age. Although the measure was developed for assessment of cognitive abilities in preschoolers and young children, some of the task demands may be challenging for children with neurodevelopmental disorders, such as ASD. It represents a downward extension of the WISC tests. This measure was normed on 1,700 children ages 2 years, 2 months to 7 years, 3 months.

The Wechsler Abbreviated Scale of Intelligence (WASI; Wechsler, 1999) is an abbreviated measure of general intelligence that is used to obtain an estimated IQ across much of the lifespan, from 6 to 89 years of age. This instrument was developed to fill the need for a shorter, yet reliable, assessment of intelligence. As this measure only takes about 30 minutes to complete, it is frequently used in research. It can be useful for lower-functioning individuals, as long as their mental age is close to 6 years or above. Four subtests (Vocabulary, Block Design, Similarities, and Matrix Reasoning) are used to calculate Verbal, Performance, and Full Scale IQ. Norms were nationally standardized with 2,245 individuals.

The Stanford–Binet Intelligence Scales, Fifth Edition (SB5; Roid, 2003) is a standardized measure of general intelligence that follows a theoretical model of a *g* factor of general intelligence, as well as secondary factors including crystallized ability, fluid ability, and short-term memory (Cattell, 1971). The SB5 is unique in that it covers a wide age span by assessing cognitive functioning from 2 years through adulthood. This makes it advantageous for following children over time; however, one should use caution in interpreting changes in some of the subtests (e.g., Comprehension), since the task demands change considerably as a child progresses. Normative data were based on 4,800 individuals from the ages of 2 to over 80. The sample was representative of the U.S. 2000 census.

The Bayley Scales of Infant and Toddler Development, Third Edition (Bayley-III; Bayley, 2005) is used to assess the mental, motor, and behavioral functioning of children from the age of 1 month to 42 months. The Mental scale provides assessment of early sensory-perceptual abilities, vocalization, early verbal communication, problem solving, memory, habituation, learning, generalization, and classification. The Motor Development scale assesses body control, gross motor coordination, fine motor manipulation, posture, and mobility. The Infant Behavior Rating Scale provides ratings of the child's attention, arousal, emotion regulation, orientation, engagement, and quality of motor control. The five subtests include measures of adaptive behavior, cognitive functioning, language, motor, and social-emotional skills. The Language domain measures both expressive and receptive communication, and both preverbal and vocabulary abilities. Specifically, behaviors such as babbling and gesturing, turn taking, and object identification are assessed. Normative data for the Bayley-III were derived from 1,700 children ages 1–42 months, and were reflective of the 2000 U.S. census.

The Kaufman Assessment Battery for Children, Second Edition (KABC-II; Kaufman & Kaufman, 2004) is grounded in two models: the Cattell–Horn–Carroll psychometric model of broad and narrow abilities and Luria's processing model. Some of the subtests on the KABC-II are very appealing to children with ASD and can keep their attention relatively well. The KABC-II covers the age range from 3 to 18 years. Normative data were based on 3,025 individuals ranging in age from 3 years, 0 months to 18 years, 11 months. The sample was representative of the 2001 U.S. census.

The Cognitive Assessment System (CAS; Naglieri & Das, 1997) is a test developed to measure planning, attention, simultaneous, and successive (PASS) processes, which are the four areas of the PASS theoretical framework. It is intended for children from 5 to 17 years of age. The CAS has been used in studies including children with mental retardation, learning disabilities, attention-deficit/hyperactivity disorder (ADHD), and other disorders (see Naglieri & Das, 2005). This test was normed on a large sample of children (including ones with autism) ages 5 through 17 (N = 2,200), who closely represented the U.S. population on a number of important demographic variables (Naglieri & Das, 1997).

The Differential Ability Scales—Second Edition (DAS-II; Elliott, 2007) includes both verbal and nonverbal measures of intelligence for children ranging in age from 2 years, 6 months to 17 years, 11 months. Many subtests are included in this measure, with several specifically developed for preschool-age children, others designed for school-age children, and still others that can be used for both age groups. Individual subtests on this measure are less multifactorial than subtests on some other widely used measures, and thus easier to interpret. For this reason, the original DAS was often used in research studies, and the DAS-II will probably be used often as well. This measure can also be used to measure performance changes over time. Its normative sample was representative of the general U.S. population.

The Mullen Scales of Early Learning (Mullen, 1995) is a measure of verbal and nonverbal abilities that utilizes five different scales (Gross Motor, Visual Reception, Fine Motor, Receptive Language, and Expressive Language) for children ages 1–68 months. Since it provides separate estimates of functioning in nonverbal problem solving (Visual Reception) and receptive and expressive language for children in infancy and toddlerhood, it is also widely used in research studies of young children with ASD. The Mullen was normed on a total sample of 1,849 children ranging from 2 to 69 months of age. It should be noted that the norms were acquired in the 1980s, with demographics similar to the 1990 U.S. census but with a slightly different geographic distribution from the U.S. population in general (Bradley-Johnson, 1997).

Adaptive Functioning

Adaptive functioning involves skills and behaviors necessary for age-appropriate day-to-day functioning; these encompass communication, socialization, self-care, community use, and independent living skills. In order for an individual to receive a diagnosis of mental retardation, both IQ and adaptive functioning must fall into the impaired range (usually a standard score < 70 on most standardized tests). Adaptive skills are often measured clinically, which is perhaps a more ecologically valid means of assessing day-to-day functioning (Volkmar, 2003). In children with ASD, adaptive functioning is often significantly impaired, despite demonstration of clear cognitive potential (Klin et al., 2007).

Measures

The Vineland Adaptive Behavior Scales, Second Edition (Vineland-II) Survey Interview Form (Sparrow, Cicchetti, & Balla, 2005) is a semistructured parent interview designed to assess a child's ability to perform daily activities required for personal and social sufficiency. The main domains covered are Communicative, Daily Living skills, Socialization, and Motor skills; Maladaptive Behavior is an optional domain that may be assessed. The Vineland is designed for children 3–18 years old, and was normed on 3,695 participants ages 0–90 years, the U.S. 2001 census. An expanded interview form is also available to obtain additional information after the initial interview. This instrument is widely used in current research on ASD (e.g., Klin et al., 2007).

The Adaptive Behavior Assessment System—Second Edition (ABAS-II; Harrison & Oakland, 2003) is another adaptive measure for ages 0–89 years that is also fairly widely used. The ABAS can be administered as an interview or questionnaire. The domains assessed are similar to those in the Vineland-II, but broken down somewhat differently; they include Communication, Community Use, Functional Academics, Health and Safety, Leisure, Self-Care, Self-Direction, Social Functioning, and Work Aptitude. The forms for children ages 0–5 were normed on a group of 3,100 children, and the teacher, parent, and adult forms for those over 5 were normed on 5,270 individuals. All standardization samples were representative of the U.S. 1999–2000 census.

Attention

Attention is a fundamental cognitive domain that includes several different skills: the ability to sustain attention; the ability to switch from one focus of attention to another or from one task to another (often referred to as "mental flexibility"); and "selective attention," or the ability to focus on one stimulus and inhibit attention to distractions. Individuals with ASD display a variety of strengths and weaknesses across the various components of attention (for a review, see Allen & Courchesne, 2001). It has been previously reported that sustained attention is usually intact for preferred activities, while sustained attention for nonpreferred activities is usually impaired (Garretson, Fein, & Waterhouse, 1990). In other words, motivational contingencies affect the level of performance, making the provision of adequate incentives crucial for good performance (Garretson et al., 1990). Children with ASD and comorbid symptoms of ADHD (a fairly common combination) also exhibit impairments in both visual and auditory attention, as well as behavioral disinhibition (Corbett & Constantine, 2006). Individuals with ASD often orient to a new stimulus much more slowly (Townsend, Harris, & Courchesne, 1996) and show impairment in their ability to shift attention (Courchesne et al., 1994). However, other studies have shown specific rather than general attention-shifting deficits, again underscoring that the level of impairment is often dependent on the specific task stimuli, as well as on distraction and motivation (Pascualvaca, Fantie, Papageorgiou, & Mirsky, 1998).

A number of fundamental or primacy theories of ASD consider attention and arousal to be central to these disorders and to involve dysfunction of the attentional systems of the frontal lobes, parietal cortex, and cerebellum. It has been reported that children with autism exhibit deficits in selective attention (Ciesielski, Courchesne, & Elmasian, 1990), as well as difficulty with rapid shifts in attention. In fact, Courchesne et al. (1994) proposed that difficulty in shifting attention may underlie the social and cognitive deficits in autism (see also Lewy & Dawson, 1992; Pierce, Glad, & Schreibman, 1997). Kinsbourne (1991) has suggested that perseverative attentional focus is a fundamental feature of autism, perhaps resulting from an attempt to defend against an unstable arousal system. Dawson, Meltzoff, Osterling, Rinaldi, and Brown (1998) showed that orienting to external stimuli is reduced in children with autism, and that orienting to social stimuli (e.g., someone clapping, someone calling a child's name) is especially impaired.

Measures

The following measures may be considered in a comprehensive neuropsychological assessment, especially when aspects of attention are impaired or comorbid symptoms of ADHD (inattention and poor inhibition) are suspected. Studies of ADHD have shown that when multiple measures are used together, prediction of ADHD status improves even if overall diagnosis is limited (Doyle, Biederman, Seidman, Weber, & Faraone, 2000).

The Integrated Visual and Auditory Continuous Performance Test (IVA-CPT; Sandford & Turner, 2000) was designed to help in the diagnosis and quantification of ADHD symptoms, but it has also been used to measure attention and self-control across a variety of neurodevelopmental and psychiatric conditions. The IVA-CPT combines measures of inattention and impulsivity in a counterbalanced design across both visual and auditory modalities. It is similar to the Test of Variables of Attention (Leark, Greenberg, Kindschi, Dupuy, & Hughes, 2007; Greenberg & Waldman, 1993), which is also a computerized test of attention. For these tasks, the child is required to press a button when a specific target stimulus is flashed on a computer screen, and to refrain from pressing the button when an alternate stimulus is presented. These tasks assess vigilance (sustained attention over time), response inhibition and impulsivity, speed of information processing, and the consistency in attentional focus over time. A recent study demonstrated that children with autism showed significant deficits in visual and auditory attention and poorer visual response inhibition, compared to children with ADHD and typically developing children (Corbett & Constantine, 2006). The authors suggest that many children with ASD present with symptoms of ADHD, and that these measures can help identify impairment in sustained attention and inhibition. The normative sample consisted of approximately 1,700 individuals, and was divided by age and gender.

The Test of Everyday Attention for Children (Manly et al., 2001) consists of a series of tasks that measure selective, focused, sustained, and divided attention (the last of which is the ability to share attention between two tasks). As the name implies, the instrument was designed to have good ecological validity (Manly et al., 2001), and it facilitates motivation by using stimuli that are inherently dynamic and interesting to children. It is designed for ages 6–16 years, and norms were developed with a group of 293 male and female participants from Australia between the ages of 6 and 16.

The Test of Auditory Discrimination (TOAD; Goldman, Fristoe, & Woodcock, 1970) is a measure of auditory attention, discrimination, and distractibility. The TOAD assesses auditory factors of attention by requiring the individual to identify speech sounds under ideal listening conditions (quiet) and under controlled background noise (distraction). The instrument has been shown to be discriminating in individuals with ADHD (Corbett & Stanczak, 1999) and may have utility for assessing auditory distractibility in individuals with ASD. The TOAD can be used with persons from the age of 3 years, 8 months through 70+ years; however, the norm sample is quite old.

A child's attention in everyday situations (such as a classroom) may not be adequately captured by tests of sustained, focused, or divided attention given in a lab, on a computer, and with one-on-one adult attention. Furthermore, the child's attention may vary considerably from one time to another (Barkley, 1991). For these reasons, it is important to gather information from teachers and parents, either informally or (preferably) using validated rating scales, such as those described below.

The Conners' Rating Scales—Third Edition (Conners, 2008) provide information about behaviors associated with attention and/or hyperactivity, as well as oppositional behavior. These scales are a standard and valid group of measures that are frequently used in the assessment of ADHD (Goldstein & Goldstein, 1998). Different versions are available that vary in terms of the respondent (parent, teacher, self), scope of questions, and length of the questionnaire. It is important to note that there is limited correlation between the Conners scales and other cognitive measures (see, e.g., Naglieri, Goldstein, Delauder, & Schwebach, 2005). Nevertheless, the parent and especially the teacher versions can assist in a comprehensive clinical evaluation to clarify the expression of symptoms across settings. The Conners norms were derived from 1,200 parents and 1,200 teachers of children and adolescents ages 6–18 years, and from 1,000 individuals ages 8–18 years for the self-report forms, all based on the 2000 U.S. census.

Sensory Functioning

Differences and deficits in sensory processing have been widely reported in children with ASD (Watling, Deitz, & White, 2001). Liss, Saulnier, Fein, and Kinsbourne (2006) have proposed an overarousal hypothesis to help explain the atypical sensory (overreactivity) and attention (overfocusing) abnormalities. Children and adults with ASD show unusual patterns in visual processing. For example, when searching for targets, individuals with autism are usually faster and more accurate than typical individuals, suggesting enhanced visual discrimination (O'Riordan, 2004; O'Riordan, Plaisted, Driver, & Baron-Cohen, 2001). Recently it was reported that children with autism showed superior auditory discrimination and comparable tactile ability when compared to control subjects (O'Riordan & Passetti, 2006). Taken together with previous findings in visual processing, these studies suggest enhanced perceptual discrimination ability in ASD. Behaviorally, one often observes that children with ASD evidence visual fascinations, often spending their free time in staring at absorbing visual stimuli (e.g., spinning wheels, lights, mirrors, and shadows), lining up toys and sighting along the lines, or squinting or looking at things out of the corners of their eyes (Liss et al., 2006). Conversely, they often seem to have difficulty tolerating tactile stimuli (e.g., being touched, getting haircuts, wearing certain clothing, and eating certain foods) and auditory stimuli, and may cover their ears as protection from auditory discomfort (Liss et al., 2006).

Measures

The Sensory Profile (Dunn, 1999) is a parent questionnaire related to sensory sensitivity across several domains, including auditory, visual, vestibular, tactile, oral, and multisensory processing. Differences on this measure have been reported for individuals with ASD in sensory seeking behavior, emotional reactivity, low endurance and muscle tone, oral sensitivity, inattention/distractibility, and more (Watling et al., 2001). The Sensory Profile is designed for ages 3–10 years; however, an infant/toddler measure is available for those under 3, and an adolescent/adult form is available for those over the age of 11. A shorter questionnaire, the Short Sensory Profile, is also available. (See Liss et al., 2006, for a description of additional, autism-specific questions.) Normative data were based on more than 1,200 children nationwide ages 3–10. Norms for adolescents and adults were based on a sample of 950 individuals ages 11–97 with and without disabilities from the midwestern United States.

Motor Functioning

Motor functioning is often an overlooked area in the assessment of individuals with ASD. However, it has been reported that children with ASD exhibit notable deficits in fine and/or gross motor functioning (Provost, Lopez, & Heimerl, 2007). In addition, early motor functioning may predict diagnostic and cognitive outcome (Sutera et al., 2007). Studies on motor abilities in children with ASD have found differences in gait (Vilensky, Damasio, & Maurer, 1981), as well as in running speed, agility, balance, and bilateral coordination (Ghaziuddin, Butler, Tsai, & Ghaziuddin, 1994). Other studies have shown significant motor delays in such children, compared to normative data (Berkeley, Zittel, Pitney, & Nichols, 2001; Manjiviona & Prior, 1995; Mari, Castiello, Marks, Marraffa, & Prior, 2003; Mayes & Calhoun, 2003). In infants, subtle motor differences have been identified, including excessive mouthing of objects (Baranek, 1999). Other studies looking at infants have found hypotonia, hypoactivity, unusual postures (Adrien et al., 1993), and movements or atypical motor patterns such as delays in head-righting reactions (Teitelbaum et al., 2004; Teitelbaum, Teitelbaum, Nye, Fryman, & Maurer, 1998). It is important to point out that some reports of intact motor skills in young children with ASD are based on parent reports of developmental milestones, such as independent walking (Gillberg et al., 1990). However, other researchers (Provost et al., 2007) argue that motor skills learned later are more complex, and thus that learning to walk at a typical age does not ensure the normal acquisition of other motor skills. Although a neurologist may be required to do a thorough motor exam, including examination of reflexes, postural abnormalities, and abnormal movements, there are excellent instruments available for neuropsychologists to use in examining motor skills.

Measures

The Purdue Pegboard Test—Revised (Lafayette Instruments, 1999; see also Tiffin & Asher, 1948) assesses fine motor speed, coordination, and finger and hand dexterity. The measure requires the individual to place pegs in holes on a fixed board using the dominant hand, the nondominant hand, and then both hands. The norms for this measure are old and are based on ages 5–16 years old for children. Norms are also available for adults.

The Nine-Hole Peg Test of Finger Dexterity (Mathiowetz, Volland, Kashman, & Weber, 1992) is a more recent measure of fine motor dexterity, with current normative data on samples of 826 elementary students (Smith, Hong, & Presson, 2000) and 406 children (Poole et al., 2005), respectively. It is highly correlated with the Purdue Pegboard Test and assesses skills for both the dominant and nondominant hands.

The Beery–Buktenica Developmental Test of Visual–Motor Integration—Fifth Edition (Beery, Buktenica, & Beery, 2004) is used to assess an individual's ability to integrate visual-perceptual skills with motor functioning. It is available in both short and long formats, and is used for children ages 2–18 and adults. The short form is commonly used for those between the ages of 2 and 8. There are also supplemental tests available to address visual perception and motor coordination abilities. Normative data were representative of the U.S. 2000 census.

Since there are few if any stand-alone measures of functioning in various domains, including motor skills, selected subtests from comprehensive batteries can be utilized to screen for strength or impairment in specific skill areas.

The Fingertip Tapping subtest from the NEPSY—Second Edition (NEPSY-II; Korkman, Kirk, & Kemp, 2007) is a test of motor speed and finger dexterity, using the index finger and thumb of each hand. The task involves repetitive and sequential tapping. It is developed for ages 3–16. Normative data for the NEPSY-II were based on a sample of 1,000 children ages 3 through 12, and are representative of children from the 2003 U.S. census.

The Imitating Hand Positions subtest from the NEPSY-II (Korkman et al., 2007) measures performance in imitating finger and hand positions in both hands within a time limit. Like the Fingertip Tapping subtest, it is intended for ages 3–16; norms came from 1,000 children ages 3 through 12.

Language

Impairments in communication, especially receptive and expressive language, are part of the diagnostic criteria for autistic disorder (American Psychiatric Association, 1994, 2000). Children with autism and related disorders exhibit a variety of early deficits in communication, including delays in comprehension, reduced attention to language, limited nonverbal communication and gesture, immediate and delayed echolalia (repetition of meaningless sounds, words, or phrases), and atypical prosody (emotional intonation in speech) (Eigsti, Bennetto, & Dadlani, 2007; Howlin, 2003; Tager-Flusberg, 1981, 1996; Tager-Flusberg & Joseph, 2003).

The numerous components of language include phonology (understanding and producing speech sounds), semantics (meaning of words), pragmatics (social aspects of communication), prosody (speech rhythm, tempo, and pitch), and grammar (which includes both word order and grammatical parts of speech). Individuals with ASD can exhibit problems in any of these areas, all of which are essential for understanding and using language. In general, though grammar and phonology tend to be relatively spared, prosody and pragmatics are almost always impaired, and semantics is variable (Kelley, Paul, Fein, & Naigles, 2006).

Typical brain development is generally characterized by left-hemispheric specialization for spoken language and gesture—findings that have been widely reported by neuroimaging, lesion, and animal studies. Some theorists (Prior, 1979; Prior & Bradshaw, 1979; Rutter, 1974, 1979; Rutter, Bartak, & Newman, 1971) view autism as primarily a disorder of language, but others hold that autism involves social impairment and repetitive behavior as well as language deficits (Bishop, 1989, 1998, 2000; Bishop & Norbury, 2002; Hollander, 1997; Hollander et al., 1999; Hollander, Dolgoff-Kaspar, Cartwright, Rawitt, & Novotny, 2001; Hollander, Phillips, & Yeh, 2003), while others document the presence of language disorders in only some children with autism (Kjelgaard & Tager-Flusberg, 2001). In general, many years of language study in ASD suggests that although many individual children will be found with deficits in any given area of language, children with ASD as a group tend to have spared phonology and syntax, impaired prosody and pragmatics, and a complex semantic picture in which basic word meanings may be a strength, but connotations are ignored and certain classes of words with social content are limited. (For an expanded review of language in ASD, see Paul & Wilson, Chapter 7, this volume.)

Measures

The Peabody Picture Vocabulary Test, Fourth Edition (PPVT-4; Dunn & Dunn, 2007) is a single-word receptive vocabulary task that can be administered to individuals from 2½ to over 90 years of age. Earlier editions of the PPVT have been frequently used measures in clinical settings and research. A companion expressive test, conormed with the PPVT-4, has also been published (the Expressive Vocabulary Test, Second Edition; Williams, 2007); the early items are useful, but the later ones require a child to produce a synonym for a common word, which can be difficult for children with ASD. Norms were based on a sample of 4,000 individuals representative of the U.S. population.

The Expressive One-Word Picture Vocabulary Test (EOWPVT; Brownell, 2000) is a measure that assesses for single word expressive vocabulary, and may be administered to those 2 through 18 years of age. The EOWPVT and similar measures are also often used in clinical practice and research. Normative data came from a sample of more than 2,000 people, and were representative of the national population. A companion receptive version, the Receptive One-Word Picture Vocabulary Test (Brownell, 2000), has been conormed with the EOWPVT.

It is essential to highlight that single-word vocabulary tests alone can overestimate language skills in children with ASD (Pellicano, Maybery, Durkin, & Maley, 2006). As such, we believe that the following more comprehensive measures, which include tests of complex language, should be used in a neuropsychological assessment when possible.

The Clinical Evaluation of Language Fundamentals—Fourth Edition (CELF-4; Semel, Wiig, & Secord, 2003) is a battery of three receptive and three expressive language measures. The subtests include tasks measuring auditory attention, classification, concept formation, syntax, word structure, and grammar. The CELF-4 has been developed for ages 5–21. Normative data came from a sample of 2,650 individuals that was representative of the 2000 U.S. census, and that included children with diagnosed language disorders and other conditions.

The Test of Language Competence (TLC; Wiig & Secord, 1989) assesses a child's ability to understand and use the abstract, figurative, ambiguous, and inferential aspects of language. As such, this is a good measure for higher-functioning children with good basic word knowledge who demonstrate difficulty with more abstract and complex language formation. It is designed for ages 5–18. In 1984, the TLC level 1 was standardized on 1,795 students ages 9–19 in 13 states. In 1987, the TLC level 2 was standardized on 2,188 students ages 5–9 in 28 states.

The Preschool Language Scale—Fourth Edition (Zimmerman, Steiner, & Pond, 2002) is designed for children from 2 weeks through 6 years, 11 months of age. It evaluates receptive and expressive language through parent interviews and direct assessment of the child. Although there are not a lot of items at any given age level, it is a widely used assessment of overall levels of expressive and receptive language. The normative sample of 1,500 children was reflective of the 2000 U.S. census and included children with disabilities.

The Comprehensive Assessment of Spoken Language (Carrow-Woolfolk, 1999) measures different aspects of spoken and written language, including the identification of antonyms and syntax, as well as figurative and pragmatic language. It is for use with ages 3–21. Normative data were developed from a nationwide sample of 1,700 individuals.

Memory

Memory, like attention, is complex and encompasses many domains, including visual, verbal, auditory, rote, short-term, nonverbal, episodic (events), and face memory. Different aspects of memory have been studied in children and adults with ASD (e.g., Bennetto, Pennington, & Rogers,

1996; Bowler, Gardiner, & Berthollier, 2004; Rogers, Bennetto, McEvoy, & Pennington, 1996), but the research findings are equivocal in regard to consistently identifying specific areas of deficit (O'Shea, Fein, Cillessen, Klin, & Schultz, 2005). Not surprisingly, verbal memory is often impaired (Kamio & Toichi, 1998); visual–spatial memory is usually intact, with the exception of memory for social stimuli such as faces and social situations (Williams, Goldstein, & Minshew, 2005b). While spatial working memory tends to be impaired (Luna et al., 2002; Williams, Goldstein, Carpenter, & Minshew, 2005a), the findings regarding working memory are varied and may depend on the type of task performed (Ozonoff & Strayer, 2001). Although it has been reported that episodic memory is often deficient in individuals with autism (Millward, Powell, Messer, & Jordan, 2000), there are many reports in the clinical literature of individuals who show exceptional, detailed memory for events to which they were motivated to attend. Source memory has been found to be impaired, but it appears that it may be influenced by the type of context information to be remembered, and may be especially impaired when it involves social information (O'Shea et al., 2005).

Measures

The California Verbal Learning Test—Children's Version (CVLT-C; Delis, Kramer, Kaplan, & Ober, 1994) requires a child to learn two lengthy "shopping lists," each of which contains several categories of items. This test assesses the strategies the child uses to learn the lists and is useful in identifying problems with encoding, retention, and retrieval of verbal information. The computerized version of the CVLT-C provides measures of additional variables: the efficiency of new learning, proactive and retroactive interference, consistency of learning over trials, the difference between recall and recognition (an indicator of retrieval problems), retention of learning over a delay period, and the degree to which the child clusters the words by meaning (an indicator of depth and automaticity of semantic processing). The CVLT-C is intended for ages 5 through 16, and has a standardization sample of 920 children based on the U.S. population (Spreen & Strauss, 1998).

The NEPSY-II Memory for Faces subtest (Korkman et al., 2007) is a measure of face recognition and memory. It requires the child to identify a series of faces after a brief exposure and following a 30-minute delay. The age range and normative sample for the NEPSY-II have been described earlier.

The Wide Range Assessment of Memory and Learning, Second Edition (WRAML2; Sheslow & Adams, 2003) is a comprehensive battery of different aspects of visual and verbal memory. The subtests can be administered individually and cover the following domains: verbal, visual, and attention and concentration. From these subtests, scores of general memory, working memory, visual memory, and attention and concentration are derived. In addition, there are recognition subtests of verbal, visual, design, and story memory. The WRAML2 is designed for ages 5–90 years, and norms were developed for this group from a national sample.

The Children's Memory Scale (CMS; Cohen, 1997) is a well-developed battery for assessing visual and verbal learning, and immediate and delayed memory. It includes tasks dependent on recall, recognition, and attentional processes, and parallels the widely used Wechsler Memory Scale for adults. Specifically, the CMS looks at working memory and learning characteristics under conditions of both short and long delay, as well as verbal and visual memory. The CMS is designed for children and adolescents 5–16 years of age, and has normative data based on a sample of 1,000 typically developing children ages 5–16, who were representative of the 1995 U.S. census.

Executive Functioning

"Executive functioning" is an umbrella term referring to mental processes that enable physical, cognitive, and emotional self-control (Denckla, 1996; Lezak, 1995; Pennington & Ozonoff, 1996), and that are necessary to maintain effective goal-directed behavior (Welsh & Pennington, 1988). Executive functions generally include response inhibition, working memory, cognitive flexibility (set shifting), planning, and fluency (Ozonoff & Strayer, 1997; Pennington & Ozonoff, 1996).

Investigations of individuals with ASD have shown deficits in various executive functions, especially set shifting and planning (Ozonoff & Jensen, 1999). More recently, impairments in switching and strategy have been reported (Kleinhans, Akshoomoff, & Delis, 2005). Some theorists have suggested that executive functioning deficits are central to ASD (Ozonoff, Pennington, & Rogers, 1991; Pennington & Ozonoff, 1996; Russell, 1997), and that the prefrontal cortex is involved in the pathophysiology of ASD. Although deficits in executive functioning may be present in several neurodevelopmental disorders, children with ASD typically demonstrate broader deficits and more impaired skills than do those with other disorders, such as ADHD or Tourette syndrome (Geurts, Verte, Oosterlaan, Roeyers, & Sergeant, 2004; Goldberg et al., 2005). Difficulty in shifting set (and, consequently, perseveration) has been noted in ASD for many years; this especially holds true for shifting attention away from preferred activities, but may also apply to shifting cognitive set away from any ongoing activity. Although deficient executive functioning may often be associated with autism, some authors would argue that it is by no means universal or directly associated with deficits in other domains of functioning, such as adaptive skills or language ability (Landa & Goldberg, 2005; Liss et al., 2001). Others, however, have indeed found executive functioning deficits to be associated with deficits in social behavior, communication, and adaptive skills in children with autism (Gilotty, Kenworthy, Sirian, Black, and Wagner, 2002). It is therefore valuable to assess executive functioning in determining a child's neuropsychological profile.

Measures

The Delis–Kaplan Executive Function System (D-KEFS; Delis, Kaplan, & Kramer, 2001) consists of nine tests that measure many aspects of executive functioning, including initiating problem-solving behavior, verbal and nonverbal problem-solving abilities, inhibition and flexibility (switching), word generation, rule learning, verbal abstraction skills, and design fluency. The subtests include Verbal Fluency, Design Fluency, Card Sorting, Trail Making, Color–Word Interference, Word Context, Twenty Questions, Proverbs, and Tower Tests. (The Verbal Fluency and Tower Tests are described in more detail below.) The D-KEFS is designed for ages 8 through 89, and its normative sample included 1,750 nonclinical individuals. The sample was based on the 2000 U.S. census (Homack, Lee, & Riccio, 2005).

Controlled Oral Word Association ("F-A-S"; Spreen & Benton, 1977) is an often used measure of speed and efficiency in producing words according to specified constraints. The letters "F," "A," and "S" are the most commonly used letters for this test. The individual is required to produce orally as many words as possible beginning with a certain letter in a limited period of time (usually 60 seconds). There are norms for ages 6 through 95; however, it should be noted that these are old.

The Verbal Fluency Test from the D-KEFS (Delis et al., 2001) is a more comprehensive verbal fluency test, in that it consists of three testing conditions: Letter Fluency (producing words beginning with a certain letter), Category Fluency (producing words from specified categories), and Category Switching (switching between different conditions). Together, these three conditions provide information regarding the individual's vocabulary knowledge, ability to fluently retrieve words beginning with the same letter, and ability to retrieve lexical items from a designated category. See the description of the D-KEFS above for age range and normative information.

The Wisconsin Card Sorting Test (WCST; Heaton, Chelune, Talley, Kay, & Curtis, 1993) is a measure of inhibition and cognitive flexibility. There are different versions, but most have conditions consisting of color naming (word finding), word reading (reading speed), and inhibition (verbal inhibition). The WCST is intended for ages 6½ to 89 years, and has normative data for 899 individuals in this age range. There are also new versions of the WCST that can be administered on a computer (e.g., Heaton & PAR Staff, 2000).

The Tower Test from the D-KEFS (Delis et al., 2001) is a measure of visual planning, working memory, and the ability to develop appropriate rule-based strategies for problem solving. This task requires the individual to determine how to move colored beads on sticks in order to create a specific pattern, using a specified number of moves. The individual's planning ability is measured by the time taken to complete the pattern and the number of moves required. Again, see the description of the D-KEFS for age range and normative information.

The Children's Color Trails Test I and II (CCTT-I and CCTT-II; Llorente, Williams, Satz, & D'Elia, 2003) are analogous to trail-making tests administered to adults, which measure alternating and sustained visual attention, sequencing ability, psychomotor speed, cognitive flexibility, and inhibition. The CCTT-I requires the individual to connect different colored circles rapidly and in the correct numerical order (1-2-3 . . .). The CCTT-II requires connecting the circles in numerical order while switching between colored numbers. Normative data are available for ages 8–16.

The Stroop Color and Word Test: Children's Version (Golden, Freshwater, & Golden, 2004) is a measure of inhibition and flexibility that exposes a child to different reading conditions. Although there are different versions of the Stroop test, it typically assesses color naming (word finding), word reading (reading speed), inhibition (verbal inhibition), and inhibition switching (cognitive flexibility). The Children's Version has normative data from 182 children ages 5–14.

As noted above in the "Attention" section, neuropsychological measures may not correlate with rating scales, especially across settings (Naglieri et al., 2005). As such, practitioners must interpret their findings cautiously and resist the temptation to generalize the findings too broadly. Nevertheless, the inclusion of questionnaires and rating scales can still provide additional valuable information regarding a child's functioning across constructs and settings.

The Behavior Rating Inventory of Executive Function (BRIEF; Gioia, Isquith, Guy, & Kenworthy, 2000) is a parent report instrument that yields separate scores for various areas of executive functioning, including initiation, working memory, planning/organizing, inhibition, emotional control, behavior regulation, and shifting. Although a group of children with ASD showed impairments on most scales, initiation and working memory were found to have particular relationships with adaptive functioning in this group (Gilotty et al., 2002). The BRIEF is designed for ages 5 through 18. Normative data samples were based on protocols from 1,419 parents and

720 teachers that were acquired from public and private school settings in the state of Maryland.

Academic Functioning

In general, children with ASD tend to perform more poorly than control subjects on achievement measures that involve a comprehension component, but perform well (and consistently with level of cognitive ability) on mechanical reading, spelling, and computational tasks (Minshew, Goldstein, Taylor, & Siegel, 1994). Reading has been examined in several studies of children with various ASD (Frith & Snowling, 1983; Goldberg, 1987; Loveland & Tunali-Kotoski, 1997; Minshew, Goldstein, & Siegel, 1995; Minshew et al., 1994; Myles et al., 2002; O'Connor & Hermelin, 1994; Patti & Lupinetti, 1993; Venter, Lord, & Schopler, 1992; Whitehouse & Harris, 1984). In general, decoding or basic word identification is an area of strength (commensurate with overall cognitive development or more advanced cognitive ability) for many children with ASD, amidst poor reading comprehension (Goldberg, 1987; O'Connor & Hermelin, 1994; Patti & Lupinetti, 1993). On the other hand, comprehension of written material can be quite impaired, especially when any nonliteral meaning must be inferred (Minshew et al., 1994). In addition, children with ASD may rely on syntactic structure, rather than on semantics combined with real-world knowledge (e.g., they will be unbothered by the sentence "The elephant was chased by the mouse"). Similarly, comprehension may be relatively good at the single-word level, but impaired for material of sentence length and beyond; therefore, assessments of single-word comprehension may overestimate reading ability (Newman et al., 2007).

A small number of children with ASD show advanced decoding at an early age (Newman et al., 2007). These "hyperlexic" children have not been well studied, and it is likely that their advanced reading skills may not be functionally useful in most cases. However, it appears that their reading skills may level off at about 10 years of age and become comparable to those of age-matched typically developing peers (Newman et al., 2007).

Fewer studies have examined the component processes of writing in children with ASD. In general, writing is an area of weakness (Gross, 1994; Mayes & Calhoun, 2003). For many children, this includes all aspects of writing: graphomotor skills, word retrieval, spelling, word spacing, alignment, formulation of sentences, and organization of longer works. Our collective clinical experience suggests that writing tends to be an area disliked by children with ASD, and that their efforts may be minimal and compositions short.

There is limited research on mathematics and ASD. It does appear, however, that a child's performance on math is closely associated with IQ

(Mayes & Calhoun, 2003). It has also been reported that high-functioning children with autism perform as well on computation tasks as typically developing peers do (Minshew et al., 1994).

Although a clear distinction can be made between measures of achievement and ability level (Naglieri & Bornstein, 2003), for the purpose of this section we include both tests of academic achievement (acquired skills) and ability (capacity) in determining the individual's level of current and potential functioning.

Measures

The Wechsler Individual Achievement Test—Second Edition (WIAT-II; Wechsler, 2001) is a measure of basic academic skills, designed for children 5–19 years of age. It consists of nine subtests: Mathematics Reasoning, Numerical Operations, Spelling, Written Expression, Basic Reading, Reading Comprehension, Pseudoword Decoding, Oral Language, and Listening Comprehension. The assessments elicit written or oral responses. One of the advantages of using this measure is that it was conormed with the WISC-IV across a nationally stratified sample including 498 participants. An abbreviated version is available that includes Basic Reading, Mathematics Reasoning, and Spelling. Recently, in a study of children with high-functioning autism, the WISC-IV (Wechsler, 2003) Full Scale IQ was determined to be the best predictor of academic achievement on the WIAT-II (Mayes & Calhoun, 2008). Normative data came from 3,600 children and adolescents in prekindergarten through 12th grade; the sample was based on the 1998 U.S. census.

The Woodcock–Johnson III (Woodcock, McGrew, & Mather, 2001) consists of an achievement and a cognitive battery, assessing reading, math, and writing skills, and is intended for ages 2 to 90+. The achievement battery can be used to measure general academic performance. Updated norms reflecting the 2005 U.S. census are available; these came from a sample of 8,782 individuals.

The Phonological Processing subtest from the NEPSY-II (Korkman et al., 2007) assesses the capacity to perceive and manipulate the phonemic elements (i.e., individual sound elements) of words, which is an important skill for lexical reading. Like the rest of the NEPSY-II, this measure is for ages 3–16; norms were based on a sample of 1,000 children ages 3 through 12.

The Test of Written Language—Third Edition (Hammill & Larsen, 1996) is a comprehensive assessment of written language designed for ages 7½ through 17. The test consists of an essay format and a traditional test format, to measure both spontaneous and contrived language. It provides an assessment of many areas of language, including syntax, spelling, vocabulary, and style. In addition, through story construction, plot and character development can be assessed. Normative data came from a sample of over 2,000 students in 26 states.

Social-Emotional/Social-Perceptual Skills

By definition, social perception and social-emotional expression are areas of significant weakness in ASD, and many consider social functioning to be the most important core deficit. As part of their difficulties in interpreting the social world, individuals with ASD often demonstrate impaired processing of emotions (Fein, Lucci, Braverman, & Waterhouse, 1992; Gepner, Deruelle, & Grynfeltt, 2001; Hobson, 1986a, 1986b; Hobson, Ouston, & Lee, 1988; Humphreys, Minshew, Leonard, & Behrmann, 2007), abnormal processing of faces (e.g., Adolphs, Baron-Cohen, & Tranel, 2002; Adolphs, Sears, & Piven, 2001; Baron-Cohen et al., 1999, 2000; Critchley et al., 2000; Schultz et al., 2003), impaired judgment of mental state (Baron-Cohen et al., 1999), and deficits in theory of mind (e.g., Baron-Cohen, Leslie, & Frith, 1985; Boucher, 1989).

These and other findings from pathology studies have implicated regions involved in social processing to include structures in the medial temporal lobe, such as the amygdala, superior temporal gyrus, superior temporal sulcus, and orbital–frontal gyrus. Social and emotional primacy theories have been proposed, emphasizing various aspects of social-perceptual abilities (Adolphs et al., 2001, 2002; Baron-Cohen et al., 1985, 1999, 2000; Critchley et al., 2000; Hobson, 1986a, 1986b; Hobson et al., 1988; Schultz et al., 2003). Children with pervasive developmental disorders (PDD) have been found to be slightly impaired on tasks of emotion perception where emotion was matched to context (Fein et al., 1992). In addition, difficulty in imitating actions, theory-of-mind deficits, and the presence of language impairments such as echolalia have led some researchers to believe that an abnormality in the development of mirror neurons, found in the frontal cortex, may exist in children with ASD (Williams, Whiten, Suddendorf, & Perrett, 2001).

Measures

Not very many measures assess social-emotional/social-perceptual skills; however, a few tests do address these abilities.

The Autism Diagnostic Observation Scale (ADOS; Lord, Rutter, DiLavore, & Risi, 1999) is a diagnostic measure of current behaviors of indicative autism, including social, communication, and behavioral domains; however, it can be used to assess social-emotional functioning. Specifically, the measure contains specific tasks eliciting social and play interactions, which can be coded on a behaviorally anchored scale.

Face Recognition (Benton, Sivan, Hamsher, Varney, & Spreen, 1994) is used as a measure of the individual's capacity to identify and discriminate photographs of unfamiliar human faces. The test requires the child to choose a target face among different distracters. The stimuli are presented in black and white, with different profiles and contrasts. This is a challenging task for many individuals, and the norms are quite old; as a result, it may not be useful for some individuals other than to document impairment. It is intended for persons over the age of 8. Normative data came from 286 typical adults and 266 children with normal intelligence ages 6–14.

The Social Perception domain from the NEPSY-II (Korkman et al., 2007) is a new addition to the NEPSY-II, released in spring 2007, and includes subtests of theory of mind and affect recognition. Again, see the earlier descriptions of NEPSY-II subtests for age range and normative information.

Visual–Spatial Skills

Visual–spatial skills are typically thought of as an area of strength in children with ASD (Bertone, Mottron, Jelenic, & Faubert, 2005; Caron, Mottron, Rainville, & Chouinard, 2004; O'Riordan, 2004; O'Riordan & Passetti, 2006; O'Riordan et al., 2001; Shah & Frith, 1993). Recently, individuals with high-functioning autism demonstrated superior accuracy in a map-learning task related to cued recall and shorter latency (Caron et al., 2004). It has been proposed that enhanced discrimination, detection, and memory for simple visual stimuli may explain the superior performance often observed on visual–spatial tasks in individuals with ASD. Such persons tend to show greater aptitude with feature detection and to perform well on measures of visual–spatial construction ability (Shah & Frith, 1993).

Frith (1989) was the first to put forth the theory of weak central coherence, proposing that individuals with autism show impairment in the ability to integrate information into a meaningful, coherent whole. This impairment thus results in a bias toward local processing rather than global processing. The weakness in central coherence may be observed on tasks that require more global processing (such as categorization tasks) and enhanced performance on other tasks (such as block design). The theory of weak central coherence has received equivocal support, however, and so should not serve as the basis of interpretation in neuropsychological testing (Jolliffe & Baron-Cohen, 2001; Mottron, Burack, Iarocci, Belleville, & Enns, 2003).

It has also been suggested that autistic symptoms are the result of a complex information-processing deficit (Minshew, Goldstein, & Siegel, 1997). Similarly, Rimland (1964) conceptualized autism as the primary result of poor integration of information. More recently, less functional connectivity has been reported in children with high-functioning autism than in typically developing children (Just, Cherkassky, Keller, & Minshew, 2004), supporting the notion of a fundamental deficit in integrating information at neural and cognitive levels.

Measures

The Arrows subtest from the NEPSY-II (Korkman et al., 2007) assesses a child's ability to judge the direction, angularity, and orientation of lines. This task requires the child to select arrows pointing to a center target. It is important to note that this test does not require a motor response. The age range and normative data for the NEPSY-II have been described earlier.

The Gestalt Closure subtest from the KABC-II (Kaufman & Kaufman, 2004) assesses the ability to "mentally fill in the gaps" on degraded pictures of familiar objects and figures. This subtest is similar to the Gestalt Completion Task (Street, 1931). The KABC-II's age range and normative information have also been provided earlier.

The Motor-Free Visual Perception Test, Third Edition (Colarusso & Hammill, 2003) is a measure of visual perception for children and adults ages 4 through 85. The tasks include matching, form discrimination, figure–ground, closure, and visual memory, and (as the test title suggests) can be completed without depending on motor skills. Standardization scores were based on a sample of 1,856 individuals from 36 states, which was representative of the U.S. population. It should be noted that age groups were not evenly distributed across the sample (McCane, 2006).

COMPREHENSIVE ASSESSMENT

Although clinicians may choose to select many instruments, the NEPSY-II offers comprehensive assessment with a single measure. This new NEPSY (Korkman et al., 2007), released in spring 2007, includes six domains: Executive Functioning and Attention, Language, Memory and Learning, Sensorimotor Functioning, Visuospatial Processing, and Social Perception. Several of the NEPSY-II subtests have been described earlier.

WORKING FROM A NEUROPSYCHOLOGICAL MODEL

As can be seen from the present review of neuropsychological assessment, research findings, and overarching theories, there is no clear neuropsychological profile for ASD. Instead, these disorders are heterogeneous, complex, and variable—all of which indicate the need for more comprehensive

TABLE 9.1. A Guide to Treatment Recommendations

Domain	Home recommendations	Educational recommendations
Cognitive functioning	• Provide a stimulating environment • Expose child to variety of activities	• Full inclusion when possible, with aide • Individualized curriculum
Adaptive functioning	• Include child in day-to-day activities • Provide opportunities to learn with supervision • Teach individual adaptive skills, broken down into small steps and reinforced	• Provide an aide when needed • Teach independent self-care skills • Teach functional academics • Reinforce home and community skills
Attention	• Structure activities • Provide visual cues and reminders • Use repetition and clarification	• Seat child near teacher • Limit extraneous visual and auditory stimuli • Provide breaks • Take apart tasks and show how information goes together • Use repetition • Provide teacher outlines • Allow increased time for tasks
Sensory functioning	• Limit extraneous stimuli, especially in child's room • Be cognizant of child's sensory issues • Prepare for stressful situations	• Use headphones • Computer-based teaching • Individualized work environment for study • Give gross motor breaks and intersperse preferred activities • Cubicle work • Reinforce increasing tolerance of stimulation
Motor functioning	• Physical exercise • Trampoline and swings • Craft activities that require fine motor skills	• Include child in general physical education class • Teach typing skills • Have another student take notes
Language	• Talk frequently to child, regardless of his/her level of language • Reinforce attempts at communication • Carry over behavioral or language therapy lessons at home for increased practice and generalization	• Speech and language therapy as needed • Augmented communication devices when necessary

(continued)

TABLE 9.1. *(continued)*

Domain	Home recommendations	Educational recommendations
Memory	• Give shorter assignments • Chunk information into groups • Shape new information by gradually introducing more information • Link new information to old • Use visual schedules	• Provide repetition as needed • Teach how things are associated, especially new knowledge • Organize information visually
Executive functioning	• Establish and maintain an organized room • Provide a structured home environment • Engage in activities (e.g., cooking) that require planning and organization • Chart chores and daily behavior • Play family concentration and word-finding games	• Provide structure • Teach basic organizational strategies • Use different-colored binders and folders • Use checklists • Highlight important information • Present information more clearly, slowly
Academic functioning	• Have good communication with teacher • Be available during homework • Find real-life examples of school lessons	• Develop individualized curriculum • Ensure that it is stimulating • Utilize areas of strength • Use visual materials • Use graph paper for math
Social-Emotional/ social-perceptual skills	• Exposure to peers for brief play dates with supervision • Video modeling • When watching TV, label emotions and social situations with child • Use social stories and comic strip conversations	• Buddy system at school • Social skills training • Structured activities • Group learning projects • After-school activities with children with shared interests
Visual–spatial skills	• Provide blocks, puzzles, and construction tasks for play	• If this is an area of strength, utilize it in teaching • Use visually cued instruction
General functioning	• Consistent behavior plan across environments	• Notebook between school and home

testing. It is also plausible that many measures may not be sensitive to the cognitive problems inherent in children with ASD, or specific enough to be helpful for an individual child. Even so, the advantage of a neuropsychological model is that it provides a framework for the assessment of abilities and deficits across many areas of functioning. Conceptualizing ASD in terms of many facets of functioning allows different and potentially more meaningful interpretation of these disorders. In other words, if one only assesses cognitive or language functioning in children with ASD, without a theoretical framework related to other domains of functioning, it is unlikely that the results will be very informative. In contrast, it is likely that expanding the measures used in clinical practice and research will provide more useful information, which may contribute to our understanding of behavioral endophenotypes of autism.

TREATMENT RECOMMENDATIONS

Perhaps a more important reason for providing a thorough neuropsychological assessment is that when specific deficits and areas of strength are identified, the results can better guide treatment. The findings can help identify the target behaviors to address, and can signal what strategies to use for comprehensive and individualized treatment planning (Batchelor & Dean, 1995). Table 9.1 is intended to be merely a guide as to how neuropsychological findings in cognitive functioning, adaptive skills, attention, and so on may result in specific recommendations across the various domains of functioning.

ACKNOWLEDGMENT

We would like to thank Howard Glidden, PhD, for his clinical insights in developmental neuropsychological assessment, which helped inspire this chapter.

REFERENCES

Adolphs, R., Baron-Cohen, S., & Tranel, D. (2002). Impaired recognition of social emotions following amygdala damage. *Journal of Cognitive Neuroscience, 14*(8), 1264–1274.

Adolphs, R., Sears, L., & Piven, J. (2001). Abnormal processing of social information from faces in autism. *Journal of Cognitive Neuroscience, 13*(2), 232–240.

Adrien, J. L., Lenoir, P., Martineau, J., Perrot, A., Hameury, L., Larmande, C., et al. (1993). Blind ratings of early symptoms of autism based upon family home movies. *Journal of the American Academy of Child and Adolescent Psychiatry, 32*(3), 617–626.

Allen, G., & Courchesne, E. (2001). Attention function and dysfunction in autism. *Frontiers in Bioscience, 6,* D105–D119.

American Psychiatric Association. (1994). *Diagnostic and statistical manual of mental disorders* (4th ed.). Washington, DC: Author.

American Psychiatric Association. (2000). *Diagnostic and statistical manual of mental disorders* (4th ed., text rev.). Washington, DC: Author.

Baranek, G. T. (1999). Autism during infancy: A retrospective video analysis of sensory–motor and social behaviors at 9–12 months of age. *Journal of Autism and Developmental Disorders, 29*(3), 213–224.

Barkley, R. A. (1991). The ecological validity of laboratory and analogue assessment methods of ADHD symptoms. *Journal of Abnormal Child Psychology, 19*(2), 149–178.

Baron, I.S. (2005). Test review: Wechsler Intelligence Scale for Children—Fourth Edition (WISC-IV). *Child Neuropsychology, 11*(5), 471–475.

Baron-Cohen, S., Leslie, A. M., & Frith, U. (1985). Does the autistic child have a "theory of mind"? *Cognition, 21*(1), 37–46.

Baron-Cohen, S., Ring, H. A., Bullmore, E. T., Wheelwright, S., Ashwin, C., & Williams, S. C. (2000). The amygdala theory of autism. *Neuroscience and Biobehavioral Reviews, 24*(3), 355–364.

Baron-Cohen, S., Ring, H. A., Wheelwright, S., Bullmore, E. T., Brammer, M. J., Simmons, A., et al. (1999). Social intelligence in the normal and autistic brain: An fMRI study. *European Journal of Neuroscience, 11*(6), 1891–1898.

Batchelor, E. S., Jr., & Dean, R. S. (1995). *Pediatric neuropsychology.* Boston: Allyn & Bacon.

Bayley, N. (2005). *Bayley Scales of Infant and Toddler Development, Third Edition (Bayley-III).* San Antonio, TX: Harcourt Assessment.

Beery, K. E., Buktenica, N. A., Beery, N. A. (2004). *Beery-Buktenica Developmental Test of Visual-Motor Integration,* (5th ed.). Bloomington, MN: Pearson Assessments.

Bennetto, L., Pennington, B. F., & Rogers, S. J. (1996). Intact and impaired memory functions in autism. *Child Development, 67*(4), 1816–1835.

Benton, A.L., Sivan, A.B., Hamsher, K. de S., Varney, N.R., & Spreen, O. (1994) *Contributions to neuropsychological assessment: A clinical manual* (2nd ed.). New York: Oxford University Press.

Berkeley, S. L., Zittel, L. L., Pitney, L. V., & Nichols, S. E. (2001). Locomotor and object control skills of children diagnosed with autism. *Adapted Physical Activity Quarterly, 18,* 405–416.

Bertone, A., Mottron, L., Jelenic, P., & Faubert, J. (2005). Enhanced and diminished visuo-spatial information processing in autism depends on stimulus complexity. *Brain, 128*(Pt. 10), 2430–2441.

Bishop, D. V. M. (1989). Autism, Asperger's syndrome and semantic–pragmatic disorder: Where are the boundaries? *British Journal of Disorders of Communication, 24*(2), 107–121.

Bishop, D. V. M. (1998). Development of the Children's Communication Checklist (CCC): A method for assessing qualitative aspects of communicative impairment in children. *Journal of Child Psychology and Psychiatry, 39*(6), 879–891.

Bishop, D. V. M. (2000). What's so special about Asperger syndrome?: The need for further exploration of the borderlands of autism. In A. Klin, F. R. Volkmar, & S. S. Sparrow (Eds.), *Asperger syndrome* (pp. 254–277). New York: Guilford Press.

Bishop, D. V. M., & Norbury, C. F. (2002). Exploring the borderlands of autistic disorder and specific language impairment: A study using standardised diagnostic instruments. *Journal of Child Psychology and Psychiatry, 43*(7), 917–929.

Boucher, J. (1989). The theory of mind hypothesis of autism: Explanation, evidence and assessment. *British Journal of Disorders of Communication, 24*(2), 181–198.

Bowler, D. M., Gardiner, J. M., & Berthollier, N. (2004). Source memory in adolescents and adults with Asperger's syndrome. *Journal of Autism and Developmental Disorders, 34*(5), 533–542.

Bradley-Johnson, S. (1997). Mullen Scales of Early Learning. *Psychology in the Schools, 34*(4), 379–382.

Brownell, R. (2000). *Expressive One-Word Picture Vocabulary Test*. Novato, CA: Academic Therapy.

Caron, M. J., Mottron, L., Rainville, C., & Chouinard, S. (2004). Do high functioning persons with autism present superior spatial abilities? *Neuropsychologia, 42*(4), 467–481.

Carrow-Woolfolk, E. (1999). *Comprehensive Assessment of Spoken Language*. Circle Pines, MN: American Guidance Service.

Cattell, R. B. (1971). *Abilities: Their structure, growth and action*. New York: Harcourt Brace Jovanovich.

Ciesielski, K. T., Courchesne, E., & Elmasian, R. (1990). Effects of focused selective attention tasks on event-related potentials in autistic and normal individuals. *Electroencephalography and Clinical Neurophysiology, 75*(3), 207–220.

Cohen, M. (1997). *Children's Memory Scale*. San Antonio, TX: Psychological Corporation.

Colarusso, R. P., Hammill, D. D. (2003) *Motor-Free Visual Perception Test (MVPT-3)*. Novato, CA: Academic Therapy.

Conners, C. K. (2008). *Conners' Rating Scales—Revised: Manual*. Tonawanda, NY: Multi-Health Systems.

Corbett, B. A., & Constantine, L. J. (2006). Autism and attention deficit hyperactivity disorder: Assessing attention and response control with the Integrated Visual and Auditory Continuous Performance Test. *Child Neuropsychology, 12*(4–5), 335–348.

Corbett, B. A., & Stanczak, D.E. (1999). Neuropsychological performance of adults evidencing attention-deficit hyperactivity disorder. *Archives of Clinical Neuropsychology, 14*(4), 373–387.

Courchesne, E., Townsend, J., Akshoomoff, N. A., Saitoh, O., Yeung-Courchesne, R., Lincoln, A. J., et al. (1994). Impairment in shifting attention in autistic and cerebellar patients. *Behavioral Neuroscience, 108*(5), 848–865.

Critchley, H. D., Daly, E. M., Bullmore, E. T., Williams, S. C., Van Amelsvoort, T., Robertson, D. M., et al. (2000). The functional neuroanatomy of social behaviour: Changes in cerebral blood flow when people with autistic disorder process facial expressions. *Brain, 123*(Pt. 11), 2203–2212.

Dawson, G., Meltzoff, A. N., Osterling, J., Rinaldi, J., & Brown, E. (1998). Children with autism fail to orient to naturally occurring social stimuli. *Journal of Autism and Developmental Disorders, 28*(6), 479–485.

Delis, D. C., Kaplan, E., & Kramer, J. H. (2001). *Delis–Kaplan Executive Function System*. San Antonio, TX: Psychological Corporation.

Delis, D. C., Kramer, J. H., Kaplan, E., & Ober, B. A. (1994). *California Verbal Learning Test—Children's Version: Manual*. San Antonio, TX: Psychological Corporation.

Denckla, M. B. (1996). Biological correlates of learning and attention: What is relevant to learning disability and attention-deficit hyperactivity disorder? *Journal of Developmental and Behavioral Pediatrics, 17*(2), 114–119.

Doyle, A. E., Biederman, J., Seidman, L. J., Weber, W., & Faraone, S. V. (2000). Diagnostic efficiency of neuropsychological test scores for discriminating boys with and without attention deficit-hyperactivity disorder. *Journal of Consulting and Clinical Psychology, 68*(3), 477–488.

Dunn, L. M., & Dunn, D. M. (2007). *Peabody Picture Vocabulary Test, Fourth Edition*. Bloomington, MN: Pearson Assessments.

Dunn, W. (1999). *Short Sensory Profile*. San Antonio, TX: Psychological Corporation.

Eigsti, I. M., Bennetto, L., & Dadlani, M. B. (2007). Beyond pragmatics: Morphosyntactic development in autism. *Journal of Autism and Developmental Disorders, 37*(6), 1007–1023.

Elliott, C. (2007). *Differential Ability Scales—Second Edition (DAS-II)*. San Antonio, TX: Harcourt Assessment.

Fein, D., Lucci, D., Braverman, M., & Waterhouse, L. (1992). Comprehension of affect in context in children with pervasive developmental disorders. *Journal of Child Psychology and Psychiatry, 33*(7), 1157–1167.

Filipek, P. A., Accardo, P. J., Baranek, G. T., Cook, E. H., Jr., Dawson, G., Gordon, B., et al. (1999). The screening and diagnosis of autistic spectrum disorders. *Journal of Autism and Developmental Disorders, 29*(6), 439–484.

Frith, U. (1989). A new look at language and communication in autism. *British Journal of Disorders of Communication, 24*(2), 123–150.

Frith, U., & Snowling, M. (1983). Reading for meaning and reading for sound in autistic and dyslexic children. *British Journal of Developmental Psychology, 1*(4), 329–342.

Garretson, H. B., Fein, D., & Waterhouse, L. (1990). Sustained attention in children with autism. *Journal of Autism and Developmental Disorders, 20*(1), 101–114.

Gepner, B., Deruelle, C., & Grynfeltt, S. (2001). Motion and emotion: A novel approach to the study of face processing by young autistic children. *Journal of Autism and Developmental Disorders, 31*(1), 37–45.

Geurts, H. M., Verte, S., Oosterlaan, J., Roeyers, H., & Sergeant, J. A. (2004). How specific are executive functioning deficits in attention deficit hyperactivity disorder and autism? *Journal of Child Psychology and Psychiatry, 45*(4), 836–854.

Ghaziuddin, M., Butler, E., Tsai, L., & Ghaziuddin, N. (1994). Is clumsiness a marker for Asperger syndrome? *Journal of Intellectual Disability Research, 38*(Pt. 5), 519–527.

Gillberg, C., Ehlers, S., Schaumann, H., Jakobsson, G., Dahlgren, S. O., Lindblom, R., et al. (1990). Autism under age 3 years: A clinical study of 28 cases referred for autistic symptoms in infancy. *Journal of Child Psychology and Psychiatry, 31*(6), 921–934.

Gilotty, L., Kenworthy, L., Sirian, L., Black, D. O., & Wagner, A. E. (2002). Adaptive skills and executive function in autism spectrum disorders. *Child Neuropsychology, 8*(4), 241–248.

Gioia, G., Isquith, P., Guy, S., & Kenworthy, L. E. (2000). *Behavior Rating Inventory of Executive Function.* Odessa, FL: Psychological Assessment Resources.

Goldberg, M. C., Mostofsky, S. H., Cutting, L. E., Mahone, E. M., Astor, B. C., Denckla, M. B., et al. (2005). Subtle executive impairment in children with autism and children with ADHD. *Journal of Autism and Developmental Disorders, 35*(3), 279–293.

Goldberg, T. E. (1987). On hermetic reading abilities. *Journal of Autism and Developmental Disorders, 17*(1), 29–44.

Golden, C. J., Freshwater, S. M., & Golden, Z. (2004). *Stroop Color and Word Test: Children's Version.* Wood Dale, IL: Stoelting.

Goldman, R., Fristoe, M., & Woodcock, R. W. (1970). *Test of Auditory Discrimination.* Circle Pines, MN: American Guidance Service.

Goldstein, S., & Goldstein, M. (1998). *Managing attention deficit hyperactivity disorder in children: A guide for practitioners.* New York: Wiley.

Greenberg, L., & Waldman, I. (1993). Developmental normative data on the Test of Variables of Attention (TOVA). *Journal of the American Academy of Child and Adolescent Psychiatry, 34,* 1019–1030.

Gross, J. (1994). Asperger's syndrome: A label worth having? *Educational Psychology, 10*(2), 104–110.

Hammill, D. D., & Larsen, S. C. (1996). *Test of Written Language—Third Edition.* Austin, TX: PRO-ED.

Harrison, P. L., & Oakland, T. (2003). *Adaptive Behavior Assessment System— Second Edition (ABAS-II).* San Antonio, TX: Psychological Corporation.

Heaton, R. K., Chelune, G. J., Talley, J. L., Kay, G. G., & Curtis, G. (1993). *Wisconsin Card Sorting Test (WCST) manual revised and expanded.* Lutz, FL: Psychological Assessment Resources.

Heaton, R. K., & PAR Staff. (2000). *WCST-64: Computer Version 2 Research Edition (WCST-64:CV2).* Lutz, FL: Psychological Assessment Resources.

Hobson, R. P. (1986a). The autistic child's appraisal of expressions of emotion. *Journal of Child Psychology and Psychiatry, 27*(3), 321–342.

Hobson, R. P. (1986b). The autistic child's appraisal of expressions of emotion: A further study. *Journal of Child Psychology and Psychiatry, 27*(5), 671–680.

Hobson, R. P., Ouston, J., & Lee, A. (1988). Emotion recognition in autism: Coordinating faces and voices. *Psychological Medicine, 18*(4), 911–923.

Hollander, E. (1997). The obsessive–compulsive spectrum disorders. *International Review of Psychiatry, 9*(1), 99–110.

Hollander, E., DelGiudice-Asch, G., Simon, L., Schmeidler, J., Cartwright, C., DeCaria, C. M., Kwon, J., Cunningham-Rundles, C., Chapman, F., & Zabriskie, J. B. (1999). B lymphocyte antigen D8/17 and repetitive behaviors in autism. *American Journal of Psychiatry, 156*(2), 317–320.

Hollander, E., Dolgoff-Kaspar, R., Cartwright, C., Rawitt, R., & Novotny, S. (2001). An open trial of divalproex sodium in autism spectrum disorders. *Journal of Clinical Psychiatry, 62*(7), 530–534.

Hollander, E., Phillips, A. T., & Yeh, C. C. (2003). Targeted treatments for symptom domains in child and adolescent autism. *Lancet, 362*(9385), 732–734.

Homack, S., Lee, D., & Riccio, C. A. (2005). Test review: Delis–Kaplan Executive Function System. *Journal of Clinical and Experimental Neuropsychology, 27*(5), 599–609.

Howlin, P. (2003). Outcome in high-functioning adults with autism with and without early language delays: Implications for the differentiation between autism and Asperger syndrome. *Journal of Autism and Developmental Disorders, 33*(1), 3–13.

Humphreys, K., Minshew, N., Leonard, G. L., & Behrmann, M. (2007). A fine-grained analysis of facial expression processing in high-functioning adults with autism. *Neuropsychologia, 45*(4), 685–695.

Jolliffe, T., & Baron-Cohen, S. (2001). A test of central coherence theory: Can adults with high-functioning autism or Asperger syndrome integrate fragments of an object? *Cognitive Neuropsychiatry, 6*(3), 193–216.

Just, M. A., Cherkassky, V. L., Keller, T. A., & Minshew, N. J. (2004). Cortical activation and synchronization during sentence comprehension in high-functioning autism: evidence of underconnectivity. *Brain, 127*(8), 1811–1821.

Kamio, Y., & Toichi, M. (1998). Affective understanding in high-functioning autistic adolescents. *Japanese Journal of Child and Adolescent Psychiatry, 39*, 340–351.

Kaufman, A. S., & Kaufman, N. L. (2004). *Kaufman Assessment Battery for Children, Second Edition.* Circle Pines, MN: American Guidance Service.

Kelley, E., Paul, J. J., Fein, D., & Naigles, L.R. (2006). Residual language deficits in optimal outcome children with a history of autism. *Journal of Autism and Developmental Disorders, 36*(6), 807–828.

Kinsbourne, M. (1991). Overfocusing: An apparent subtype of attention deficit hyperactivity disorder. In N. Amir, I. Rapin, & D. Branski (Eds.), *Pediatric neurology: Vol. 1. Behavior and cognition of the child with brain dysfunction* (pp. 18–35). Basel: Karger.

Kjelgaard, M. M., & Tager-Flusberg, H. (2001). An investigation of language impairment in autism: Implications for genetic subgroups. *Language and Cognitive Processes, 16*(2–3), 287–308.

Kleinhans, N., Akshoomoff, N., & Delis, D. C. (2005). Executive functions in autism and Asperger's disorder: Flexibility, fluency, and inhibition. *Developmental Neuropsychology, 27*(3), 379–401.

Klin, A., Saulnier, C. A., Sparrow, S. S., Cicchetti, D. V., Volkmar, F. R., & Lord, C. (2007). Social and communication abilities and disabilities in higher functioning individuals with autism spectrum disorders: The Vineland and the ADOS. *Journal of Autism and Developmental Disorders, 37*(4), 748–459.

Korkman, M., Kirk, U., & Kemp, S. (2007). *NEPSY—Second Edition.* San Antonio, TX: Harcourt Assessment.

Lafayette Instruments. (1999). *Purdue Pegboard Test—Revised Edition.* Lafayette, IN: Author.

Landa, R. J., & Goldberg, M. C. (2005). Language, social, and executive functions in high functioning autism: A continuum of performance. *Journal of Autism and Developmental Disorders, 35*(5), 557–573.

Leark, R. A., Greenberk, L. K., Kindschi, C. L., Dupuy, T. R., & Hughes, S. J. (2007). Test of Variables of Attention: Professional Manual. Los Alamitos, CA: The Tova Company.

Lewy, A. L., & Dawson, G. (1992). Social stimulation and joint attention in young autistic children. *Journal of Abnormal Child Psychology, 20*(6), 555–566.

Lezak, M. (1995). *Neuropsychological assessment* (3rd ed.). New York: Oxford University Press.

Liss, M., Fein, D., Allen, D., Dunn, M., Feinstein, C., Morris, R., et al. (2001). Executive functioning in high-functioning children with autism. *Journal of Child Psychology and Psychiatry, 42*(2), 261–270.

Liss, M., Saulnier, C., Fein, D., & Kinsbourne, M. (2006). Sensory and attention abnormalities in autistic spectrum disorders. *Autism, 10*(2), 155–172.

Llorente, A. M., Williams, J., Satz, P., & D'Elia, L. F. (2003). *Children's Color Trails Test.* Lutz, FL: Psychological Assessment Resources.

Lord, C., Rutter, M., DiLavore, P., & Risi, S. (1999). *Autism Diagnostic Observation Schedule—WPS Edition.* Los Angeles, CA: Western Psychological Services.

Loveland, K. A., & Tunali-Kotoski, B. (1997). The school age child with autism. In D. J. Cohen & F. R. Volkmar (Eds.), *Handbook of autism and pervasive developmental disorders* (2nd ed., pp. 283–308). New York: Wiley.

Luna, B., Minshew, N. J., Garver, K. E., Lazar, N. A., Thulborn, K. R., Eddy, W. F., et al. (2002). Neocortical system abnormalities in autism: An fMRI study of spatial working memory. *Neurology, 59*(6), 834–840.

Manjiviona, J., & Prior, M. (1995). Comparison of Asperger syndrome and high-functioning autistic children on a test of motor impairment. *Journal of Autism and Developmental Disorders, 25*(1), 23–39.

Manly, T., Anderson, V., Nimmo-Smith, I., Turner, A., Watson, P., & Robertson, I. H. (2001). The differential assessment of children's attention: The Test of Everyday Attention for Children (TEA-Ch), normative sample and ADHD performance. *Journal of Child Psychology and Psychiatry, 42*(8),1065–1081.

Mari, M., Castiello, U., Marks, D., Marraffa, C., & Prior, M. (2003). The reach-to-grasp movement in children with autism spectrum disorder. *Philosophical Transactions of the Royal Society of London, Series B, 358*(1430), 393–403.

Mathiowetz, V., Volland, G., Kashman, N., & Weber, K. (1992). Nine Hole Peg Test (NHPT). In D. Wade (Ed.), *Measurement in neurological rehabilitation* (p. 171). New York: Oxford University Press.

Mayes, S.D., & Calhoun, S.L. (2003). Ability profiles in children with autism: Influence of age and IQ. *Autism, 7*(1), 65–80.

Mayes, S. D., & Calhoun, S. L. (2008). WISC-IV and WIAT-II profiles in children with high-functioning autism. *Journal of Autism and Developmental Disorders, 38*(3), 428–439.

McCane, S. J. (2006). Test review: Motor-Free Visual Perception Test. *Journal of Psychoeducational Assessment, 24*(3), 265–272.

Millward, C., Powell, S., Messer, D., & Jordan, R. (2000). Recall for self and other in autism: Children's memory for events experienced by themselves and their peers. *Journal of Autism and Developmental Disorders, 30*(1), 15–28.

Minshew, N. J., Goldstein, G., & Siegel, D. J. (1995). Speech and language in high functioning autistic individuals. *Neuropsychology, 9*, 255–261.

Minshew, N. J., Goldstein, G., & Siegel, D. J. (1997). Neuropsychologic functioning in autism: Profile of a complex information processing disorder. *Journal of the International Neuropsychological Society, 3*(4), 303–316.

Minshew, N. J., Goldstein, G., Taylor, H. G., & Siegel, D. J. (1994). Academic achievement in high functioning autistic individuals. *Journal of Clinical and Experimental Neuropsychology, 16*(2), 261–270.

Mottron, L., Burack, J. A., Iarocci, G., Belleville, S., & Enns, J. T. (2003). Locally oriented perception with intact global processing among adolescents with high-functioning autism: Evidence from multiple paradigms. *Journal of Child Psychology and Psychiatry, 44*(6), 904–913.

Mullen, E. M. (1995). *Mullen Scales of Early Learning* (AGS ed.). Circle Pines, MN: American Guidance Service.

Myles, B. S., Hilgenfeld, T. D., Barnhill, G. P., Griswold, D. E., Hagiwara, T., & Simpson, R. L. (2002). Analysis of reading skills in individuals with Asperger syndrome. *Focus on Autism and Other Developmental Disabilitites, 17*(1), 44–47.

Naglieri, J. A., & Bornstein, B. T. (2003). Intelligence and achievement: Just how correlated are they? *Journal of Psychoeducational Assessment, 21*(3), 244.

Naglieri, J. A., & Das, J. P. (1997). *Cognitive Assessment System.* Itasca, IL: Riverside.

Naglieri, J. A., & Das, J. P. (2005). Planning, attention, simultaneous, successive (PASS) theory: A revision of the concept of intelligence. In D. P. Flanagan & P. L. Harrison (Eds.), *Contemporary intellectual assessment* (2nd ed., pp. 136–182). New York: Guilford Press.

Naglieri, J. A., Goldstein, S., Delauder, B. Y., & Schwebach, A. (2005). Relationships between the WISC-III and the Cognitive Assessment System with Conners' Rating Scales and continuous performance tests. *Archives of Clinical Neuropsychology, 20*(3), 385–401.

Newman, T. M., Macomber, D., Naples, A. J., Babitz, T., Volkmar, F., & Grigorenko, E. L. (2007). Hyperlexia in children with autism spectrum disorders. *Journal of Autism and Developmental Disorders, 37*(4), 760–774.

O'Connor, N., & Hermelin, B. (1994). Two autistic savant readers. *Journal of Autism and Developmental Disorders, 24*(4), 501–515.

O'Riordan, M. A. (2004). Superior visual search in adults with autism. *Autism, 8*(3), 229–248.

O'Riordan, M. A., & Passetti, F. (2006). Discrimination in autism within different sensory modalities. *Journal of Autism and Developmental Disorders, 36*(5), 665–675.

O'Riordan, M. A., Plaisted, K. C., Driver, J., & Baron-Cohen, S. (2001). Superior visual search in autism. *Journal of Experimental Psychology: Human Perception and Performance, 27*(3), 719–730.

O'Shea, A. G., Fein, D. A., Cillessen, A. H., Klin, A., & Schultz, R. T. (2005). Source memory in children with autism spectrum disorders. *Developmental Neuropsychology, 27*(3), 337–360.

Ozonoff, S., & Jensen, J. (1999). Brief report: Specific executive function profiles in three neurodevelopmental disorders. *Journal of Autism and Developmental Disorders, 29*(2), 171–177.

Ozonoff, S., Pennington, B. F., & Rogers, S. J. (1991). Executive function deficits in high-functioning autistic individuals: Relationship to theory of mind. *Journal of Child Psychology and Psychiatry, 32*(7), 1081–1105.

Ozonoff, S., & Strayer, D. L. (1997). Inhibitory function in nonretarded children with autism. *Journal of Autism and Developmental Disorders, 27*(1), 59–77.

Ozonoff, S., & Strayer, D. L. (2001). Further evidence of intact working memory in autism. *Journal of Autism and Developmental Disorders, 31*(3), 257–263.

Pascualvaca, D. M., Fantie, B. D., Papageorgiou, M., & Mirsky, A. F. (1998). Attentional capacities in children with autism: Is there a general deficit in shifting focus? *Journal of Autism and Developmental Disorders, 28*(6), 467–478.

Patti, P. J., & Lupinetti, L. (1993). Brief report: Implications of hyperlexia in an autistic savant. *Journal of Autism and Developmental Disorders, 23*(2), 397–405.

Pellicano, E., Maybery, M., Durkin, K., & Maley, A. (2006). Multiple cognitive capabilities/deficits in children with an autism spectrum disorder: "Weak" central coherence and its relationship to theory of mind and executive control. *Development and Psychopathology, 18*(1), 77–98.

Pennington, B. F., & Ozonoff, S. (1996). Executive functions and developmental psychopathology. *Journal of Child Psychology and Psychiatry, 37*(1), 51–87.

Pierce, K., Glad, K. S., & Schreibman, L. (1997). Social perception in children with autism: An attentional deficit? *Journal of Autism and Developmental Disorders, 27*(3), 265–282.

Poole, J. L., Burtner, P. A., Torres, T. A., McMullen, C. K., Markham, A., Marcum, M. L., et al. (2005). Measuring dexterity in children using the Nine-Hole Peg Test. *Journal of Hand Therapy, 18*(3), 348–351.

Prior, M. R. (1979). Cognitive abilities and disabilities in infantile autism: A review. *Journal of Abnormal Child Psychology, 7*(4), 357–380.

Prior, M. R., & Bradshaw, J. L. (1979). Hemisphere functioning in autistic children. *Cortex, 15*(1), 73–81.

Provost, B., Lopez, B. R., & Heimerl, S. (2007). A comparison of motor delays in young children: Autism spectrum disorder, developmental delay, and developmental concerns. *Journal of Autism and Developmental Disorders, 37*(2), 321–328.

Rimland, B. (1964). *Infantile autism: The syndrome and its implications for a neural theory of behavior.* New York: Appleton-Century-Crofts.

Rogers, S. J., Bennetto, L., McEvoy, R., & Pennington, B. F. (1996). Imitation and pantomime in high-functioning adolescents with autism spectrum disorders. *Child Development, 67*(5), 2060–2073.

Roid, G. H. (2003). *Stanford–Binet Intelligence Scales, Fifth Edition.* Itasca, IL: Riverside.

Russell, J. (1997). *Autism as an executive disorder.* New York: Oxford University Press.

Rutter, M. (1974). The development of infantile autism. *Psychological Medicine, 4,* 147–163.

Rutter, M. (1979). Language, cognition and autism. *Annals of the Academy of Medicine, Singapore, 8*(3), 301–311.

Rutter, M., Bartak, L., & Newman, S. (1971). Autism—a central disorder of cognition and language. In M. Rutter (Ed.), *Infantile autism: Concepts, characteristics and treatment* (pp. 148–171). London: Churchill Livingstone.

Sandford, J. A., & Turner, A. (2000). *Integrated Visual and Auditory Continuous Performance Test manual.* Richmond, VA: Brain Train.

Schultz, R. T., Grelotti, D. J., Klin, A., Kleinman, J., Van der Gaag, C., Marois, R., et al. (2003). The role of the fusiform face area in social cognition: implications for the pathobiology of autism. *Philosophical Transactions of the Royal Society of London, Series B, 358*(1430), 415–427.

Semel, E., Wiig, E. H., & Secord, W. A. (2003). *Clinical Evaluation of Language Fundamentals–Fourth Edition.* San Antonio, TX: Harcourt Assessment.

Shah, A., & Frith, U. (1993). Why do autistic individuals show superior performance on the Block Design task? *Journal of Child Psychology and Psychiatry, 34*(8), 1351–1364.

Sheslow, D., & Adams, W. (2003). *Wide Range Assessment of Memory and Learning, Second Edition (WRAML2).* San Antonio, TX: Harcourt Assessment.

Smith, Y. A., Hong, E., & Presson, C. (2000). Normative and validation studies of the Nine-Hole Peg Test with children. *Perceptual and Motor Skills, 90*(3, Pt. 1), 823–843.

Sparrow, S. S., Cicchetti, D. V., & Balla, D. A. (2005). *Vineland Adaptive Behavior Scales, Second Edition (Vineland-II).* Circle Pines, MN: American Guidance Service.

Spreen, O., & Benton, A. L. (1977). *Neurosensory Center Comprehensive Examination for Aphasia (NCCEA).* Victoria, British Columbia, Canada: University of Victoria Neuropsychology Laboratory.

Stevens, M. C., Fein, D. A., Dunn, M., Allen, D., Waterhouse, L. H., Feinstein, C., et al. (2000). Subgroups of children with autism by cluster analysis: A longitudinal examination. *Journal of the American Academy of Child and Adolescent Psychiatry, 39*(3), 346–352.

Street, R. F. (1931). *A Gestalt Completion Test.* New York: Teachers College, Columbia University.

Sutera, S., Pandey, J., Esser, E. L., Rosenthal, M. A., Wilson, L. B., Barton, M., et al. (2007). Predictors of optimal outcome in toddlers diagnosed with autism spectrum disorders. *Journal of Autism and Developmental Disorders, 37*(1), 98–107.

Tager-Flusberg, H. (1981). On the nature of linguistic functioning in early infantile autism. *Journal of Autism and Developmental Disorders, 11*(1), 45–56.

Tager-Flusberg, H. (1996). Brief report: Current theory and research on language and communication in autism. *Journal of Autism and Developmental Disorders, 26*(2),169–172.

Tager-Flusberg, H., & Joseph, R. M. (2003). Identifying neurocognitive phenotypes in autism. *Philosophical Transactions of the Royal Society of London, Series B, 358*(1430), 303–314.

Teitelbaum, O., Benton, T., Shah, P. K., Prince, A., Kelly, J. L., & Teitelbaum, P. (2004). Eshkol–Wachman movement notation in diagnosis: The early detection of Asperger's syndrome. *Proceedings of the National Academy of Sciences USA, 101*(32), 11909–11914.

Teitelbaum, P., Teitelbaum, O., Nye, J., Fryman, J., & Maurer, R. G. (1998). Movement analysis in infancy may be useful for early diagnosis of autism. *Proceedings of the National Academy of Sciences USA, 95*(23), 13982–13987.

Tiffin, J., & Asher, E. J. (1948). The Purdue Pegboard: Norms and studies of reliability and validity. *Journal of Applied Psychology, 32,* 234–247.

Townsend, J., Harris, N. S., & Courchesne, E. (1996). Visual attention abnormalities in autism: Delayed orienting to location. *Journal of the International Neuropsychological Society, 2*(6), 541–550.

Turkheimer, E. (1989). Techniques of quantitative measurement of morphological structures of the central nervous system. In R. A. Yeo, E. D. Bigler, & E. Turkheimer (Eds.), *Neuropsychological function and brain imaging* (pp. 47–64). New York: Plenum Press.

Venter, A., Lord, C., & Schopler, E. (1992). A follow-up study of high-functioning autistic children. *Journal of Child Psychology and Psychiatry, 33*(3), 489–507.

Vilensky, J. A., Damasio, A. R., & Maurer, R. G. (1981). Gait disturbances in patients with autistic behavior: A preliminary study. *Archives of Neurology, 38*(10), 646–649.

Volkmar, F. R. (2003). Adaptive skills. *Journal of Autism and Developmental Disorders, 33*(1), 109–110.

Waterhouse, L., Morris, R., Allen, D., Dunn, M., Fein, D., Feinstein, C., et al. (1996). Diagnosis and classification in autism. *Journal of Autism and Developmental Disorders, 26*(1), 59–86.

Watling, R. L., Deitz, J., & White, O. (2001). Comparison of Sensory Profile scores of young children with and without autism spectrum disorders. *American Journal of Occupational Therapy, 55*(4), 416–423.

Wechsler, D. (1999). *Wechsler Abbreviated Scale of Intelligence.* San Antonio, TX: Psychological Corporation.

Wechsler, D. (2001). *Wechsler Individual Achievement Test—Second Edition.* San Antonio, TX: Harcourt Assessment.

Wechsler, D. (2002). *Wechsler Preschool and Primary Scale of Intelligence—Third Edition.* San Antonio, TX: Psychological Corporation.

Wechsler, D. (2003). *Wechsler Intelligence Scale for Children—Fourth Edition.* San Antonio, TX: Psychological Corporation.

Welsh, M. C., & Pennington, B. F. (1988). Assessing frontal lobe functioning in children: View from developmental psychology. *Developmental Neuropsychology, 4,* 199–230.

Whitehouse, D., & Harris, J. C. (1984). Hyperlexia in infantile autism. *Journal of Autism and Developmental Disorders, 14*(3), 281–289.

Wiig, E. H., & Secord, W. (1989). *Test of Language Competence—Expanded Edition.* San Antonio, TX: Psychological Corporation.

Williams, D. L., Goldstein, G., Carpenter, P. A., & Minshew, N. J. (2005a). Verbal and spatial working memory in autism. *Journal of Autism and Developmental Disorders, 35*(6), 747–756.

Williams, D. L., Goldstein, G., & Minshew, N. J. (2005b). Impaired memory for faces and social scenes in autism: Clinical implications of memory dysfunction. *Archives of Clinical Neuropsychology, 20*(1), 1–15.

Williams, J. H., Whiten, A., Suddendorf, T., & Perrett, D. I. (2001). Imitation, mirror neurons and autism. *Neuroscience and Biobehavioral Reviews, 25*(4), 287–295.

Williams, K. T. (2007). *Expressive Vocabulary Test, Second Edition.* Bloomington, MN: Pearson Assessments.

Woodcock, R. W., McGrew, K. S., & Mather, N. (2001). *Woodcock–Johnson III.* Itasca, IL: Riverside.

Zimmerman, I. L., Steiner, V. G., & Pond, R. E. (2002). *Preschool Language Scale, Fourth Edition (PLS-4).* San Antonio, TX: Harcourt Assessment.

CHAPTER TEN

Assessment of Comorbid Psychiatric Conditions in Autism Spectrum Disorders

Lesley Deprey

Sally Ozonoff

The occurrence of two or more clinical diagnoses, known as "comorbidity," has received much attention in the child psychopathology literature in recent years (Matson & Nebel-Schwalm, 2006). Co-occurrence of disorders within the same time interval can be defined narrowly, more broadly, or even with reference to the entire lifetime (e.g., "concurrent" vs. "successive" comorbidity; Angold, Erkanli, Costello, & Rutter, 1996; Costello, Foley, & Angold, 2006). The issue of comorbidity and autism spectrum disorders (ASD) has become increasingly important, as it has been recognized that ASD can co-occur with a number of other conditions, and that these additional problems have a substantial negative impact on functioning (Lecavalier, 2006). Two recent large studies found that over 70% of children with ASD were above diagnostic thresholds for another emotional or behavioral disorder (Leyfer et al., 2006; Tonge & Einfeld, 2003). Thus this is an area that must be addressed in any comprehensive evaluation of a child with an ASD. Comorbidity should be considered whenever there are signs of psychiatric problems that are not part of ASD; when there are marked changes in functioning from baseline, or an existing problem is markedly exacerbated; or when an individual with an ASD does not respond as expected to interventions that are traditionally effective (Lainhart, 1999).

Assessment of comorbidity is inherently complex. Children may present with mixed symptoms that may stem from a single disorder with unusual presentation or from the simultaneous occurrence of multiple disorders (Caron & Rutter, 1991). Although students and clinicians are often taught to make a single diagnosis whenever possible, comorbidity is very common in epidemiological studies of many child psychiatric disorders. Conversely, there are a variety of ways in which an apparent picture of comorbidity can be falsely created. In a seminal paper, Caron and Rutter (1991) remind us that detection artifacts, such as referral biases, can distort impressions of the frequency of comorbidity. It is also possible that a disorder has been misconceived, so that overlapping diagnostic criteria, artificial subdivisions of syndromes, or one disorder representing an early manifestation of another disorder may present a false picture of comorbidity. Beyond such artifactual comorbidities, these authors describe the mechanisms that may underlie true comorbidity, such as shared risk factors or one disorder creating a risk for another disorder.

Developmental specialists involved in both clinical and research endeavors must be knowledgeable about the interplay between neurodevelopment and mental health issues, as the presentation of comorbid conditions results in more challenging assessments. The complexity of diagnosing ASD, with their different subtypes and broad range of intellectual functioning, is already a difficult task. Differences in clinical presentation associated with comorbidity add to the challenges of diagnostic assessment. Although differential diagnosis is difficult, it is essential, as treatment of the ASD symptoms alone will usually not result in improvement in the other behavioral or emotional problems that coexist. Undertreatment or partial treatment can result in significant functional impairment.

This chapter begins with a discussion of theoretical and methodological issues associated with comorbidity in ASD. We use the term "ASD" to encompass autistic disorder, Asperger's disorder, and pervasive developmental disorder not otherwise specified (PDD-NOS). We then discuss specific psychiatric conditions known to co-occur with ASD, including mood disorders, anxiety disorders, attention-deficit/hyperactivity disorder (ADHD), tic disorders, and psychotic disorders. Each section reviews the literature on prevalence rates, differential diagnosis, and differences in symptom expression when the disorder or disorders co-occur with ASD. After this, we discuss different instruments that can be helpful in the assessment of possible comorbidities and the differential diagnostic process. We end the chapter with directions for future research.

CHALLENGES IN ASSESSING
COMORBID CONDITIONS

Clinicians encounter several difficulties when assessing children with ASD whose functioning may also be affected by other forms of psychopathology.

Standardization and Norming Issues

Standardized assessment instruments should be utilized to evaluate impairment and range of possible diagnosable disorders (Kazdin, 1993). Unfortunately, most behavior checklists and diagnostic interview tools were standardized without children with ASD, making interpretation of scores challenging. It is not clear that norms developed for children without developmental disorders and with average cognitive functioning are relevant for children with ASD, with or without mental retardation. Thus it is sometimes hard to know whether a child is scoring in the clinical range on an instrument because he or she has ASD, or because he or she is experiencing the particular difficulties that the tool measures.

Insight and Self-Report Problems

A second set of difficulties in assessing potential psychiatric problems in children with ASD and/or mental retardation is limitations in the ability to process and talk about emotions and internal experiences (Sovner, 1996). In the assessment of psychopathology, the gold standard method is self-report, which captures "the experiencing self"—the individual centered in the phenomenon (Derogatis, 1983). Unfortunately, limitations in insight and mentalizing pose considerable challenges to obtaining accurate, clinically useful information when self-report is utilized in individuals with ASD. Many studies have demonstrated the difficulties individuals with ASD experience in attributing mental and emotional states to others (Baron-Cohen, O'Riordan, Stone, Jones, & Plaisted, 1999b; Jolliffe & Baron-Cohen, 1999; Sicotte & Stemberger, 1999). Such difficulties are also proposed to cause these individuals impairments in recognizing and describing their own emotional and mental states (Baron-Cohen, Tager-Flusberg, & Cohen, 2000; Ben Shalom et al., 2006; Berthoz & Hill, 2005). Individuals with ASD tend to focus on physical, concrete characteristics rather than on inner abstract experiences (Hill, Berthoz, & Frith, 2004). It has been suggested that children with ASD lack an "inner language" to describe their socioemotional difficulties (Walters, Barrett, & Feinstein, 1990). Functional communication and pragmatic language skills may be limited. Response perseveration can also have an impact on self-report ratings (Ben Shalom et al., 2006). For all these reasons, self-reporting of internal phenomena—essential to most assessments of psychopathology—may be less useful with children with ASD, especially those who are younger or lower-functioning. Higher functioning adolescents and adults may be able to provide more useful self-reports. One study found that adolescents and adults with Asperger's syndrome did not differ from comparison subjects on a measure of "private self-consciousness," defined as attention to the private aspects of the self, such as feelings and motives (Blackshaw, Kinderman, Hare, & Hatton, 2001). Autobiographical writings of adults with Asperger syndrome reveal awareness of their interpersonal and socioemotional difficulties (Happé, 1991; Spicer, 1998). A recent paper found that self-report using the Minnesota Multiphasic Personality Inventory–2 yielded profiles very consistent with the ASD phenotype, with elevations on scales measuring social isolation, introversion, and rigidity; these findings indicated that the adult participants were able to describe their difficulties validly (Ozonoff, Garcia, Clark, & Lainhart, 2005a). A case study of a young adult with high-functioning autism suggested that he had "accurate knowledge of his traits" (Klein, Chan, & Loftus, 1999, p. 413). Although such evidence is indirect, this collective body of work suggests that there may be some capacity for introspection, and therefore for accurate self-reporting on dimensions of psychopathology, in older and higher-functioning individuals on the autism spectrum. Nevertheless, we believe that self-report measures should still be used cautiously with the ASD population.

Differences in Symptom Manifestation

A third complication in the assessment of comorbidities in ASD is that differences in clinical expression can influence the range and quality of symptoms displayed. Symptoms of another condition may look different in the context of ASD, and symptom expression may be influenced by lowered cognitive capacity (Sovner, 1996). Individuals with ASD may not demonstrate certain symptoms, such as the feelings of guilt often seen in depression or the grandiosity and inflated self-esteem typical of mania, due to cognitive limitations, lack of understanding of certain concepts, or reduced social and peer comparison. Anxiety may be manifested as obsessive questioning or insistence on sameness, rather than as rumination or somatic complaints. Emotional problems and oppositionality may present when minor changes are made to routines. The ASD alone involve differences in socioemotional expression (such as reductions in reciprocity, joint attention, and coordination of gaze and gesture) that will affect social responsiveness during an assessment, as well as overall clinical impressions. Changes in sleep and/or eating behaviors may be less obvious because of the motivation of individuals with ASD to follow routines (Lainhart, 1999). In the sections on specific comorbid conditions below, we review what is known for each disorder about potential differences between typical symptom manifestation and manifestation within the context of ASD.

Solutions to Assessment Challenges

One of the best ways to evaluate the presence of comorbidities in ASD is to focus on changes in behavior from baseline. Significant changes in behavior from how the individual was described in the past—such as increases in social withdrawal, repetitive motor movements, aggression/outbursts, resistance to change, irritability, and avoidance of novelty; or decreases in activities that once brought pleasure—can be crucial to making an accurate diagnosis (Lainhart, 1999). For example, a decrease in the amount of time spent discussing a special interest (e.g., the solar system or Canadian Prime Ministers) may be helpful in evaluating anhedonia and the onset of a mood disorder. In addition, the appearance of new challenging behaviors that have not been part of the clinical picture in the past, such as self-injury or aggression, will indicate the need for further evaluation. Unexplained decreases in self-care and other everyday living skills may also present diagnostic clues related to comorbidities in ASD. A comorbidity should be suspected when such changes from baseline are accompanied by significant clinical impairment in functioning and decreased adaptive behavior. Evaluations of risk factors (especially family history of comorbid conditions) and of environmental factors (e.g., appropriate access to services and support) are other key elements to making an accurate differential diagnosis.

Differential Diagnosis versus Comorbidity

So far, we have discussed psychiatric problems that may coexist with ASD. However, it is of course also possible that a child has another disorder alone, and that in fact the diagnosis of an ASD is inaccurate. Thus another important part of the process of case formulation is differential diagnosis: Does the child have both an ASD and another disorder, or just another disorder? The rest of this chapter will help clinicians address the first half of this question, but how can an evaluator tell whether it would be more parsimonious to ascribe difficulties to just one condition? For example, poor eye contact and low social initiative may be indicative of an ASD, but also of depression. How does a clinician go about deciding whether the difficulties are due to one or the other of these explanations, rather than comorbidity? The answer is deceptively simple. Examining the developmental history for the consistency of symptoms over time and pervasiveness across situations will help the clinician immensely in the process of differential diagnosis. Children with depression alone, for example, do not exhibit the widespread and long-term difficulties in social interaction, communication, and behavior that are characteristic of ASD. Children who present with a restricted range of facial expressions, poor eye contact, and low social initiative, and who also display limited empathy, few gestures, pedantic speech, or unusual interests, are likely to have both ASD and a mood disorder. The package of social and communication limitations, combined with odd or repetitive behaviors, expressed consistently throughout the lifetime, should alert the clinician that ASD must be part of the differential diagnosis. No other condition includes all of these difficulties. Then, if additional problems not encompassed by the ASD criteria are present, if there are changes from baseline indicating onset of new difficulties, or if the individual is not responding as expected to treatment, comorbidity should be considered (Lainhart, 1999). If, however, the social and communication difficulties are limited to behaviors that might plausibly stem from depression and do not extend to pragmatic communication, symbolic activities, empathy, or stereotyped behaviors, or have not been part of the developmental history but are of recent onset, then the differential diagnosis is more likely to include just the mood disorder.

In the next section, we consider specific disorders that commonly co-occur with ASD.

ASD AND SPECIFIC COMORBIDITIES

ASD and Depression

Prevalence

The Methods for the Epidemiology of Mental Disorders in Children and Adolescents study estimated that the prevalence rate of mood disorders in U.S. children ages 9–17 years is 6.2% (Lahey et al., 1996), with the rate of major depression estimated at 5% (Shaffer et al., 1996). Depression and other mood disorders are among the most commonly reported mental health problems in individuals with ASD (Howlin, 1997). No epidemiological studies have yet been conducted to help estimate prevalence, but the occurrence of depression in clinic-based samples has been reported to range from 2% to 38% (Ghaziuddin, Tsai, & Ghaziuddin, 1992; Lainhart & Folstein, 1994). Thus rates in persons with ASD may be even higher than the general population risk, particularly in higher-functioning adolescent and young adult samples (Brereton, Tonge, & Einfeld, 2006; Ghaziuddin, Ghaziuddin, & Greden, 2002; Kim, Szatmari, Bryson, Streiner, & Wilson, 2000). Leyfer et al. (2006) reported that 10% of their sample with ASD had experienced major depressive disorder, with subsyndromal cases reaching a rate of 24%. In a large sample with ASD (N = 241), approximately 3% of school-age children also met criteria for major depression, and 11% met criteria for dysthymia (Gadow, DeVincent, Pomeroy, & Azizian, 2005). Unlike the general population, persons with ASD have been found to show few gender differences in the rate of depression (Ghaziuddin et al., 2002). Among close relatives of individuals with ASD, rates of depression have also been found to be increased (Piven & Palmer, 1999). As in the general population, children with ASD who suffer from depression are more likely to have a family history of depression (Ghaziuddin & Greden, 1998).

Diagnostic Criteria and Symptom Expression

Diagnostic and Statistical Manual of Mental Disorders, fourth edition, text revision (DSM-IV-TR) criteria for a major depressive episode include depressed and/or irritable mood or loss of interests for at least 2 weeks, accompanied by at least four additional symptoms; these may include changes in weight, sleep patterns, activity level, psychomotor agitation or retardation, suicidal ideation, self-injurious behavior, feelings of worthlessness, and unwarranted feelings of guilt (American Psychiatric Association, 2000).

Several studies have examined the phenomenology of depression in individuals with ASD, and differences in symptom expression are often found. Lainhart (1999; Lainhart & Folstein, 1994) has remarked that the presenting complaint is often not mood-related, but new or worsened aggression, agitation, self-injurious behavior, increased compulsive behaviors, hypoactivity, or an overall deterioration in everyday functioning across environments. Similarly, Ghaziuddin et al. (2002) have noted that although higher-functioning individuals with ASD are better able than lower-functioning persons to communicate their feelings, the expression of sadness remains difficult. In a summary of published case studies of ASD and depression, depressed mood was a frequently cited symptom, but in only one case was the affected individual able to report the change in mood directly (Stewart, Barnard, Pearson, Hasan, & O'Brien, 2006). Increases in irritability and sleep disturbances were frequently reported, however. Symptoms that may be specific to depression when it is comorbid with ASD and that were also common in this case series included losing interest in a special topic, evidencing a decrease in adaptive functioning, a loss of bowel control, and an increase in maladaptive behaviors (particularly aggression and self-injury) (Stewart et al., 2006).

ASD and Bipolar Disorder

Prevalence

Approximately 1% of adolescents in the general population meet criteria for bipolar I disorder (Lewinsohn, Klein, & Seeley, 1995), hereafter referred to as simply bipolar disorder. The prevalence of bipolar disorder in ASD remains unknown (Jan et al., 1994; Stahlberg, Soderstrom, Rastam, & Gillberg, 2004), with no epidemiological studies yet performed to estimate rates of comorbidity. Reported rates of mania in selected clinical samples of individuals with ASD range from 2% to 21% (Ghaziuddin, Weidmer-Mikhail, & Ghaziuddin, 1998; Wozniak et al., 1997). One of the larger multisite studies (N = 109 individuals with ASD) found that 2.8% met criteria for some form of manic episode (Leyfer et al., 2006).

Diagnostic Criteria and Symptom Expression

A manic episode is characterized by elevated or irritable mood, grandiosity, decreased need for sleep, pressured speech, flight of ideas, distractibility, increases in goal-directed activity or psychomotor agitation, and involvement in dangerous or risky activities (American Psychiatric Association, 2000). Symptoms of hypomania present with a shorter duration (lasting 4 days or less) than those associated with a full manic episode (i.e., 1-week duration). Mania and hypomania can be difficult to diagnose in ASD, due to superficial similarities in presentation or overlap of symptoms. Nonspecific behaviors that often occur in children with ASD, such as irritability, overactivity, lack of fear, and overtalkativeness (Lainhart, 1999; Stahlberg et al., 2004), may be quite difficult to differentiate from bipolar symptoms. Sleep disturbance, particularly decreased need for sleep, is already common among children with ASD (Oyane & Bjorvatn, 2005; Polimeni, Richdale, & Francis, 2005; Wiggs & Stores, 2004). Only when clear changes from an individual's typical pattern are evident might sleep disturbances be indicative of mania, so obtaining a detailed sleep history and examining it for clear changes are critical. Leyfer et al. (2006) have commented that children with ASD (without bipolar disorder) often demonstrate poorly modulated, fluctuating mood and overreactive emotions. They may speak at an abnormal rate, describe preoccupations or ideas in an excited manner, or laugh for no apparent reason, all of which could be confused with symptoms of mania. Children with ASD may engage in dangerous activities, as do individuals experiencing mania, but for very different reasons. Depending on a child's mental age, he or she may not comprehend that particular activities are unsafe or may not link cause and effect, resulting in participation in potentially dangerous experiences. According to Leyfer et al. (2006), both their empirical results and clinical experience suggest that the comorbidity of ASD and bipolar disorder is relatively rare. Thus, in most cases, care must be taken to differentiate core symptoms of ASD from comorbid symptoms of mania (e.g., flight of ideas, pressured speech). As with depression, the key to identifying bipolar disorder in individuals with ASD is to evaluate mood relative to baseline behavior. That is, did these persons generally display positive affect before, but at present do they seem grouchy, cranky, or angry most of the time? Did they typically have a mild reaction to interruptions in activities, but have they become explosive and uncontrollable when interrupted?

ASD and Anxiety Disorders

Prevalence

The estimated prevalence rate of anxiety disorders in U.S. children ages 9–17 is 13% (Shaffer et al., 1996). There are several studies evaluating anxiety disorders in ASD. A large-scale study (N = 301 children) of consecutive ASD referrals to a developmental disabilities specialty clinic found the following prevalence rates for 3- to 5-year-olds and 6- to 12-year-olds, respectively: generalized anxiety disorder (6%, 24%), separation anxiety disorder (6%, 7%), and specific phobia (18%, 59%) (Weisbrot, Gadow, DeVincent, & Pomeroy, 2005). An epidemiological, community-based sample of children with ASD diagnoses from 37 school districts across Ohio found that between 14% and 21% exhibited anxiety symptoms (Lecavalier, 2006). A smaller (N = 44) clinically ascertained sample of school-age children with ASD found that 84% met DSM-IV criteria for at least one anxiety disorder (Muris, Steerneman, Merckelbach, Holdrinet, & Meesters, 1998). Studies have also shown an increased rate of anxiety among first-degree relatives of individuals with ASD (Bolton, Pickles, Murphy, & Rutter, 1998).

Diagnostic Criteria and Symptom Expression

The anxiety disorders included in DSM-IV-TR that may co-occur with ASD are generalized anxiety disorder (i.e., persistent and excessive anxiety about a number of issues or activities), panic disorder (i.e., recurrent sudden onset of intense fear), agoraphobia (i.e., fear and avoidance of situations where escape may be difficult), specific phobia (i.e., fear and avoidance of a specified object or situation), social phobia (i.e., fear and avoidance of social or performance situations), separation anxiety disorder (OCD; i.e., anxiety about separation from caregivers), and obsessive–compulsive disorder (OCD; i.e., involuntary thoughts that cause marked anxiety and actions that serve to neutralize the anxiety).

Anxiety seems to increase with age in ASD (Gadow, DeVincent, Pomeroy, & Azizian, 2004). Symptoms are reported at about the same rate as the general population in preschool-age children with ASD, but appear to increase above population rates in school-age children and adolescents with ASD (Weisbrot et al., 2005). Children with PDD-NOS and Asperger's disorder tend to show more severe anxiety symptoms than children with autistic disorder (Weisbrot et al., 2005). Two studies have found that specific phobias are the most common anxiety disorders in ASD (Leyfer et al., 2006; Muris et al., 1998). One study found that children with ASD were more fearful of thunderstorms, large crowds, and dark places than were same-age peers (Matson & Love, 1990). Another study found a higher rate of medical, animal, and situational phobias in children with ASD than in children with Down syndrome or typically developing controls (Evans, Canavera, Kleinpeter, Maccubbin, & Taga, 2005). Lainhart (1999) suggested that individuals with ASD may be at greater risk for anxiety disorders because of cognitive impairments—for example, not understanding certain phenomena (e.g., thunderstorms) and therefore experiencing inordinate anxiety about them. Leyfer et al. (2006) have indicated that anxiety varies less over time in children with ASD than in anxious peers without ASD, appearing more trait-like than state-like. Anxiety was more likely to focus on one rather than multiple things and was often associated with transitions or environmental changes. For these reasons, few children with ASD in this study met criteria for generalized anxiety disorder.

Key issues remain unresolved regarding the relationship between core ASD symptoms and OCD (Bejerot, 2007). The need for sameness, cognitive inflexibility, sensory seeking behavior, and repetitive use of objects often seen in ASD can be confused with OCD, although the diagnostic criteria for OCD do not include these symptoms. Differentiating the common ritualistic behaviors seen in ASD from the compulsions of OCD is more difficult. One differentiating feature is the prominent anxiety if a ritual is not completed that is part of OCD; rituals in ASD often appear to bring pleasure, or at least are much less ego-dystonic than those in OCD. The repeated touching or tapping of objects, which is sometimes seen in ASD as a sensory-seeking or self-stimulating behavior, could also be viewed as a compulsive behavior. In most cases of ASD, although it can be difficult to assess because of self-report problems, this behavior is not performed to counteract intrusive thoughts or reduce anxiety. Therefore, it should be a rare child who is diagnosed with comorbid ASD and OCD, and this should only be done when obsessions and compulsions that are similar in form to children without ASD are present and cannot be accounted for by the third set of symptoms in ASD (stereotyped and repetitive behaviors).

In summary, there is ample evidence that anxiety symptoms are elevated in persons with ASD and therefore are important targets of intervention to improve well-being and overall functioning. There are also clear overlaps between core behaviors of ASD and some anxiety disorders, such as OCD and social phobia; such overlaps require clinicians to weigh carefully whether additional diagnoses are required. The bottom line is that meeting diagnostic criteria for an anxiety disorder, in addition to ASD, does not necessarily warrant an additional diagnosis.

ASD and ADHD

Prevalence

The prevalence of ADHD in U.S. children is estimated to be 3–7% (American Psychiatric Association, 2000; Shaffer et al., 1996). At the current time, dual diagnoses of ADHD and any pervasive developmental disorder are excluded by DSM-IV-TR diagnostic rules. Despite this, many studies have noted the high rate of ADHD symptoms in children with ASD (Frazier et al., 2001; Goldstein & Schwebach, 2004; Matson & Nebel-Schwalm, 2006)—near 50% in some large and/or epidemiological, community-based studies (Gadow et al., 2004; Lecavalier, 2006; Leyfer et al., 2006). A recent large-scale study of consecutive referrals to a developmental disabilities clinic found lower but still substantial rates, with 6.1% of a school-age sample with ASD meeting criteria for the inattentive subtype, 6.3% for the hyperactive–impulsive subtype, and 11.0% for the combined subtype (Gadow et al., 2005).

Diagnostic Criteria and Symptom Expression

Core features of ADHD include inattention (e.g., failing to pay attention to detail, not listening, difficulty with organization), hyperactivity (e.g., fidgeting, difficulty playing quietly), and impulsivity (e.g., blurting out responses, difficulty waiting a turn), with symptoms present before age 7 (American Psychiatric Association, 2000). Despite the DSM-IV-TR algorithmic rules, comorbid diagnoses of ASD and ADHD are commonly made in clinical practice—in part because the symptoms can be quite impairing, are not improved by standard treatments for ASD, and have effective treatments. Since the overlap between attentional issues and ASD is covered in detail elsewhere in this book (see Corbett, Carmean, & Fein, Chapter 9), we only briefly discuss a few key issues in the differential diagnosis.

Common features of ADHD in ASD include difficulties in listening to and following instructions, keeping things organized, sitting still, taking turns, talking excessively, and interrupting others. Many of these difficulties can be challenging to differentiate from the core impairments of ASD; for example, turn-taking deficits, excessive talking, and interrupting may be secondary to social impairments, while poor organization may be an executive function difficulty. It is critical to examine the pervasiveness of symptoms across settings. It has been suggested that the attention problems that occur in the context of ASD are qualitatively different from those found in ADHD. "Overfocus" of attention and internal distractibility are said to be more characteristic of ASD, whereas underfocused attention and distractibility by external events and stimuli are the hallmarks of ADHD (Hendren, 2003; Jensen, Larrieu, & Mack, 1997). It has also been suggested that hyperactivity may be more prominent in children with ASD at younger ages, but that it diminishes with age, so that only inattention and distractibility remain in adulthood (Klin, Sparrow, Marans, Carter, & Volkmar, 2000; Tantum, 2003). Others have found that occasionally children present with symptoms of ASD in preschool, but appear to "grow out" of their social symptoms and present very much like children with primary ADHD later in childhood (Fein, Dixon, Paul, & Levin, 2005). Conducting additional tests of attention will provide clarity to differential diagnosis.

Please refer to Chapter 9 for useful assessment measures.

ASD and Tic Disorders

Prevalence

The general population prevalence of Tourette's disorder and other tic disorders varies considerably, with 5–20% of school-age children experiencing a simple or complex motor or vocal tic during their lifetime (Shapiro, Shapiro, Young, & Feinberg, 1988). In a sample of 553 elementary school children, monthly point prevalence of motor tics ranged from 3.2% to 9.6% (Snider et al., 2002). Rates of Tourette's disorder may be even higher in ASD than in the general population. In an epidemiological study of Asperger's disorder conducted in Sweden, using DSM-III-R criteria, one-fifth of the sample met criteria for Tourette's disorder, while three-fifths demonstrated some motor and/or vocal tics (Ehlers & Gillberg, 1993). In a recent large Italian study of 105 children with ASD, 11% met criteria for Tourette's disorder, while 11% had chronic motor tics (Canitano & Vivanti, 2007).

Diagnostic Criteria and Symptom Expression

The childhood onset (mean age 6–7 years) of multiple motor and one or more vocal tics is the hallmark of Tourette's disorder. Tics are sudden, recurrent, stereotyped movements or vocalizations that can be simple (e.g., head or shoulder jerks, eye blinking, throat clearing, sniffing, grunting) or complex (touching, saying words or phrases, echolalia), with a variable course. For full criteria for Tourette's disorder to be met, symptoms must occur often throughout the day for a period of more than 1 year, without a tic-free period of more than 3 consecutive months. Chronic motor or vocal tic disorder is characterized by the presence of either motor or vocal tics, but not both (American Psychiatric Association, 2000).

Common features of autistic stereotypies and tic disorders include abnormal motor movements, echolalia, need for sameness, and behavioral rigidity (Baron-Cohen, Mortimore, Moriarty, Izaguirre, & Robertson, 1999a). This may make the two conditions appear hard to distinguish, but in fact the similarities are largely superficial. In short, the topography of tics, which are rapid, involuntary, and nonrhythmic, is quite different from the stereotypies of ASD, which tend to be rhythmic (e.g., hand flapping, pacing, rocking), longer in duration, and under some voluntary control. Tics are sudden and rapid, lack a purposeful quality, may interrupt the flow of speech and behavior, and often are preceded by an unpleasant sensation or premonitory urge (Jankovic, 1997; Lainhart, 1999). Whereas complex stereotypies are rhythmical, complex tics are spasmodic. Other features that may assist in differentiating symptoms include the following: (1) ASD motor mannerisms tend to involve the hands, fingers, and whole body, while tics typically involve the face, neck, arms, and shoulders; (2) individuals with tics may seem distressed by the behaviors, whereas individuals performing autistic stereotypies are not; and (3) stereotyped movements are less variable over time (not waxing and waning) and less influenced by psychosocial factors (Lainhart, 1999). However, when movements or sounds that are rapid, nonrhythmic or spasmodic, and difficult to control are present in a child with ASD, then the additional diagnosis of a tic disorder is warranted.

Although it has been suggested that children with comorbid Tourette's disorder are higher-functioning (Burd, Fisher, Kerbeshian, & Arnold, 1987), Canitano and Vivanti (2007) found a positive relationship between the degree of cognitive impairment and the severity of tics, with higher rates in individuals with moderate to severe mental retardation.

ASD and Psychosis

Prevalence

The prevalence of schizophrenia across the lifespan is about 1% (American Psychiatric Association, 2000). Several studies have shown that ASD and psychotic disorders can co-occur, but not at a rate elevated beyond what would be predicted by the general population prevalence (Stahlberg et al., 2004; Volkmar & Cohen, 1991). Lainhart (1999) compiled data from 11 studies to determine a rate of schizophrenia of 1.08% in autism and 2.2% in Asperger's disorder, but cautioned that these rates might be elevated, since they were determined from studies in which individuals were referred for psychiatric care.

Diagnostic Criteria and Symptom Expression

Psychotic disorders include schizophrenia and the schizophrenia spectrum disorders, such as schizoaffective disorder, schizophreniform disorder, and delusional disorder. Symptoms and duration vary from condition to condition, but core symptoms include positive symptoms (e.g., delusions, hallucinations, disorganized speech and thought) and negative symptoms (e.g., alogia, flat affect, avolition) (American Psychiatric Association, 2000). Differential diagnosis of the two conditions is often straightforward, relying heavily on the developmental history, age of onset, and specific form of symptoms. Individuals with ASD rarely display positive symptoms of psychosis (Konstantareas & Hewitt, 2001), such as delusions and hallucinations, and when these are present in the context of ASD, it is clear that a comorbid diagnosis of a psychotic disorder is warranted. However, for examiners unfamiliar with ASD, there are superficial similarities between ASD and psychosis that might make comorbidity seem more common than it is. The pragmatic language abnormalities in ASD (including poor topic maintenance and reciprocity) may present like thought disorder; the highly focused interests may present like delusions; the unusual sensory interests or sensitivities may appear superficially similar to hallucinations; and the poor social judgment and theory-of-mind skills may present in a manner similar to paranoia. Moreover, lack of motivation and independent initiation of activities can be mistaken for the negative symptoms of schizophrenia (Lainhart, 1999).

An additional challenging differential exists between conditions at the boundaries of both the autism spectrum and the schizophrenia spectrum, where there may be true overlap of symptoms. Specifically, the prodrome of schizophrenia may include features that are part of the clinical picture of PDD-NOS, which by definition is an atypical or partial presentation of autistic behavior. Both groups may present with ritualistic behaviors, unusual verbalizations, affective flattening, and social withdrawal. Consistent with this, a recent study of 75 children with childhood-onset schizophrenia found that 25% had a lifetime diagnosis of ASD (mostly PDD-NOS; Sporn et al., 2004). It is not clear whether this indicates that PDD-NOS can be a risk factor for later development of psychosis, or whether the diagnostic criteria for PDD-NOS are just sufficiently broad to encompass heterogeneous clinical presentations that are consistent with both the autism spectrum and the emerging schizophrenia spectrum; however, we believe that the latter explanation is more likely (see Caron & Rutter, 1991). The key to differentiation may again lie in the developmental history, as symptoms consistent with ASD should be evident before the third birthday, while even prodromal symptoms of psychosis are rarely present in the preschool period and typically develop gradually and insidiously during childhood.

USEFUL INSTRUMENTS FOR ASSESSMENT OF PSYCHIATRIC COMORBIDITIES IN ASD

In this section, we first discuss broad-based instruments that measure several different areas of psychopathology, and then present specific tools that may be useful for particular comorbid conditions. In each section, we begin with instruments that have already been used with the ASD population in published studies; we then suggest other measures that may be useful because of certain attributes of each instrument, but have not yet been used in published studies with individuals on the autism spectrum.

General Measures of Psychopathology

The Achenbach System of Empirically Based Assessment (ASEBA) evaluates behavior across the lifespan and includes forms for reporting by the self, parents, and teachers (Achenbach, Howell, Quay, & Conners, 1991; Achenbach & Rescorla, 2001). It measures symptoms of depression and anxiety, somatic complaints, obsessive–compulsive behaviors, attention problems, social difficulties, aggressive behavior, and atypicalities in thinking. The version for children ages 1½–5 years also provides diagnostic information specifically related to ASD. Although the developers of the ASEBA did not specifically include children with ASD in their normative sample, its measures have been used in ASD research. Two studies demonstrated that the Child Behavior Checklist (CBCL), the ASEBA's caregiver report form for school-age children, can be used to differentiate ASD from other psychiatric conditions (Duarte, Bordin, de Oliveira, & Bird, 2003; Petersen, Bilenberg, Hoerder, & Gillberg, 2006). Of more relevance to this chapter, the CBCL has also been used to study comorbid psychiatric conditions in ASD. One recent study using the CBCL found high rates of ADHD in ASD (Holtmann, Bolte, & Poustka, 2007). The CBCL has also been used to study psychopathology in children on the autism spectrum who were also displaying manic symptoms (Wozniak et al., 1997).

The Behavior Assessment System for Children, Second Edition (BASC-2; Reynolds & Kamphaus, 2004) has also been used in children with ASD. Similar to the ASEBA, the BASC-2 evaluates symptoms related to major depressive disorder, generalized anxiety disorder, ADHD, behavior disorders, psychosis, and tic disorders. It also provides clinical information specific to autistic disorder and Asperger's disorder. The BASC-2 can be completed by parents, teachers, or the self. Lindner and Rosén (2006) found that children with Asperger's disorder had a distinct parent-reported profile on the original BASC—with high scores on the Atypicality and Withdrawn scales, and low scores on Social Skills—when compared to children with other conditions or typical development. Although we have cautioned against high reliance on self-report measures with children with ASD, the new BASC-2 self-report form for ages 6–7 (Reynolds & Kamphaus, 2004) may be appropriate to use, as the simple response format (i.e., yes–no answers) is more concrete than the Likert-type scales often used on other self-report forms.

The Aberrant Behavior Checklist—Community (ABC-Community; Aman & Singh, 1994) is a 58-item behavior checklist completed by parents, teachers, or clinicians to evaluate problem behaviors in the past 4 weeks. It was initially designed for use with adults in an institutionalized setting, but was later revised for individuals ages 6 years and older residing in the community. The ABC-Community includes five subscales: Irritability, Socially Withdrawn Behavior and Lethargy, Stereotyped Behavior, Hyperactivity and Noncompliance, and Inappropriate Speech Patterns. The factor structure is similar in ASD samples (Brinkley et al., 2006), and it has been utilized in a number of studies, often as a measure of inclusion or change in clinical trials (Akhondzadeh et al., 2004; King et al., 2001; Linday, Tsiouris, Cohen, Shindledecker, & DeCresce, 2001; Sponheim, Oftedal, & Helverschou, 2002). The Irritability subscale in particular is often used to identify patients with elevated symptoms needing psychopharmacological intervention (Arnold et al., 2000).

The Nisonger Child Behavior Rating Form (NCBRF; Aman, Tasse, Rojahn, & Hammer, 1996) is a parent and teacher rating form that was developed to use with children with developmental disabilities. It evaluates symptoms associated with depression, mania, anxiety, behavioral noncompliance, self-injury, ADHD, and tic disorders. It has 66 items rated on a 4-point scale, grouped into six subscales: Conduct Problems, Insecure/Anxious, Hyperactive, Self-Isolated/Ritualistic, Self-Injury/Stereotypic, and Overly Sensitive (parent version) or Irritable (teacher version). It has been used in a large community sample of children with ASD, with findings of elevated irritability, temper tantrums, and depressive symptoms (Lecavalier, 2006). It has also been used, along with the ABC-Community, to evaluate symptom improvement in a clinical trial of risperidone (Shea et al., 2004).

The Schedule for Affective Disorders and Schizophrenia for School-Age Children—Present and Lifetime version (K-SADS-PL) is considered a gold standard in evaluating psychiatric disorders in childhood and adolescents (Kaufman et al., 1997). The current edition consists of a 2- to 3-hour parent and child interview. It initially screens for a number of DSM-IV disorders, including major depression, bipolar disorder, anxiety disorders, ADHD, tic disorders, and psychotic disorders, and then follows up on specific issues to clarify clinical diagnoses. Recently, the K-SADS-PL has been adapted specifically for use with children on the autism spectrum, and this version is called the Autism Comorbidity Interview—Present and Lifetime Version (ACI-PL; Leyfer et al., 2006). Unlike the original K-SADS-PL, the ACI-PL is conducted via parent interview only. It has been shown to have excellent psychometric properties (Leyfer et al., 2006). It was adapted for use with this population in several ways: There is an emphasis on examining baseline behavior and changes from baseline that might signal the onset of another psychiatric condition; there is explicit acknowledgment of the ways in which symptom manifestation may be different in ASD; and certain symptoms that may require specific cognitive capacities not found in some children with ASD (e.g., guilt) are only probed if a child is capable of demonstrating such symptoms.

Version IV of the Diagnostic Interview Schedule for Children (DISC-IV; Shaffer et al., 1996; Shaffer, Fisher, Lucas, Dulcan, & Schwab-Stone, 2000) evaluates a range of diagnostic conditions in childhood, including mood and anxiety disorders, ADHD, tic disorders, and psychosis by interviewing the parent (DISC-IV-P for children ages 6–17) and/or the child (DISC-IV-Y for ages 9–17). There are few open-ended responses, with most responses limited to "yes," "no," "sometimes," or "somewhat." Muris et al. (1998), using an earlier version of the DISC, found high rates of anxiety symptoms in ASD.

The Early Childhood Inventory-4 (Sprafkin, Volpe, Gadow, Nolan, & Kelly, 2002) is a behavior rating scale that evaluates emotional and behavioral disorders in children ages 3–5 years; the Child Symptom Inventory-4 (Gadow & Sprafkin, 2002) evaluates similar symptoms in children ages 5–12, by either parent or teacher report. In research using these measures, children with ASD were found to exhibit more psychiatric symptoms than other children in regular and special education settings (Gadow et al., 2004, 2005).

Another measure that has not yet been used specifically with individuals with ASD in published studies, but that may be useful, is the Dominic-R (Valla, Bergeron, Bidaut-Russell, St.-Georges, & Gaudet, 1997). It utilizes pictures to evaluate phobias, separation anxiety disorder, generalized anxiety disorder, depression/dysthymia, ADHD, oppositional defiant disorder, and conduct disorder in children ages 6–11 years. Given the concrete nature of the questions asked and the format of the instrument, the Dominic-R may be especially helpful for those with cognitive immaturity.

Specific Measures of Psychopathology

In addition to the general measures of psychopathology just reviewed, a few instruments focus on specific forms of psychiatric disorder have been used successfully with individuals on the autism spectrum.

Depression

The Children's Depression Inventory (CDI; Kovacs, 1992) taps into five key areas of depression: negative mood, interpretation problems, ineffectiveness, anhedonia, and negative self-esteem. Hedley and Young (2006) used the CDI to examine depressive symptoms in children with Asperger's disorder. The CDI was also used to assess mood issues before and after treatment in children ages 8–12 years participating in a social skills group (Solomon, Goodlin-Jones, & Anders, 2004). Although the format of the CDI is self-report, it seems less challenging for children to answer than other self-report instruments, because it provides concrete examples of abstract concepts. It also allows a clinician to read the items (if necessary) to a child while the child follows along.

Obsessive–Compulsive Disorder

The various versions of the Yale–Brown Obsessive Compulsive Scale (Goodman et al., 1989; Scahill et al., 1997)—including a newly developed form specifically for children on the autism spectrum, the Children's Yale–Brown Obsessive Compulsive Scale for Pervasive Developmental Disorders (CYBOCS-PDD; McDougle et al., 2005; Scahill et al., 2006)—have been used widely. Children ages 6 and up and their parents are interviewed in a semistructured fashion to evaluate a range of possible OCD phenomena, including symptoms related to contamination, aggression, hoarding/saving, magical thoughts/superstitions, and possible obsessive thoughts (somatic, religious, and other). Symptoms are rated on a scale from "none" to "extremely problematic" in terms of time spent, level of distress, resistance, interference with functioning, and degree of control. The CYBOCS-PDD has an additional 5-item severity scale for repetitive and ritualistic behaviors, which helps determine whether symptom clusters are more closely associated with OCD or with ASD. For this reason, it is a very promising instrument for making this difficult differential diagnosis.

Attention-Deficit/Hyperactivity Disorder

A number of widely used instruments exist that were designed specifically to assess symptoms of ADHD. Some, such as the Conners' Rating Scales, have been used successfully with children on the autism spectrum (Posey et al., 2006). Please see Chapter 9 for more information about instruments useful in the assessment of ADHD in ASD.

Tic Disorders

The Yale Global Tic Severity Scale is a semistructured interview that collects information from both parents and children on number, frequency, intensity, complexity, and interference of vocal and motor tics (Leckman et al., 1989). It has been used to evaluate tics in a pediatric ASD sample, with ratings based primarily on parent report and clinical observation, due to limited language and self-reporting skills in the children (Canitano & Vivanti, 2007).

Psychosis

The Brief Psychiatric Rating Scale (BPRS; Ventura, Green, Shaner, & Liberman, 1993), the child version of the BPRS (Lachar et al., 2001), the Scale for the Assessment of Negative Symptoms (SANS; Andreasen, 1984a), and the Positive and Negative Syndrome Scale (PANSS; Kay, Opler, & Fiszbein, 1992) all involve conducting an interview with the patient and the patient's family members/caregivers to evaluate a range of positive and negative symptoms. The SANS, PANSS, and BPRS were used in one clinical trial of children with Asperger's disorder (Rausch et al., 2005) to measure change in negative symptoms (e.g., social withdrawal, affective flattening, and avolition) after treatment with risperidone. The SANS, along with the Scale for the Assessment of Positive Symptoms (SAPS; Andreasen, 1984b) and measures of ASD symptomatology, was helpful in differential diagnosis of psychosis and ASD in another study (Konstantareas & Hewitt, 2001). The Rorschach (Exner, 1986) has been used to examine thought-disorder-like symptoms in individuals with ASD (Dykens, Volkmar, & Glick, 1991); however, it is not recommended for differential diagnosis, given the elevated scores that may be produced by the pragmatic language impairments of ASD. In our opinion, the differential diagnosis of ASD and schizophrenia is best made on the basis of the presence of positive symptoms, since superficial similarities between core symptoms of ASD and negative symptoms of schizophrenia may cause individuals with ASD to score high on measures of negative symptoms.

CONCLUDING REMARKS

Evaluation of comorbidity in ASD challenges the best of clinicians. Functioning is already impaired in individuals with ASD, meaning that a change in behavior may have to be marked to be identifiable (Ozonoff, Goodlin-Jones, & Solomon, 2005b). Teasing out core symptoms of ASD from other conditions is a complex matter, for several reasons: the fact that many assessment tools have not been standardized on the population with ASD; the limitations of insight in this population; and the need for reliance on observation and parent/caregiver report. Selection artifacts were likely in many of the studies cited in this chapter, as most used clinically ascertained samples that may well have had higher rates of comorbidity than unselected community-based samples of individuals with ASD. Clinicians must remember that apparent comorbidity may arise from overlapping criteria, artificial subdivision of syndromes, or one disorder's representing an early manifestation of another disorder (Caron & Rutter, 1991). Care must be taken not to overdiagnose comorbidity. Conversely, it is likely that many instances of true comorbidity are missed, resulting in undertreatment or only partial treatment of the individual's difficulties. Emotional and behavioral problems influence family functioning, impacting levels of parental stress (Herring et al., 2006). With new research demonstrating the efficacy of both behavioral and psychopharmacological interventions for psychiatric disorders seen in individuals with ASD (e.g., Reaven & Hepburn, 2003; Shea et al., 2004; Sofronoff, Attwood, & Hinton, 2005), it is critically important to identify and treat additional behavioral or emotional issues.

Measurement remains a central issue, given both the limited normative data and the inadequacies of measurement formats for people on the autism spectrum. Difficulties with insight and self-report are coupled with the inherent difficulty of truly understanding the internal emotional experience of someone else. The development of better methods of assessing comorbid symptoms in an "ASD-friendly" manner is needed. Self-report measures might be administered along with picture cards presenting specific, easy-to-identify emotions (such as the Webber Photo Cards for Emotions; Webber, 2005). Such changes from standardized administration need to be studied, to examine the validity and reliability of the assessment process.

Better understanding of comorbid presentations in ASD may also improve our knowledge of the causes of ASD and etiological heterogeneities (Leyfer et al., 2006). Children who demonstrate multiple disorders may represent subtypes that should be studied separately. Conditions that commonly co-occur may provide clues about shared risk factors or shared underlying neuropathological processes.

It is our hope in writing this chapter that accurate indentification of the primary and/or secondary problems that affect the functioning of individuals with ASD will result in improved treatment planning and treatment outcomes. Given the complexities detailed in this chapter, it is clear that additional training and expertise in both traditional mental health conditions and neurodevelopmental disorders are critical in providing the best clinical care possible.

REFERENCES

Achenbach, T. M., Howell, C. T., Quay, H. C., & Conners, C. K. (1991). National survey of problems and competencies among four- to sixteen-year-olds: Parents' reports for normative and clinical samples. *Monographs of the Society for Research in Child Development, 56*(3), 1–131.

Achenbach, T. M., & Rescorla, L. A. (2001). *Manual for the ASEBA: School-age forms and profiles.* Burlington: University of Vermont, Research Center for Children, Youth, and Families.

Akhondzadeh, S., Erfani, S., Mohammadi, M. R., Tehrani-Doost, M., Amini, H., Gudarzi, S. S., et al. (2004). Cyproheptadine in the treatment of autistic disorder: A double-blind placebo-controlled trial. *Journal of Clinical Pharmacy and Therapeutics, 29*(2), 145–150.

Aman, M. G., & Singh, N. N. (1994). *Aberrant Behavior Checklist—Community.* East Aurora, NY: Slosson.

Aman, M. G., Tasse, M. J., Rojahn, J., & Hammer, D. (1996). The Nisonger CBRF: A child behavior rating form for children with developmental disabilities. *Research in Developmental Disabilities, 17,* 41–57.

American Psychiatric Association. (2000). *Diagnostic and statistical manual of mental disorders* (4th ed., text rev.). Washington, DC: Author.

Andreasen, N. C. (1984a). *Scale for the Assessment of Negative Symptoms (SANS).* Iowa City: University of Iowa.

Andreasen, N. C. (1984b). *Scale for the Assessment of Positive Symptoms (SAPS).* Iowa City: The University of Iowa.

Angold, A., Erkanli, A., Costello, E. J., & Rutter, M. (1996). Precision, reliability and accuracy in the dating of symptom onsets in child and adolescent psychopathology. *Journal of Child Psychology and Psychiatry, 37*(6), 657–664.

Arnold, L. E., Aman, M. G., Martin, A., Collier-Crespin, A., Vitiello, B., Tierney, E., et al. (2000). Assessment in multisite randomized clinical trials of patients with autistic disorder: The Autism RUPP Network. *Journal of Autism and Developmental Disorders, 30,* 99–111.

Baron-Cohen, S., Mortimore, C., Moriarty, J., Izaguirre, J., & Robertson, M. (1999a). The prevalence of Gilles de la Tourette's syndrome in children and adolescents with autism. *Journal of Child Psychology and Psychiatry, 40*(2), 213–218.

Baron-Cohen, S., O'Riordan, M., Stone, V., Jones, R., & Plaisted, K. (1999b). Recognition of faux pas by normally developing children and children with Asperger syndrome or high-functioning autism. *Journal of Autism and Developmental Disorders, 29*(5), 407–418.

Baron-Cohen, S., Tager-Flusberg, H., & Cohen, D. (2000). *Understanding other minds: Perspectives from developmental cognitive neuroscience.* New York: Oxford University Press.

Bejerot, S. (2007). An autistic dimension: A proposed subtype of obsessive–compulsive disorder. *Autism, 11,* 101–110.

Ben Shalom, D., Mostofsky, S. H., Hazlett, R. L., Goldberg, M. C., Landa, R. J., Faran, Y., et al. (2006). Normal physiological emotions but differences in expression of conscious feelings in children with high-functioning autism. *Journal of Autism and Developmental Disorders, 36*(3), 395–400.

Berthoz, S., & Hill, E. L. (2005). The validity of using self-reports to assess emotion regulation abilities in adults with autism spectrum disorder. *European Psychiatry, 20*(3), 291–298.

Blackshaw, A. J., Kinderman, P., Hare, D. J., & Hatton, C. (2001). Theory of mind, causal attribution and paranoia in Asperger syndrome. *Autism, 5*(2), 147–163.

Bolton, P. F., Pickles, A., Murphy, M., & Rutter, M. (1998). Autism, affective and other psychiatric disorders: Patterns of familial aggregation. *Psychological Medicine, 28*(2), 385–395.

Brereton, A. V., Tonge, B. J., & Einfeld, S. L. (2006). Psychopathology in children and adolescents with autism compared to young people with intellectual disability. *Journal of Autism and Developmental Disorders, 36*(7), 863–870.

Brinkley, J., Nations, L., Abramson, R. K., Hall, A., Wright, H. H., Gabriels, R., et al. (2007). Factor analysis of the Aberrant Behavior Checklist in individuals with autism spectrum disorders. *Journal of Autism and Developmental Disorders, 37*(10), 1949–1959.

Burd, L., Fisher, W. W., Kerbeshian, J., & Arnold, M. E. (1987). Is development of Tourette disorder a marker for improvement in patients with autism and other pervasive developmental disorders? *Journal of the American Academy of Child and Adolescent Psychiatry, 26*(2), 162–165.

Canitano, R., & Vivanti, G. (2007). Tics and Tourette syndrome in autism spectrum disorders. *Autism, 11*(1), 19–28.

Caron, C., & Rutter, M. (1991). Comorbidity in child psychopathology: Concepts, issues and research strategies. *Journal of Child Psychology and Psychiatry, 32*(7), 1063–1080.

Costello, E. J., Foley, D. L., & Angold, A. (2006). 10-year research update review: The epidemiology of child and adolescent psychiatric disorders: II. Developmental epidemiology. *Journal of the American Academy of Child and Adolescent Psychiatry, 45*(1), 8–25.

Derogatis, L. R. (1983). *Symptom Checklist 90—Revised (SCL-90-R).* Minneapolis: National Computer Systems.

Duarte, C. S., Bordin, I. A., de Oliveira, A., & Bird, H. (2003). The CBCL and the identification of children with autism and related conditions in Brazil: Pilot findings. *Journal of Autism and Developmental Disorders, 33*(6), 703–707.

Dykens, E., Volkmar, F., & Glick, M. (1991). Thought disorder in high-functioning autistic adults. *Journal of Autism and Developmental Disorders, 21*(3), 291–301.

Ehlers, S., & Gillberg, C. (1993). The epidemiology of Asperger syndrome: A total population study. *Journal of Child Psychology and Psychiatry, 34*(8), 1327–1350.

Evans, D. W., Canavera, K., Kleinpeter, F. L., Maccubbin, E., & Taga, K. (2005). The fears, phobias and anxieties of children with autism spectrum disorders and Down syndrome: Comparisons with developmentally and chronologically age matched children. *Child Psychiatry and Human Development, 36*(1), 3–26.

Exner, J. (1986). *The Rorschach: A comprehensive system*. New York: Wiley-Interscience.

Fein, D., Dixon, P., Paul, J., & Levin, H. (2005). Pervasive developmental disorder can evolve into ADHD: Case illustrations. *Journal of Autism and Developmental Disorders, 35*(4), 525–534.

Frazier, J. A., Biederman, J., Bellordre, C. A., Garfield, S. B., Geller, D. A., Coffey, B. J., et al. (2001). Should the diagnosis of attention deficit/hyperactivity disorder be considered in children with pervasive developmental disorder? *Journal of Attention Disorders, 4*(4), 203–211.

Gadow, K. D., DeVincent, C. J., Pomeroy, J., & Azizian, A. (2004). Psychiatric symptoms in preschool children with PDD and clinic and comparison samples. *Journal of Autism and Developmental Disorders, 34*(4), 379–393.

Gadow, K. D., DeVincent, C. J., Pomeroy, J., & Azizian, A. (2005). Comparison of DSM-IV symptoms in elementary school-age children with PDD versus clinic and community samples. *Autism, 9*(4), 392–415.

Gadow, K. D., & Sprafkin, J. (2002). *Child Symptom Inventory-4: Screening and norms manual*. Stony Brook, NY: Checkmate Plus.

Ghaziuddin, M., Ghaziuddin, N., & Greden, J. (2002). Depression in persons with autism: Implications for research and clinical care. *Journal of Autism and Developmental Disorders, 32*(4), 299–306.

Ghaziuddin, M., & Greden, J. (1998). Depression in children with autism/pervasive developmental disorders: A case–control family history study. *Journal of Autism and Developmental Disorders, 28*(2), 111–115.

Ghaziuddin, M., Tsai, L., & Ghaziuddin, N. (1992). Comorbidity of autistic disorder in children and adolescents. *European Child and Adolescent Psychiatry, 1*, 209–213.

Ghaziuddin, M., Weidmer-Mikhail, E., & Ghaziuddin, N. (1998). Comorbidity of Asperger syndrome: A preliminary report. *Journal of Intellectual Disability Research, 42*(Pt. 4), 279–283.

Goldstein, S., & Schwebach, A. J. (2004). The comorbidity of pervasive developmental disorder and attention deficit hyperactivity disorder: Results of a retrospective chart review. *Journal of Autism and Developmental Disorders, 34*(3), 329–339.

Goodman, W. K., Price, L. H., Rasmussen, S. A., Mazure, C., Fleischmann, R. L., Hill, C. L., et al. (1989). The Yale–Brown Obsessive Compulsive Scale: I. Development, use, and reliability. *Archives of General Psychiatry, 46*(11), 1006–1011.

Happé, F. (1991). The autobiographical writings of three Asperger syndrome adults: Problems of interpretation and implications for theory. In U. Frith (Ed.), *Autism and Asperger syndrome* (pp. 207–242). New York: Cambridge University Press.

Hedley, D., & Young, R. (2006). Social comparison processes and depressive symptoms in children and adolescents with Asperger syndrome. *Autism, 10*(2), 139–153.

Hendren, R. L. (2003). Contributions of the psychiatrist. In S. Ozonoff, S. J. Rogers, & R. L. Hendren (Eds.), *Autism spectrum disorders: A research review for professionals* (pp. 37–53). Arlington, VA: American Psychiatric Publishing.

Herring, S., Gray, K., Taffe, J., Tonge, B., Sweeney, D., & Einfeld, S. (2006). Behaviour and emotional problems in toddlers with pervasive developmental disorders and developmental delay: Associations with parental mental health and family functioning. *Journal of Intellectual Disability Research, 50*(Pt. 12), 874–882.

Hill, E., Berthoz, S., & Frith, U. (2004). Brief report: Cognitive processing of own emotions in individuals with autistic spectrum disorder and in their relatives. *Journal of Autism and Developmental Disorders, 34*(2), 229–235.

Holtmann, M., Bolte, S., & Poustka, F. (2007). Attention deficit hyperactivity disorder symptoms in pervasive developmental disorders: Association with autistic behavior domains and coexisting psychopathology. *Psychopathology, 40,* 172–177.

Howlin, P. (1997). *Autism: Preparing for adulthood.* London: Routledge.

Jan, J. E., Abroms, I. F., Freeman, R. D., Brown, G. M., Espezel, H., & Connolly, M. B. (1994). Rapid cycling in severely multidisabled children: A form of bipolar affective disorder? *Pediatric Neurology, 10*(1), 34–39.

Jankovic, J. (1997). Tourette syndrome: Phenomenology and classification of tics. *Neurologic Clinics, 15*(2), 267–275.

Jensen, V. K., Larrieu, J. A., & Mack, K. K. (1997). Differential diagnosis between attention-deficit/hyperactivity disorder and pervasive developmental disorder—not otherwise specified. *Clinical Pediatrics, 36*(10), 555–561.

Jolliffe, T., & Baron-Cohen, S. (1999). The Strange Stories Test: A replication with high-functioning adults with autism or Asperger syndrome. *Journal of Autism and Developmental Disorders, 29*(5), 395–406.

Kaufman, J., Birmaher, B., Brent, D., Rao, U., Flynn, C., Moreci, P., et al. (1997). Schedule for Affective Disorders and Schizophrenia for School-Age Children—Present and Lifetime Version (K-SADS-PL): Initial reliability and validity data. *Journal of the American Academy of Child and Adolescent Psychiatry, 36*(7), 980–988.

Kay, S. R., Opler, L. A., & Fiszbein, A. (1992). *Positive and Negative Syndrome Scale (PANSS).* Toronto: Multi-Health Systems.

Kazdin, A. E. (1993). Replication and extension of behavioral treatment of autistic disorder. *American Journal of Mental Retardation, 97,* 377–378.

Kim, J., Szatmari, P., Bryson, S., Streiner, D., & Wilson, F. (2000). The prevalence of anxiety and mood problems among children with autism and Asperger syndrome. *Autism, 4*(2), 117–132.

King, B. H., Wright, D. M., Handen, B. L., Sikich, L., Zimmerman, A. W., McMahon, W., et al. (2001). Double-blind, placebo-controlled study of amantadine hydrochloride in the treatment of children with autistic disorder. *Journal of the American Academy of Child and Adolescent Psychiatry, 40*(6), 658–665.

Klein, S. B., Chan, R. L., & Loftus, J. (1999). Independence of episodic and semantic self-knowledge: The case from autism. *Social Cognition, 17,* 413–436.

Klin, A., Sparrow, S. S., Marans, W. D., Carter, A., & Volkmar, F. R. (2000). Assessment issues in children and adolescents with Asperger syndrome. In A. Klin, F. R. Volkmar, & S. S. Sparrow (Eds.), *Asperger syndrome* (pp. 309–339). New York: Guilford Press.

Konstantareas, M. M., & Hewitt, T. (2001). Autistic disorder and schizophrenia: Diagnostic overlaps. *Journal of Autism and Developmental Disorders, 31*(1), 19–28.

Kovacs, M. (1992). *Children's Depression Inventory (CDI)*. North Tonawanda, NY: Multi-Health Systems.

Lachar, D., Randle, S. L., Harper, R. A., Scott-Gurnell, K. C., Lewis, K. R., Santos, C. W., et al. (2001). The Brief Psychiatric Rating Scale for Children (BPRS-C): Validity and reliability of an anchored version. *Journal of the American Academy of Child and Adolescent Psychiatry, 40*(3), 333–340.

Lahey, B. B., Flagg, E. W., Bird, H. R., Schwab-Stone, M. E., Canino, G., Dulcan, M. K., et al. (1996). The NIMH Methods for the Epidemiology of Child and Adolescent Mental Disorders (MECA) Study: Background and methodology. *Journal of the American Academy of Child and Adolescent Psychiatry, 35*(7), 855–864.

Lainhart, J. E. (1999). Psychiatric problems in individuals with autism, their parents and siblings. *International Review of Psychiatry, 11,* 278–298.

Lainhart, J. E., & Folstein, S. E. (1994). Affective disorders in people with autism: A review of published cases. *Journal of Autism and Developmental Disorders, 24,* 587–601.

Lecavalier, L. (2006). Behavioral and emotional problems in young people with pervasive developmental disorders: Relative prevalence, effects of subject characteristics, and empirical classification. *Journal of Autism and Developmental Disorders, 36*(8), 1101–1114.

Leckman, J. F., Riddle, M. A., Hardin, M. T., Ort, S. I., Swartz, K. L., Stevenson, J., et al. (1989). The Yale Global Tic Severity Scale: Initial testing of a clinician-rated scale of tic severity. *Journal of the American Academy of Child and Adolescent Psychiatry, 28*(4), 566–573.

Lewinsohn, P. M., Klein, D. N., & Seeley, J. R. (1995). Bipolar disorders in a community sample of older adolescents: Prevalence, phenomenology, comorbidity, and course. *Journal of the American Academy of Child and Adolescent Psychiatry, 34*(4), 454–463.

Leyfer, O. T., Folstein, S. E., Bacalman, S., Davis, N. O., Dinh, E., Morgan, J., et al. (2006). Comorbid psychiatric disorders in children with autism: Interview development and rates of disorders. *Journal of Autism and Developmental Disorders, 36*(7), 849–861.

Linday, L. A., Tsiouris, J. A., Cohen, I. L., Shindledecker, R., & DeCresce, R. (2001). Famotidine treatment of children with autistic spectrum disorders: Pilot research using single subject research design. *Journal of Neural Transmission, 108*(5), 593–611.

Lindner, J. L., & Rosén, L. A. (2006). Decoding of emotion through facial expression, prosody and verbal content in children and adolescents with Asperger's syndrome. *Journal of Autism and Developmental Disorders, 36*(6), 769–777.

Matson, J. L., & Love, S. R. (1990). A comparison of parent-reported fear of autistic and non-handicapped age-matched children and youth. *Australian and New Zealand Journal of Developmental Disabilities, 16*, 349–357.

Matson, J. L., & Nebel-Schwalm, M. S. (2007). Comorbid psychopathology with autism spectrum disorder in children: An overview. *Research in Developmental Disabilities, 28*(4), 341–352.

McDougle, C. J., Scahill, L., Aman, M. G., McCracken, J. T., Tierney, E., Davies, M., et al. (2005). Risperidone for the core symptom domains of autism: Results from the study by the Autism Network of the Research Units on Pediatric Psychopharmacology. *American Journal of Psychiatry, 162*(6), 1142–1148.

Muris, P., Steerneman, P., Merckelbach, H., Holdrinet, I., & Meesters, C. (1998). Comorbid anxiety symptoms in children with pervasive developmental disorders. *Journal of Anxiety Disorders, 12*(4), 387–393.

Oyane, N. M., & Bjorvatn, B. (2005). Sleep disturbances in adolescents and young adults with autism and Asperger syndrome. *Autism, 9*(1), 83–94.

Ozonoff, S., Garcia, N., Clark, E., & Lainhart, J. E. (2005a). MMPI-2 personality profiles of high-functioning adults with autism spectrum disorders. *Assessment, 12*(1), 86–95.

Ozonoff, S., Goodlin-Jones, B. L., & Solomon, M. (2005b). Evidence-based assessment of autism spectrum disorders in children and adolescents. *Journal of Clinical Child and Adolescent Psychology, 34*(3), 523–540.

Petersen, D. J., Bilenberg, N., Hoerder, K., & Gillberg, C. (2006). The population prevalence of child psychiatric disorders in Danish 8- to 9-year-old children. *European Child and Adolescent Psychiatry, 15*(2), 71–78.

Piven, J., & Palmer, P. (1999). Psychiatric disorder and the broad autism phenotype: Evidence from a family study of multiple-incidence autism families. *American Journal of Psychiatry, 156*(4), 557–563.

Polimeni, M. A., Richdale, A. L., & Francis, A. J. (2005). A survey of sleep problems in autism, Asperger's disorder and typically developing children. *Journal of Intellectual Disability Research, 49*(Pt. 4), 260–268.

Posey, D. J., Wiegand, R. E., Wilkerson, J., Maynard, M., Stigler, K. A., & McDougle, C. J. (2006). Open-label atomoxetine for attention-deficit/hyperactivity disorder symptoms associated with high-functioning pervasive developmental disorders. *Journal of Child and Adolescent Psychopharmacology, 16*(5), 599–610.

Rausch, J. L., Sirota, E. L., Londino, D. L., Johnson, M. E., Carr, B. M., Bhatia, R., et al. (2005). Open-label risperidone for Asperger's disorder: Negative symptom spectrum response. *Journal of Clinical Psychiatry, 66*(12), 1592–1597.

Reaven, J., & Hepburn, S. (2003). Cognitive-behavioral treatment of obsessive–compulsive disorder in a child with Asperger syndrome: A case report. *Autism, 7*, 145–164.

Reynolds, C. R., & Kamphaus, R. W. (2004). *Behavior Assessment System for Children, Second Edition (BASC-2) manual.* Circle Pines, MN: American Guidance Service.

Scahill, L., McDougle, C. J., & Williams, S. K., Dimitropoulos, A., Aman, A. G., McCracken, J. T., et al. (2006). The Children's Yale–Brown Obsessive Compulsive Scales modified for pervasive developmental disorders. *Journal of the American Academy of Child and Adolescent Psychiatry, 45*(9), 1114–1123.

Scahill, L., Riddle, M. A., McSwiggin-Hardin, M., Ort, S. I., King, R. A., Goodman, W. K., et al. (1997). Children's Yale–Brown Obsessive Compulsive Scale: Reliability and validity. *Journal of the American Academy of Child and Adolescent Psychiatry, 36*(6), 844–852.

Shaffer, D., Fisher, P., Dulcan, M. K., Davies, M., Piacentini, J., Schwab-Stone, M. E., et al. (1996). The NIMH Diagnostic Interview Schedule for Children Version 2.3 (DISC-2.3): Description, acceptability, prevalence rates, and performance in the MECA Study. Methods for the Epidemiology of Child and Adolescent Mental Disorders Study. *Journal of the American Academy of Child and Adolescent Psychiatry, 35*(7), 865–877.

Shaffer, D., Fisher, P., Lucas, C. P., Dulcan, M. K., & Schwab-Stone, M. E. (2000). NIMH Diagnostic Interview Schedule for Children Version IV (NIMH DISC-IV): Description, differences from previous versions, and reliability of some common diagnoses. *Journal of the American Academy of Child and Adolescent Psychiatry, 39*(1), 28–38.

Shapiro, A. K., Shapiro, S. E., Young, J., & Feinberg, T. E. (1988). *Gilles de la Tourette syndrome* (2nd ed.). New York: Raven Press.

Shea, S., Turgay, A., Carroll, A., Schulz, M., Orlik, H., Smith, I., et al. (2004). Risperidone in the treatment of disruptive behavioral symptoms in children with autistic and other pervasive developmental disorders. *Pediatrics, 114*(5), 634–641.

Sicotte, C., & Stemberger, R. M. (1999). Do children with PDDNOS have a theory of mind? *Journal of Autism and Developmental Disorders, 29*(3), 225–233.

Snider, L. A., Seligman, L. D., Ketchen, B. R., Levitt, S. J., Bates, L. R., Garvey, M. A., et al. (2002). Tics and problem behaviors in schoolchildren: Prevalence, characterization, and associations. *Pediatrics, 110*(2, Pt. 1), 331–336.

Sofronoff, K., Attwood, T., & Hinton, S. (2005). A randomised controlled trial of a CBT intervention for anxiety in children with Asperger syndrome. *Journal of Child Psychology and Psychiatry, 46*, 1152–1160.

Solomon, M., Goodlin-Jones, B. L., & Anders, T. F. (2004). A social adjustment enhancement intervention for high functioning autism, Asperger's syndrome, and pervasive developmental disorder NOS. *Journal of Autism and Developmental Disorders, 34*(6), 649–668.

Sovner, R. (1996). Behavioral and affective disturbances in persons with mental retardation: A neuropsychiatric perspective. *Seminars in Clinical Neuropsychiatry, 1*(2), 90–93.

Spicer, D. (1998). Autistic and undiagnosed: A cautionary tale. In E. Schopler, G. B. Mesibov, & L. J. Kunce (Eds.), *Asperger syndrome or high-functioning autism?* (pp. 377–382). New York: Plenum Press.

Sponheim, E., Oftedal, G., & Helverschou, S. B. (2002). Multiple doses of secretin in the treatment of autism: A controlled study. *Acta Paediatrica, 91*(5), 540–545.

Sporn, A. L., Addington, A. M., Gogtay, N., Ordonez, A. E., Gornick, M., Clasen, L., et al. (2004). Pervasive developmental disorder and childhood-onset schizophrenia: Comorbid disorder or a phenotypic variant of a very early onset illness? *Biological Psychiatry, 55*(10), 989–994.

Sprafkin, J., Volpe, R. J., Gadow, K. D., Nolan, E. E., & Kelly, K. (2002). A DSM-

IV-referenced screening instrument for preschool children: The Early Childhood Inventory-4. *Journal of the American Academy of Child and Adolescent Psychiatry, 41*(5), 604–612.

Stahlberg, O., Soderstrom, H., Rastam, M., & Gillberg, C. (2004). Bipolar disorder, schizophrenia, and other psychotic disorders in adults with childhood onset AD/HD and/or autism spectrum disorders. *Journal of Neural Transmission, 111*(7), 891–902.

Stewart, M. E., Barnard, L., Pearson, J., Hasan, R., & O'Brien, G. (2006). Presentation of depression in autism and Asperger syndrome: A review. *Autism, 10*(1), 103–116.

Tantum, D. (2003). The challenge of adolescents and adults with Asperger syndrome. *Child and Adolescent Psychiatric Clinics of North America, 12,* 143–163.

Tonge, B., & Einfeld, S. (2003). Psychopathology and intellectual disability: The Australian Child to Adult Longitudinal Study. In L. M. Glidden (Ed.), *International review of research in mental retardation* (Vol. 26, pp. 61–91). San Diego, CA: Academic Press.

Valla, J. P., Bergeron, L., Bidaut-Russell, M., St.-Georges, M., & Gaudet, N. (1997). Reliability of the Dominic-R: A young child mental health questionnaire combining visual and auditory stimuli. *Journal of Child Psychology and Psychiatry, 38*(6), 717–724.

Ventura, M. A., Green, M. F., Shaner, A., & Liberman, R. P. (1993). Training and quality assurance with the Brief Psychiatric Rating Scale: "The drift buster." *International Journal of Methods in Psychiatric Research, 3,* 221–244.

Volkmar, F. R., & Cohen, D. J. (1991). Comorbid association of autism and schizophrenia. *American Journal of Psychiatry, 148*(12), 1705–1707.

Walters, A. S., Barrett, R. P., & Feinstein, C. (1990). Social relatedness and autism: Current research, issues, directions. *Research in Developmental Disabilities, 11*(3), 303–326.

Webber, S. (2005). *Webber Photo Cards: Emotions.* Greenville, SC: Super Duper.

Weisbrot, D. M., Gadow, K. D., DeVincent, C. J., & Pomeroy, J. (2005). The presentation of anxiety in children with pervasive developmental disorders. *Journal of Child and Adolescent Psychopharmacology, 15*(3), 477–496.

Wiggs, L., & Stores, G. (2004). Sleep patterns and sleep disorders in children with autistic spectrum disorders: Insights using parent report and actigraphy. *Developmental Medicine and Child Neurology, 46*(6), 372–380.

Wozniak, J., Biederman, J., Faraone, S. V., Frazier, J., Kim, J., Millstein, R., et al. (1997). Mania in children with pervasive developmental disorder revisited. *Journal of the American Academy of Child and Adolescent Psychiatry, 36*(11), 1552–1559.

CHAPTER ELEVEN

From Assessment to Intervention

Kerry Hogan
Lee M. Marcus

This chapter focuses on how assessment information can be used to help in the individualized programming for students and older persons with autism spectrum disorders (ASD). Historically, formal assessment has been used to generate data about an individual's level of functioning and, at times, to identify a pattern of abilities. There has been less emphasis on the process of translating evaluation data into both general and specific educational suggestions and plans. In this chapter, we address from a conceptual and practical framework what is involved in using assessment information as a starting point for developing meaningful interventions. This framework is grounded in the experience of the Treatment and Education of Autistic and related Communication-handicapped CHildren (TEACCH) program, one of the first ASD programs to integrate developmental assessment into treatment decision making and planning.

The chapter is organized into the following sections: (1) a brief review of assessment approaches in ASD and how they have been applied to interventions; (2) an overview of the TEACCH approach to assessment; (3) a discussion of using the Psychoeducational Profile (PEP), the primary developmental–behavioral–educational instrument in the TEACCH program, as a vehicle for intervention planning, together with a case example demonstrating the use of the PEP-3; (4) a description and case example of informal assessment, an especially valuable approach in classroom and other nonclinic settings; (5) a brief review of assessment methods and strategies for adolescents and adults, where the emphasis is on functionality of skills in applied settings; and (6) concluding comments.

For the purposes of this chapter, "assessment" is defined as the formal or informal process of gathering data on behavioral and learning/developmental functioning as an aid in developing an initial program and continuing to evaluate its effects over time and settings. This perspective differs from the data-based assessment process. A data-based process focuses on specific goals and objectives, whereas our view of assessment is intended to be broad-based and comprehensive. Although data-based monitoring can and should have a role in ASD intervention programs, this chapter addresses the assessment of skills, learning patterns/styles, and ASD-specific behaviors that serve as the basis for individualized programming.

In general, once diagnosis (and, in some cases, prognostic clarification) has been established for a child with an ASD, there is a need to understand the child's levels of developmental functioning, including his or her unique pattern of strengths and weaknesses. With a younger child, the assessment profile should be based primarily on guidelines derived from developmental norms; should use developmentally sequenced materials and activities; and should reflect concepts derived from well-established developmental models and themes (such as means–end reasoning, causality, and role-taking perspective). At the adolescent age level and beyond, strictly developmental guidelines may need to be gradually replaced by criterion-based assessment of specific, pragmatic skills. The shift from the more developmentally based approaches to those concerned with assessment of behavior and competence in a functional environment reflects the current efforts of special educators in establishing appropriate secondary-level programs for individuals with severe ASD. Regardless of the fundamental assumptions of the assessment approach, the evaluation and analysis of both abilities and disabilities within and across specific skill areas should be basic objectives.

OVERVIEW OF ASSESSMENT APPROACHES IN INTERVENTION IN ASD

Historically, the link between assessment and intervention in ASD has reflected the philosophical and methodological bases of the treatment model. Not all intervention approaches value assessment—or, at least, not all require a formal or informal assessment process to guide treatment planning. For example, psychodynamic therapies typically operate from a theoretical framework that does not rely on or require an initial systematic assessment leading to a specific treatment plan. Although individualization is possible and adjustments can be made, the intervention is largely based on its conceptual framework. The role and importance of assessment in treatment planning vary: Assessment may be valued as a core, integral, and ongoing part of the intervention process; it may be viewed as a means to jump-start the treatment process, but carried out in either a limited way or not systematically; or it may not be done at all.

In general, tests and other assessment measures that have been standardized on a typical general population have not addressed the unique characteristics of individuals with ASD; nor have they been designed to lead to comprehensive treatment planning. For example, standardized cognitive and achievement tests, although valuable in assessing functioning levels and patterns of strengths and weaknesses, do not lend themselves to being translated into meaningful, individualized intervention goals. These tests were not designed for individuals with ASD, although certain subtest patterns may emerge in those who function in the average range or higher. Such patterns may suggest educational intervention strategies (e.g., for someone with a low verbal score, emphasizing visual methods of instruction), but this test analysis approach is not specific to ASD and is usually secondary to the purpose of the testing.

Researchers have devoted considerable effort to identifying and developing assessment measures that evaluate developmental and behavioral functioning in ASD, especially in the areas of social and communication skills (e.g., Carter, Davis, Klin, & Volkmar, 2005; Tager-Flusberg, Paul, & Lord, 2005; Watson, Lord, Schaffer, & Schopler, 1989). The past few years have seen increasing agreement on and endorsement of many of these measures, based on the factors of validity, reliability, and relevance for the subject population. Some developmental and cognitive tests, such as the Mullen Scales of Early Learning (Mullen, 1995) and the original Differential Ability Scales (Elliott, 1990), have been widely used and are highly regarded in the ASD research field. However, these and other assessment measures used in research are less valuable in generating teaching ideas and strategies, primarily because they were not designed for this purpose and are not specific to ASD. Similarly, widely used and well-standardized diagnostic instruments for ASD, such as the Autism Diagnostic Observation Schedule (Lord, Rutter, DiLavore, & Risi, 2002) and the Childhood Autism Rating Scale (Schopler, Reichler, & Renner, 1988) are used both clinically and in research; they yield valuable information on all aspects of behavioral characteristics seen in ASD across the entire age range. However, they are not intended to serve as a basis for treatment planning, beyond the classification of an individual as having an ASD diagnosis or not.

There are many model ASD intervention programs, which have been reviewed in previous publications (e.g., Dawson & Osterling, 1997; Handleman & Harris, 2001). All incorporate assessment information to some degree, although with considerable variation in comprehensiveness and in description of how assessment information is organized and translated into treatment goals. All of these, and others not cited, employ explicit data collection methods and have clearly defined philosophies and frameworks, as well as specific approaches. Two groups emerge from among these programs. The first group fully integrates assessment data and considers the assessment process a critical component of intervention planning; the second group appears to be less wedded to assessment as a core component (to judge by published reports), but makes use of these data in treatment planning. Three programs fall into the first group: TEACCH (Mesibov, Shea, & Schopler, 2005), Social Communication, Emotional Regulation, and Transactional Supports (SCERTS) (Prizant, Wetherby, Rubin, Laurent, & Rydell, 2006), Developmental, Individual Differences, Relationship-Based Model (DIR) (Greenspan & Wieder, 2006). Six programs fall into the second group: the Denver Model (Rogers & Lewis, 1989), the Young Child Project (Lovaas, 1987), the Douglass Developmental Disabilities Center (Harris, Handleman, Arnold, & Gordon, 2001; see Harris, Bruey, Palmieri, & Handleman, Chapter 12, this volume), Pivotal Response Training (Koegel, Koegel, & McNerney, 2001), Learning Experiences Alternative Program (LEAP) (Strain & Cordisco, 1994), and the Walden School (McGee, Morrier, Daly, & Jacobs, 2001). As noted earlier, these nine programs are intended to be representative of the range of ASD-specific models cited by the field. They reflect a diversity of frameworks, including developmental, behavioral, eclectic, and social-emotional. The reader is encouraged to review the programs' descriptions in the literature for detailed information about how they incorporate assessment information into treatment and educational planning. The balance of this chapter focuses on the formal and informal assessment methods used in the TEACCH program.

OVERVIEW OF THE TEACCH APPROACH TO ASSESSMENT

Individualized assessment has always been an integral part of the TEACCH program. The rationale for the first version of the PEP included the need for an assessment tool that could reliably measure developmental skills at a time when most professionals believed that autistic children were "untestable," as well as the need to find a systematic method for individualizing educational programs that would meet the needs of children whose learning patterns varied, though they showed the common criteria defining autism (Schopler & Reichler, 1979). The PEP demonstrated that a test that reduced language demands and could be flexibly administered resulted in more accurate developmental information and could help in program planning. By the late 1980s more children were being identified at the preschool age, so the PEP was revised (becoming the PEP-R) to better assess children under age 3. Most recently, the PEP-3 revision (Schopler, Lansing, Reichler, & Marcus, 2005) has brought the test further in line with current concepts of cognitive functioning and psychometric properties. The strengths of the PEP include its ability to be used with the entire range of preschool-age and elementary-school-age children with ASD (regardless of the severity of their disorders), its integration of the behavioral and the developmental domains, and its value for educational and home programming. In our work with teachers, we demonstrate how the basic features of the formal PEP assessment instrument can be translated into informal assessment methods in the classroom, and urge them to use these methods to help with day-to-day decision making regarding curriculum and behavior management issues. Specifically, we emphasize the concept of "emerging skills" and the importance of noting each child's interests and learning style, spotting possibly interfering ASD characteristics, and recognizing parents' priorities as they pertain to various curriculum areas.

As a student moves out of childhood and preadolescence and into the teenage years, assessment shifts from the developmental to the functional as the curriculum emphasis changes. The assessment process remains critical, but the focus and location of assessment moves from the classroom to other in-school settings (such as the office or cafeteria) and to actual life space areas in the community (such as work sites). Even for those students who can continue on an academic track, there is a need for functional assessment of communication, social, and work behavior skills. The Adolescent and Adult Psychoeducational Profile (AAPEP; Mesibov, Schopler, Schaffer, & Landrus, 1988) was designed to provide a functional assessment for adolescents and adults with ASD and mental retardation. It has been recently revised to serve more explicitly as a tool to help with transition planning, becoming the TEACCH Transition Assessment Profile (TTAP; Mesibov, Thomas, Chapman, & Schopler, 2007). An important feature of the AAPEP/TTAP is that it enables a direct and consistent evaluation of a person's skills in a number of functional domains, across home, school, and work settings. In addition to the formal assessment instrument that constituted the older AAPEP, the newer TTAP includes an informal measure for older adolescents and adults who are candidates for supported employment services. This instrument, which has been developed and fine-tuned for nearly two decades through our TEACCH Supported Employment program, evaluates the skills and behaviors that are needed in actual work settings (Keel, Mesibov, & Woods, 1997).

The information gathered with these two assessment instruments is used to help with job placement decisions and determining strategies for on-the-job instructional programs. For high-functioning individuals, traditional psychological and achievement tests may also be used to clarify cognitive patterns and strengths and weaknesses. These are supplemented by tasks from neuropsychological tests, as well as by measures of social understanding and expression, theory of mind, and central coherence. Observations and results from all of these measures help pinpoint subtle social and communication problems and specific thinking and learning issues (e.g., literalness, difficulties with perspective taking, and cognitive inflexibility) that may need to be specially addressed in a job setting.

A very important aspect of assessment is gathering and sharing information from and with parents. At the preschool level, the initial assessment process is usually geared to determining a diagnosis and answering questions about its implications (Marcus & Stone, 1993). This time is also used to introduce the parents to our philosophy, approach, and commitment to ongoing support. Because we provide direct follow-up (see below), the initial evaluation serves as a relationship-building experience rather than as the end of an assessment process. Seeking and using parents' observations and opinions are integral to the assessment process, as well as to making such treatment decisions as appropriate school placement, need for medication, and future residential and vocational placements.

THE PEP-3: DESCRIPTION AND CASE EXAMPLE

As noted above, the PEP-3, the most recent revision of the PEP, is a developmental test that helps with diagnosis and individualized programming. The test normally can be given in 45–90 minutes and provides multiple opportunities for informal observations of behavior. Covering a developmental age range from about 6 months to 7 years, the PEP-3 includes a direct test and observation scale and a Caregiver Report. The child test scale yields age scores in six developmental areas, three focusing on language skills and the other three focusing on motor skills. Composite scores for these skill areas can be calculated. There are four behavior areas specific to ASD, and the derived standard and percentile scores are based on a sample with ASD. The Caregiver Report allows for an assessment of adaptive skills and specific behaviors. Information from both parts of the instrument can be integrated in formulating a treatment and education plan.

In reviewing the data, the clinician should consider various levels of analysis: examining the child's overall pattern of strengths and weaknesses, analyzing the individual items that were passed or where an "emerging" score was obtained, reviewing the pattern of maladaptive behaviors, and considering the parent's or caregiver's information. Below is a case example based on a PEP-3 assessment.

As part of his 3-year reevaluation, the school psychologist administered the PEP-3 to Sam. Sam was a 5-year-old child with a previous diagnosis of autistic disorder. Previous developmental testing suggested that his level of cognitive development was behind his chronological age by 12–24 months, depending on the area of functioning assessed. According to his performance on the PEP-3, his Communication Skills age equivalent was at the 40-month level. His Expressive score was higher than his Receptive score;

this pattern was related to his strengths in labeling objects and repeating words. His Cognitive Verbal/Preverbal score was at the 48-month level, due to strengths in matching skills and to several emerging skills related to preschool concepts (e.g., identifying numbers, letters, shapes, and colors). Sam's Motor Skills were more developed than his Communication Skills. His overall Motor Skills score was 41 months; although this was a lower score than his Communication Skills score, he was at ceiling in Gross Motor Skills. He was at the 45-month level in Fine Motor Skills. He was not able to write his name or color in the lines of pictures, but he had emerging skills in copying shapes. He had numerous difficulties with visual–motor imitation tasks because of his limited attention to the examiner.

On the behavioral scales of the PEP-3, Sam's Social Relating Skills were more impaired than those of other children on the autism spectrum. He had a percentile score of 35 in this domain, reflecting his tendency to ignore others, his lack of reciprocity in interactions, and his difficulty in expressing affect appropriate to a situation. By contrast, Sam's Communication Skills (percentile score of 70) were less impaired than those of other children with ASD. Although he demonstrated some unusual uses of language, such as occasional immediate and delayed echolalia, his language development was otherwise delayed but not unusual. Sam's percentile score on the Characteristic Motor Behaviors domain was 75, indicating that he demonstrated fewer unusual motor behaviors than other children with ASD. On the Caregiver Report, Sam's parents noted Personal Self-Care at the 41-month level. His mother reported that she had not previously expected much independence from him in his self-care, and that she would now like to focus on developing these skills at home. His Problem Behaviors outside of school were not severe. In this area he was at the 80th percentile relative to other children with ASD, and his Adaptive Behavior as measured on the Caregiver Report was also a strength relative to other children with ASD.

Sam's teacher reviewed his PEP-3 developmental performance and noted that he had strengths in visual skills such as matching, communication skills such as labeling, and gross motor skills. To determine appropriate teaching goals, she decided to focus on emerging skills—particularly in Sam's areas of strength, as he was likely to make quicker progress in these areas, which could then be used to develop his areas of weakness. He demonstrated the following emerging abilities: matching letters, counting, naming shapes and colors, and labeling pictures. He had mastered some skills, such as matching objects to picture outlines, and he was interested in books (especially books about vehicles). However, Sam's teacher was concerned about his difficulty in relating to others, especially his lack of attention to other people, as she felt that this difficulty was delaying his development in other areas. For example, she was having a hard time teaching him fine motor movements, such as using scissors, because he did not attend to her demonstrations and resisted physical prompts. She had also discussed Sam's delayed self-care skills with his mother, and had agreed to try to help him develop more independence in daily living activities.

Sam's teacher used all this information to assist her in developing many goals for his individualized education program (IEP). One developmental goal for Sam was to increase his awareness of the math concept of quantity. The teacher planned to use his mastered skill of matching objects to picture outlines to develop his emerging skill of counting. She created several activities to teach him during instructional time, which he could, then practice throughout the day. For example, she taught him to attach blocks to cards containing the same number of squares as the numeral written on the card. She also taught him to match pictures of his peers to a number jig with circles matching the size of the pictures. Once he had mastered these tasks, he could practice the block activity during his independent work time and the picture activity during circle time, to help the children count how many students were in class that day.

One of Sam's social goals was to pay more attention to people. Again, the teacher used his mastered skills in matching and his interest in books and vehicles to teach this skill. During her instructional time, she taught Sam several activities. She took pictures of the classroom staff in their cars and the other students in their parents' cars or the buses they rode to school. Using these photographs, she created an adapted book about the people in Sam's school environment and their cars. When looking at the book, Sam had a selection of pictures identical to those in the book, and he matched the pictures to each page in the book so that he had looked at pictures of each person. The teacher also attached pictures of each student to the placemats they used for snacks and to the table at the place they usually sat. Sam's job was to pass out placemats, first using the picture cues on the table and then, once he mastered this task, matching each placemat to the person sitting at that place. Sam's teacher also showed this activity to his mother as an example of how she could teach him to be more independent at home.

Sam's teacher thus used the information from the PEP-3 to formulate both social and developmental goals, and to create activities that would allow him to practice these goals throughout his day. Once Sam mastered these goals, she used informal assessment to create new goals. For example, as he mastered the activities created to help him learn the concept of quantity, she began to assess whether he could match blocks to cards with numerals but no outlines. She also assessed whether she could use a number line, so that Sam could match objects to the outlines on the line and then choose the numeral matching that amount. In this way, she combined formal and informal assessment to determine her student's pattern of learning, strengths, and weaknesses. She also used the concept of emerging abilities to identify areas of readiness, and then based her teaching on all these types of information.

USING INFORMAL ASSESSMENT
TO DEVELOP EDUCATIONAL PLANS

The results of standardized intellectual assessments can be used to develop an IEP that is based on an understanding of a student's learning profile. Developmental, vocational, adaptive, and achievement testing are perhaps more directly related to developing intervention goals. But even with the guidance of formal assessment data, teachers are often required to "fill in the gaps" in order to develop effective IEPs. For many reasons, standardized assessments may have limited use for educators. Teachers are often faced with writing goals for students whose records have relatively little assessment information. They may only have access to outdated evaluations. Developmental testing or adaptive assessments contain items that might directly apply to educational goals, but test protocols that indicate performance on specific items are not available to teachers. The general scores in a psychoeducational report provide information about learning profiles that teachers can use to infer goals, but the uneven performance of students with ASD may not be reflected in those goals. All these limitations of formal assessments leave teachers with a need for a method of ongoing assessment to facilitate educational planning throughout the school year. This type of evaluation is called "informal assessment." Informal assessment is based on the student's present performance in the classroom as opposed to his or her performance on a test with standardized administration and scoring.

Informal assessment is a process of presenting novel tasks to a student in order to determine that student's readiness to learn those tasks. Readiness is determined by observing those areas in which a student demonstrates emerging skills. This type of assessment is intended to be a supplement to, but not a replacement for, formal assessments such as intellectual or achievement testing. In fact, standardized assessment can be a useful starting point for determining the types of skills that might be included in an informal assessment. By identifying a student's current level of performance through informal assessment, a teacher can begin developing specific goals for an IEP.

The advantages of informal assessment in developing an IEP are several. In the TEACCH program, we have observed that activities that have a clear purpose are more readily acquired than tasks where the purpose is not meaningful or is unclear (Mesibov et al., 2005). In informal assessment, a teacher can assess real-life activities or skills presented in a way that is more meaningful to a student than those activities administered in most standardized test instruments. For example, achievement tests may assess reading comprehension by using sentences or paragraphs that have no relation to a student's interests or daily activities. Informal assessment does not have the restrictions of standardized administration, so a teacher can assess comprehension by using materials related to a student's special interest, or sentences with instructions the student would follow in daily life.

Informal assessment also gives the teacher the opportunity to focus on emerging skills where the student is demonstrating readiness to learn. This is one of the most significant advantages of informal assessment over formal educational assessment. Other than the PEP-3 and TTAP, there are no standardized assessment measures that account for emerging abilities. Some measures of adaptive behavior (e.g., the Vineland Adaptive Behavior Scales, Second Edition [Vineland-II]; Sparrow, Cicchetti, & Balla, 2005) provide scores for items that are performed inconsistently. For the most part, though, an examiner is required to identify skills that may be potential learning goals based on items that the student failed during testing, even though the student may not be ready to learn those skills.

Following is a description of how to plan, administer, and interpret informal assessments in order to implement educational goals. The case example that follows this description details the process from start to finish as it might be implemented for a young child with an ASD. Figure 11.1 is a graphic representation of this process—beginning with formal assessment; progressing to informal assessment, goal development, and intervention; and then returning to assessment.

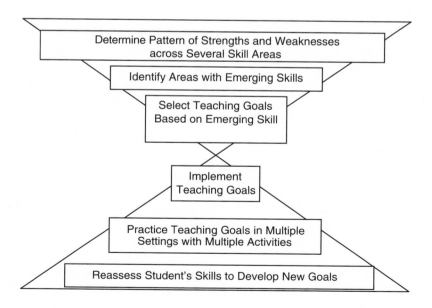

FIGURE 11.1. Process of developing goals from assessment to intervention and back to assessment.

Planning an Informal Assessment

For most teachers, determining which activities to assess is the most difficult aspect of informal assessment. This process can be greatly enhanced by a good knowledge of typical development, especially for teachers of young children. Understanding developmental norms across a range of skill areas will allow a teacher to determine possible next steps based on developmental test results. Standardized educational and developmental curricula can also provide useful direction to the teacher planning an informal assessment. Norms related to the development of typical students, however, should be used with caution, as the development of students with ASD is likely to be uneven (Joseph, Tager-Flusberg, & Lord, 2002). Teachers should expect that prerequisite skills may not have been mastered even when more advanced skills are present, or that a concept may not have been generalized even if it is demonstrated in one context.

Another source of ideas for informal assessment is task analysis. Teachers of older students should especially have experience with detailed task analysis. During an informal assessment of an adaptive skill, task analysis will assist the teacher in finding those aspects of a task that reflect emerging skills.

Informal assessment should not consist only of tasks that the teacher expects that the student has not learned. Skills that have been acquired in one context should be assessed across a range of contexts. This will assist the teacher in determining whether a skill has generalized to other activities or has only been mastered within the tasks that have been taught. For example, if a student with an ASD has been successfully sorting blocks by color, the teacher may want to assess whether the child can sort other objects by color or match pictures according to color. Until the student has demonstrated competency with that concept in a range of ways, the teacher cannot be confident that the student has mastered that concept. Skills that may have been mastered, therefore, should still be included in informal assessment.

Skills that the teacher suspects the student would fail are still worth assessing during the informal assessment. This is especially the case if the teacher is aware of particular interests and strengths the student has demonstrated in the past. The uneven skill development of students with ASD results in some students' mastering skills even though they appear not to have mastered prerequisite skills. For example, a number of young children with ASD develop some reading skills before they have learned to speak (Craig & Telfer, 2005). A teacher who plans assessments based only on skills expected for a child with a similar developmental level may miss important strengths that were not previously assessed because the child had already met ceiling criteria before reaching that skill in a formal assessment.

Administering the Assessment

Informal assessment can be done at any time. Observation of a child's initiations on the playground could be considered an informal assessment of social skills, for example. But informal assessment, despite its name, is not intended to be administered without planning or some structure. It is important for the teacher to be clear about the goals of the assessment and the criteria for passing, emerging, or failing scores. These need not be standardized criteria, but they should be specific enough for the teacher to determine whether skills can be considered as mastered, as emerging, or as absent.

When the informal assessment is administered, thought should be given to the student's expectations. If the assessment makes use of tabletop activities, then it should be done at a time and place where the student usually works with a teacher, so that it takes place within a familiar work routine. In this way, the student is more likely to be able to give his or her best performance. When the teacher is planning the assessment, a hierarchy of prompts should be considered along with the scoring criteria. For example, a verbal student might be presented with the materials and given a brief demonstration. If this prompt is ineffective, then the teacher might give a short verbal instruction. Additional prompts can be used in a systematic fashion. If the teacher is aware of the prompts being used, it will be easier to score the assessment and easier to make decisions about the best teaching techniques.

Monitoring the level of prompting helps the teacher plan a goal, given the student's present performance. The teacher should not, however, confuse exploring prompts with teaching. The assessment is not instructional time, and the teacher should not become sidetracked by teaching. Teaching will not be effective until the emerging skills are identified, and this must be done at the conclusion of the assessment, not during the assessment.

Scoring the Informal Assessment

Identifying "emerging skills," or those skills that a child is most ready to learn, is the goal of informal assessment. If the criterion for each activity is clear, then the student may pass the task, fail it, or complete it partially or with help. If the child can do some part of the task or can complete it with help, this task should be considered an emerging skill. When the teacher is scoring the informal assessment, the primary goal should be to identify emerging abilities.

In addition to identifying emerging abilities, informal assessment is an opportunity for a teacher to observe other aspects of the student's learning style. Because most activities in an informal assessment will be new, the teacher is able to observe the student's problem-solving skills. As in a formal psychoeducational evaluation, all behavior during the assessment is useful information about the student's responses to a variety of materials, his or her patience and persistence with difficult tasks, the student's organizational abilities, and the cues that the student responds to best.

Developing Goals Based on the Informal Assessment

Once the assessment is completed and the teacher has determined which skills reflect emerging abilities, the teacher's task is to design teaching activities that will develop the identified skills. It is important to avoid the trap of designing only one activity to develop each skill. The strengths of students with ASD in the area of memory, and their weaknesses in generalization, often lead to mastery of specific activities through memorization without actually learning the underlying principle.

To develop goals, the teacher should think of times throughout the day when each skill would be used, and then teach activities that correspond to those times of day. Repeated practice in multiple contexts will make the skill more meaningful to a student with an ASD and will ensure that when the skill is reassessed, the student will have mastered the concept rather than memorizing a specific task.

Monitoring Goals Based on Informal Assessment

Teachers are required to monitor students' progress on all IEP goals, although planning goals in the manner described above may require types of monitoring that are unfamiliar to some teachers. We suggest that teachers continue to make use of the concepts of "pass," "emerge," and "fail" to assess a students' progress. Some teachers group all the activities related to a single goal on one data sheet, in order to be able to compare progress on related activities. Most teachers we have worked with prefer to keep activities on data sheets in the order in which they would occur during the day, to promote ease of data collection. With this format, a teacher can record data at the times during the day when memory of a student's performance is freshest. For example, the teacher can keep a record form for each student that has the schedule written in a column on the left, and specific activities related to IEP goals listed to the right of the time of day each one occurs. Following a morning group, a member of the classroom staff can pick up the data sheet for some of the students and circle "pass," "emerge," or "fail" for the skills that were practiced during that time.

After a few days, the teacher may transfer the daily data for each child onto a sheet that groups the activities by goal or curriculum area, to see whether the child is mastering the goal in a variety of areas. Then the teacher is able to observe whether some activities are mastered while others are not. The teacher will also be able to see whether some activities need to be modified because the student's readiness was not what it appeared to be during the original informal assessment. We often find that a teacher needs to restructure activities related to a goal, to help promote more timely progress. Or, if performance is quite different from what the original data suggested, the teacher may need to repeat the assessment.

As the teacher's daily data indicate that a child is consistently passing (or consistently failing) items related to a teaching concept, then the teacher will plan a new informal assessment in order to keep the student's goals in line with his or her progress. Informal assessment, then, is not considered an annual event, but one that will continue throughout the year as the student makes progress. As reflected in Figure 11.1, assessment is always both the beginning and the end of the teaching development process.

Case Example

Susan was a 10-year-old with autism who completed her mandated reevaluation with the school psychologist. Results indicated that her Wechsler Intelligence Scale for Children—Fourth Edition (WISC-IV) Full Scale IQ was in the mild range of mental retardation, with strengths in Perceptual Reasoning. She particularly excelled at WISC-IV Block Design and Matrix Reasoning. On the Woodcock–Johnson III she generally performed at the first-grade level, but was at the third-grade level on Math Calculation, Spelling, and Decoding. Her Reading Comprehension, Writing, and Applied Problems were significant weaknesses. The psychologist also completed the Vineland-II with her parents. Susan's Adaptive Behavior Composite was well below her age level, with a standard score of 54. Scores were relatively even across Communication, Daily Living, and Socialization.

Susan's parents were especially interested in seeing that her reading skills advance. Her teacher had observed that, despite her decoding ability, Susan understood words best when they were associated with a practical task or visual image. She decided, therefore, to complete an informal assessment with particular emphasis on Susan's reading comprehension. In the informal assessment, Susan's teacher presented a variety of activities; these included sorting identical words and matching single words to familiar pictures (such as those on her picture schedule or pictures of favorite foods). She also showed Susan sentences and asked her to match the sentences to a picture. To assess her understanding of writing without visual cues, she gave Susan a list of simple written directions, such as "Stand up," to see whether she could follow these directions in a written format. She also gave Susan a list of words and several objects, and asked her to collect all the objects that matched the words on the list. Using simple picture books, Susan's teacher assessed whether she could match pictures to pages of the book containing the same picture, and whether she could match words to pages containing the same word.

During the informal assessment, Susan's teacher observed emerging abilities in the following tasks: matching words to pictures, choosing objects to correspond to a list, matching pictures to sentences, and matching words to pages in a book. Susan's teacher also noticed that she was especially interested in books and pictures about animals. She had observed in the past that Susan enjoyed playing the role of a "helper" at school, and Susan's parents reported that the same was true at home.

Based on this assessment, Susan's teacher planned for her to improve her comprehension skills throughout the day by completing the following activities. During morning group, Susan would match the written names of each student to the picture of each student, to assist in taking attendance. During Susan's work time, her teacher would present file folder activities requiring her to match pictures to words and pictures to short sentences. As Susan mastered these activities, she could practice them during independent work time. Depending on her progress, the teacher could present new folder activities with additional vocabulary and sentence comprehension items during instructional time. Her teacher would make sure that at least a few of the activities involved animals, to maintain Susan's interest in and enjoyment of reading. During her work time with the teacher, Susan would also use adapted books. These books would require her to match words to pictures in the book. The teacher selected several easy books with topics of interest to Susan, in order to expand her repertoire of leisure activities. Once Susan had mastered this skill using these adapted books, her teacher would keep them in the classroom reading center, where Susan could complete them during her free time. All the students in Susan's class took turns completing chores. Susan's teacher had labeled the shelves in the play area, and when it was Susan's turn to clean up, she would practice matching the toys to the written labels. At snacktime, Susan would collect supplies to set the table by following brief written directions accompanied by a picture. For example, a direction might be "Put the plates on the table," and there would be a drawing of a person putting plates on the table. Finally, when she was preparing to go home, Susan would pack her school bag, using a written list of single words and checking off each word as she placed that object in the bag.

As indicated by this list of activities, Susan's teacher was following the recommendation of developing a skill by using several activities and having the student practice that skill throughout the day. The specific skills being developed were the comprehension of single written words and short sentences. Rather than learning and practicing this skill in a reading book, Susan would be learning these skills by using her visual strengths. Ideally, Susan's acquisition of these skills would also be promoted by including some of Susan's interests and utilizing her motivation to be helpful to her teacher.

As the teacher taught and then allowed Susan to practice the activities she had created, she noticed that Susan had an exceptional memory and that her performance on some tasks might not reflect her actual comprehension. In particular, she had memorized most of the directions associated with snacktime, and she had also memorized where the toys in the play area belong. To accommodate these observations, Susan's teacher changed the position of the toys and their labels once a week, and had Susan begin to practice using written directions for other chores and for a "Simon Says" game that the students played during their social group.

As Susan progressed, her teacher noted consistent passing performance on those tasks involving single words and a visual cue. All the words that had been used so far were from the first-grade curriculum. Susan's performance on tasks that included sentences was still inconsistent. So her teacher performed another informal assessment, this time presenting similar tasks with more difficult vocabulary words, longer written checklists, and adapted books that required matching sentences to pictures rather than single words. As the year ended, Susan's teacher noted at the IEP meeting that Susan's reading comprehension had improved, though it was still delayed relative to her decoding skills. Also, because her teacher had selected emerging skills that were within Susan's ability to master without excessive frustration, Susan was more motivated to read and was spending more time in the reading center with her adapted books. She had also begun to explore books that weren't adapted. Susan's parents reported that they had been able to use some of these skills at home. She was now able to follow a written checklist to complete her morning routine independently before school, and to clean up her room. They had also noticed Susan's increased interest in reading, and now saw reading as a potential leisure interest for Susan in the future.

The final step in this process was for Susan's teacher to identify future goals that would build on Susan's newly mastered skills. Susan's teacher planned yet another informal assessment, adding reading activities that were somewhat lengthier and that included number concepts. This allowed her to assess whether Susan was ready to learn adaptive skills such as following a simple recipe.

ASSESSING ADOLESCENTS AND ADULTS

Although the bulk of this chapter examines assessment as it relates to educational goals for younger students with ASD, it is still important to briefly summarize assessment instruments available for those working with older students, and to review their applicability to students with ASD. Not many tests are available for the assessment of adolescents and adults with ASD;

those that exist are, however, more closely tied to intervention goals than are many instruments used to test younger children. As students become older, there is more emphasis on adaptive skills within the special education curriculum. Furthermore, the Individuals with Disabilities Education Improvement Act of 2004 (IDEA, 2004) requires that transition plans be developed in adolescence, and this constitutes a legal imperative to assess functional community and vocational skills. Given the functional nature of assessments used with older students, the transition between assessment and intervention is somewhat smoother than it seems with younger students. Although these measures appear to be more practical, they may not always account for the learning styles of individuals with ASD. This shortcoming may lead to educational plans that do not include important goals for students with ASD who are making the transition to adulthood. For example, vocational assessments that focus on basic work skills (e.g., packaging or office work) may neglect work behaviors that limit vocational success in individuals with ASD, such as the ability to cope with transitions or follow verbal instructions.

The instruments most commonly used with adolescents and adults are adaptive interviews, such as the Vineland-II (Sparrow et al., 2005), or adaptive checklists, such as the Adaptive Behavior Assessment System—Second Edition (Harrison & Oakland, 2003). Although these provide general information about adaptive functioning, they do not assess issues specific to adolescent and adult curriculum planning. They also require information from a limited number of sources. Curriculum development for adolescents and adults with ASD requires knowledge about performance across a range of settings; limiting information to one or two settings may lead to an incomplete assessment. Checklists that are more specific to the curriculum for adolescents and adults include the Transition Planning Inventory—Updated Version (TPI-UV; Clark & Patton, 2006) and the Becker Work Adjustment Profile:2 (Becker, 2005). These instruments measure skills related to daily living abilities, community, and vocational functioning. Both instruments also enable information to be obtained from at least two sources. Although interviews and checklists are a useful means of gathering information from multiple sources, their ability to identify emerging skills that are most amenable to instruction is limited. The TPI-UV does contain information for teachers concerning informal assessment. This link between the checklist and specific goals, however, is not a formal component of the assessment.

Some direct assessments also exist, including the Independent Living Scales (ILS; Loeb, 1996), and the Street Survival Skills Questionnaire (SSSQ; Linkenhoker & McCarron, 1993). The ILS contains items that simulate actual living skills, such as using a telephone book, while the SSSQ uses pictures of real-life events to complete the assessment. Both scales assess specific skills that could be easily translated into a transition plan, and the SSSQ has a curriculum guide to facilitate this process. The learning styles of individuals with ASD include poor generalization and difficulties in drawing inferences from abstract stimuli (Mesibov et al., 2005). Assessment instruments containing "real-world" materials are, for individuals with ASD, more likely to provide meaningful information that can be directly transformed into teaching goals.

The only assessment instruments specifically designed for students with ASD who are adolescents or older are the Autism Screening Instrument for Educational Planning—Third Edition (ASIEP-3; Krug, Arick, & Almond, 2008) and the TTAP, described earlier in this chapter (Mesibov et al., 2007). The ASIEP-3 contains items appropriate for adolescents and adults, but was designed for the entire age range from preschool through adults. The ASIEP-3's application to intervention planning for older students is limited by the wide range of skills it is designed to assess. As noted earlier, the TTAP is based on the AAPEP (Mesibov et al., 1998), so it was specifically designed to assess curriculum-related skills for adolescents and adults with ASD. The TTAP has expanded on the AAPEP by adding components that provide for direct assessment in work environments, giving suggestions for developing goals based on test performance, expanding the range of items included in order to facilitate assessment of individuals with a wide range of cognitive abilities, and providing mechanisms for measuring progress as an individual develops his or her skills. The TTAP specifically addresses the characteristics of ASD that can make other assessment instruments less effective when instructors are developing teaching goals for this population. Specifically, it provides for both direct assessment and obtaining interview information from other sources, including caregivers and teachers or work supervisors. Assessing skills across a range of environments and gathering information from other observers will help teachers to determine whether a skill has been acquired and whether it has generalized to a variety of settings. The TTAP also assesses an individual's ability to use a variety of visual supports, such as schedules or visual rules, to determine how the person's visual strengths can be used to improve performance across settings. As with the PEP-3 (Schopler et al., 2005), there are no basal or ceiling rules in administration; this allows for full assessment of the uneven patterns of learning in individuals with ASD. Finally, the TTAP incorporates informal assessment in a variety of school and work environments, to facilitate observation of how different types of job demands interact with the individual's skills and personality. Assessment and instruction in real-world environments will also allow the individual to experience different types of work directly. People with ASD have difficulty making decisions based on abstract or descriptive information; they are better able to make decisions about job preferences when they have experienced different placements firsthand. Making choices based on written or pictured information is less likely to be valid, although this is the typical approach to assessing vocational interests (e.g., the Wide Range Interest and Occupation Test—Second Edition; Glutting & Wilkinson, 2003).

The process of developing curriculum goals based on the TTAP is much like that outlined in Figure 11.1. The pattern of strengths and weaknesses in skill and behavioral development is assessed by direct observation, as well as via caregiver and teacher interviews. From this understanding of the individual's learning profile, and from the identification of emerging skills, specific goals are developed. Those goals are assessed in a variety of environments through the use of informal assessment. Finally, instruction is provided for emerging abilities throughout the areas assessed, and assessment is repeated as skills are mastered. The primary difference when this process is applied to adolescents and adults rather than children is that instruction is more likely to take place in real-life settings than in the classroom. Teaching across several settings is more heavily emphasized, because of the need to prepare adolescents and adults for using their skills in the community.

CONCLUDING COMMENTS

In this chapter, we have described both formal and informal assessment approaches as a basis for planning individualized treatment and education goals and activities for students with ASD. These approaches are largely derived from our experience with the TEACCH model; however, regardless of the model used, psychologists, educators, and other professionals need to view assessment as a continuing process rather than an annual event. Moreover, assessment should be seen as a means of integrating child, home, and school information not just to understand a child's levels of functioning and basic problems, but to help determine general and specific needs, and then generate intervention ideas. Being able to communicate with the "end users" (parents, teachers, and other service providers) requires knowledge not only of assessment tools and strategies, but also of developmental and educational instruction methods, curricula, and activities. Individuals with ASD and their families, and the professionals who help them, will all be beneficiaries of this effort.

REFERENCES

Becker, R. L. (2005). *Becker Work Adjustment Profile:2*. Columbus, OH: Elbern.

Carter, A., Davis, N. O., Klin, A., & Volkmar, F. R. (2005). Social development in autism. In F. R. Volkmar, R. Paul, A. Klin, & D. J. Cohen (Eds.), *Handbook of autism and pervasive developmental disorders* (3rd ed., Vol. 1, pp. 312–334). Hoboken, NJ: Wiley.

Clark, G. M., & Patton, J. R. (2006). *Transition Planning Inventory—Updated Version: Administration and resource guide*. Austin, TX: PRO-ED.

Craig, H. K., & Telfer, A. S. (2005). Hyperlexia and autism spectrum disorder: A case study of scaffolding language development over time. *Topics in Language Disorders, 25, 253–269.*

Dawson, G., & Osterling, J. (1997). Early intervention in autism: Effectiveness and common elements of current approaches. In M. J. Guralnick (Ed.), *The effectiveness of early intervention: Second generation research* (pp. 307–326). Baltimore: Brookes.

Elliott, C. D. (1990). *Differential Ability Scales*. San Antonio, TX: Psychological Corporation.

Glutting, J. J., & Wilkinson, G. (2003). *Wide Range Interest and Occupation Test—Second Edition*. Austin, TX: PRO-ED.

Greenspan, S. I., & Wieder, S. (2006). *Engaging autism: Helping children relate, communicate and think with the DIR Floortime approach*. Cambridge, MA: Da Capo Press.

Handleman, J. S., & Harris, S. L. (Eds.). (2001). *Preschool education programs for children with autism* (2nd ed). Austin, TX: PRO-ED.

Harris, S. L., Handleman, J. S., Arnold, M. S., & Gordon, R. (2001). The Douglass Developmental Center. In J. S. Handleman & S. L. Harris (Eds.), *Preschool education programs for children with autism* (2nd ed., pp. 233–260). Austin, TX: PRO-ED.

Harrison, P. L., & Oakland, T. (2003). *Adaptive Behavior Assessment System—Second Edition*. San Antonio, TX: Psychological Corporation.

Individuals with Disabilities Education Improvement Act of 2004, Pub. L. No. 108-446, 118 Stat. 2647 (2004).

Joseph, R. M., Tager-Flusberg, H., & Lord, C. (2002). Cognitive profiles and social-communicative functioning in children with autism spectrum disorder. *Journal of Child Psychology and Psychiatry, 43, 807–821.*

Keel, J. H., Mesibov, G. B., & Woods, A. (1997). TEACCH-supported employment programs. *Journal of Autism and Developmental Disorders, 27, 3–9.*

Koegel, R. L., Koegel, L. K., & McNerney, E. K. (2001). Pivotal areas in intervention for autism. *Journal of Clinical Child Psychology, 30, 19–32.*

Krug, D., Arick, J. R., & Almond, P. (2008). *Autism Screening Instrument for Educational Planning—Third Edition*. Austin, TX: PRO-ED.

Linkenhoker, D., & McCarron, L. (1993). *Street Survival Skills Questionnaire*. San Antonio, TX: Psychological Corporation.

Loeb, P.A. (1996). *Independent Living Scales*. San Antonio, TX: Psychological Corporation.

Lord, C., Rutter, M., DiLavore, P. C., & Risi, S. (2002). *Autism Diagnostic Observation Schedule*. Los Angeles: Western Psychological Services.

Lovass, O. J. (1987). Behavioral treatment and normal educational and intellectual functioning in young autistic children. *Journal of Consulting and Clinical Psychiatry, 55, 3–9.*

Marcus, L. M., & Stone, N. L. (1993). Assessment of the young autistic child. In
   E. Schopler, M. E. van Bourgondien, & M. Bristol (Eds.). *Preschool issues
   in autistic and related development of handicaps* (pp. 149–173). New York:
   Plenum.
McGee, G. G., Morrier, M. J., Daly, T., & Jacobs, H. A. (2001). The Walden Early
   Childhood Programs. In J. S. Handleman & S. L. Harris (Eds.), *Preschool
   education programs for children with autism* (2nd ed., pp. 157–190). Austin,
   TX: PRO-ED.
Mesibov, G. B., Schopler, E., Schaffer, B., & Landrus, R. (1988). *Adolescent and
   Adult Psychoeducational Profile.* Austin, TX: PRO-ED.
Mesibov, G. B., Shea, V., & Schopler, E. (2005). *The TEACCH approach to autism
   spectrum disorders.* New York: Kluwer Academic/Plenum.
Mesibov, G., Thomas, J. B., Chapman, S. M., & Schopler, E. (2007). *TEACCH
   Transition Assessment Profile—Second Edition.* Austin, TX: PRO-ED.
Mullen, E. M. (1995). *Mullen Scales of Early Learning* (AGS ed.). Circle Pines,
   MN: American Guidance Service.
Prizant, B. M., Wetherby, A. M., Rubin, E., Laurent, A. C., & Rydell, P. J. (2006).
   *The SCERTS® model: A comprehensive educational approach for children
   with autism spectrum disorders.* Baltimore: Brookes.
Rogers, S. J., & Lewis, H. (1989). An effective day treatment model for young
   children with pervasive developmental disorders. *Journal of the American
   Academy of Child and Adolescent Psychiatry, 28,* 207–214.
Schopler, E., Lansing, M. D., Reichler, R. J., & Marcus, L. M. (2005). *Psychoeducational Profile—Third Edition.* Austin, TX: PRO-ED.
Schopler, E., & Reichler, R. J. (1979). *Individualized assessment and treatment for
   developmentally disabled children: Vol. 1. Psychoeducational Profile.* Baltimore, MD: University Park Press.
Schopler, E., Reichler, R. J., & Renner, B. R. (1988). *The Childhood Autism Rat-
   ing Scale (CARS).* Los Angeles: Western Psychological Services.
Sparrow, S. S., Cicchetti, D. V., & Balla, D. A. (2005). *Vineland Adaptive Behavior Scales, Second Edition (Vineland-II).* Circle Pines, MN: American Guidance Service.
Strain, P. S., & Cordisco, L. K. (1994). LEAP Preschool. In S. Harris & J. S.
   Handleman (Eds.), *Preschool education programs for children with autism*
   (pp. 225–252). Austin, TX: PRO-ED.
Tager-Flusberg, H., Paul, R., & Lord, C. (2005). Language and communication in
   autism. In F. R. Volkmar, R. Paul, A. Klin, & D. J. Cohen (Eds.), *Handbook
   of autism and pervasive developmental disorders* (3rd ed., pp. 335–364).
   Hoboken, NJ: Wiley.
Watson, L., Lord, C., Schaffer, B., & Schopler, E. (1989). *Teaching spontaneous
   communication to autistic and developmentally handicapped children.* Austin, TX: PRO-ED.

CHAPTER TWELVE

Assessment of Students with Autism Spectrum Disorders in the Schools

Sandra L. Harris

Carolyn Thorwarth Bruey

Mark J. Palmieri

Jan S. Handleman

The assessment of autism spectrum disorders (ASD) in the schools requires psychologists, behavior analysts, and other service providers not only to know the technical nuances of the specific assessment procedures, but to possess a sophisticated understanding of the ways schools operate as systems, the pressure school administrators and educators find themselves under to offer empirically supported assessment and instructional methods for their students, and the need to demonstrate accountability for educational outcomes based on these interventions. Schools are complex places in which to operate because of the multiple demands the people working in them face from their many constituents—including students, parents, teachers, taxpayers, school board members, district superintendents, state education officials, and state and national legislators. The consultant or staff member who assesses the needs of a student with an ASD for special services in the public schools needs to understand not only the needs of the child, but the educational system and community in which that child is to be served.

The current chapter introduces the reader to some of the issues faced by individuals with ASD in schools, by schools as systems, and by schools within their larger social-systemic context. We also consider the need for empirically supported assessment and intervention methods to educate students with ASD in schools. The chapter describes the psychological assessment methods currently being employed in a variety of model programs that serve learners with ASD in public, university-operated, and private settings. We offer an overview of the assessment practices in one such public school model program through the close examination of a single case. We also move beyond traditional psychological diagnostic and assessment methods to include a discussion of the use of functional assessment procedures within the schools, and suggestions for how these often-time consuming procedures might be made more time-efficient and user-friendly when adapted for application in classrooms. A case example from a recent study (Palmieri, 2007) illustrates the potential time savings that such an assessment process might provide for many of the problem behaviors arising in the classroom.

THE PUBLIC SCHOOL AS A SYSTEM

As school administrators, classroom teachers, school psychologists, and other professionals who work in schools know well, public schools have their own cultures. In order to be an effective innovator within any school, one must understand how the system of that school operates. A consultant or staff member who fails to join effectively with the teaching staff will find the process of innovation difficult if not impossible to accomplish. The failure to appreciate the nature of the leadership roles in schools and the political and interpersonal demands that play out in these settings (such as the pressures on principals and other senior managers) has scuttled more than one effort to introduce new teaching or assessment methods that seem to their innovators to offer substantial contributions to students' welfare, and that have sound empirical data to back them up. Factors such as "organizational climate" (Glisson & Hemmelgarn, 1998) have a substantial impact on how one goes about introducing change, including new assessment methods, to a school system.

Ringeisen, Henderson, and Hoagwood (2003) discuss the complexities of introducing empirically supported mental health services to children in the public schools. Although their target population, children with mental health challenges, is different from that of children on the autism spectrum, some of the same systemic issues arise in trying to serve both populations. They note that the past 20 years have seen major advances in the empirical knowledge base for identifying and serving children with mental health needs (e.g., Lonigan, Elbert, & Johnson, 1998). A parallel can be seen in the education of children with ASD, where the past several decades have witnessed major advances in our knowledge of how to assess and support the learning of these youngsters (e.g., National Research Council, 2001). In both cases, researchers have made major advances in both understanding the needs of the population and determining how to serve it effectively; however, broad-scale implementation of services in the public schools lags behind our empirical knowledge. This gap between empirically based knowledge and broadly disseminated implementation is costly to children, their families, their schools, and the wider community.

The assessment and treatment of children with ASD, like those of children with mental health needs, have shifted from specialized programs and residential settings to community-based programs, especially the public schools (Ringeisen et al., 2003). In recognition of the growing disconnection between our knowledge of empirically supported treatments for children and the practices often available in community settings, especially the public schools, several federal government reports have offered recommendations for closing this troubling gap between what researchers know and what practitioners do in treating children's mental health needs (e.g., U.S. Public Health Service, 2000) and for evaluating and educating youngsters on the autism spectrum (e.g., National Research Council, 2001). As Ringeisen et al. (2003) note, these national reports on evidence-based and/ or empirically supported practices have paid insufficient attention to the context of the schools and the influence of this environment on the delivery of services. There has been a lack of sensitivity on the part of researchers to the outcomes that are most salient for schools, including, for example, the academic achievements of students or the need for ongoing special education services. If we are to effectively introduce research-based methods for the assessment of children with ASD, we need to be attuned to the needs of the school and ensure that the methods we offer address the needs of educators, not just those of researchers.

In their reflection on the school as a system, Ringeisen et al. (2003) adopt a three-level model of how schools operate. These key factors are the individual, the organization, and the state and national levels of influence. They give examples of child factors at the individual level, including the child's achievements and peer relationships. Teacher variables such as job-related stress, extent of professional training, and relationships within the school are also individual factors. In addition to the children, their teachers, and their parents, and others (including administrators and school board members) should be considered at this level, as they all may have a role to play in supporting high-quality assessment services.

At the organizational level, there are such factors as the size of the school and the number of children with ASD who require specialized services. Ringeisen et al. (2003) highlight such organizational factors as creating a caring environment with strong cooperation among the students, teachers, and family members, and the availability of technical knowledge, resources, and emotional support for all participants. At the state and national levels, we find such variables as political issues that may underlie educational funding and standards, and the state and national legislation that influences access to services and imposes demands for educational accountability. Ringeisen et al. (2003) also discuss the need for an ongoing feedback loop in which new practices are implemented and the outcomes provide feedback for modifications that may be essential to allowing an innovative model to work in a public school setting. As they note, the sooner practitioners (including teachers, school psychologists, and principals) become part of the conversation about the development of an educational intervention or assessment method, the easier it will be to introduce that model into the schools.

An important aspect of implementing effective educational practices for children with ASD is ensuring the involvement of the school psychologists and teaching staff in the planning. These psychologists and educators know when methods are too complex for them to use without enhanced training in teaching or assessment methods. Later in this chapter, we describe one program for involving classroom teachers in doing functional assessments during the school day. The use of these assessment methods is a very good example of a situation where a well-trained teaching staff, supervised by a behavior analyst or psychologist, can be crucial to the in-depth assessment of a child's challenging behaviors.

EMPIRICALLY SUPPORTED ASSESSMENT AND INTERVENTION IN THE SCHOOLS

One of the important events of recent years has been the extended discussion of the need for empirically supported assessment and intervention methods in every sphere of psychological and educational services. There is growing understanding that the work in clinics, mental health centers, and schools requires a database to support its implementation. One offshoot of this focus on using methods that have research support is the work of the Task Force on Evidence-Based Interventions in School Psychology consisting of the Division of School Psychology of the American Psychological Association, the National Association of School Psychologists, and the Society for the Study of School Psychology (Kratochwill & Shernoff, 2003). This Task Force was established to "identify, review and code studies of psychological and educational interventions for behavioral, emotional, and academic problems and disorders for school-aged children and their families" (Kratochwill & Shernoff, 2003, pp. 389–390). One of its objectives is to ensure that school psychologists understand this approach to developing intervention and can identify and employ research-based methods in the schools where they work. Kratochwill and Shernoff (2003) note that one of the challenges the field of school psychology faces is that of moving research-based interventions from the lab to the school setting.

CLASSROOM-BASED FUNCTIONAL ANALYSIS

An excellent example of the need to translate a well-studied and effective assessment tool from a research setting to a typical classroom is found in the challenge of adapting functional analysis methods to the realities of the public schools. Assessing challenging behavior through data-based collection procedures is a necessary component of applied behavior analysis (Cooper, Heron, & Heward, 1987). Functional analysis utilizes defined environmental manipulations to reliably identify the variables that maintain challenging behavior. These procedures then inform treatment development, facilitating an empirical evaluation of a reliable relationship between the intervention and behavior change. The original research on functional analysis procedures was conducted in highly controlled treatment settings (Carr & Durand, 1985; Cooper & Harding, 1993; Iwata, Dorsey, Slifer, Bauman, & Richman, 1982/1994; Iwata, Pace, Kalsher, Cowdery, & Cataldo, 1990). Recently, research attention has shifted toward evaluating the use of functional analysis in outpatient settings with less precise and sustained control (Cooper & Harding, 1993; Cooper, Wacker, Sasso, Reimers, & Donn, 1990; Harding, Wacker, Cooper, Millard, & Jensen-Kovalan, 1994; Northup et al., 1991). This research has provided a great deal of support for brief functional analysis as a means of assessing challenging behavior (e.g., Cooper et al., 1992; Derby et al., 1992, 1994).

One potential result of the type of functional analysis done in controlled settings, where stimuli from the participant's natural environment are expected to have minimal influence on assessment conditions, is that the functional analysis may suggest a relationship that does not exist in the natural environment (Hanley, Iwata, & McCord, 2003). This phenomenon may compromise the ecological validity of functional analysis findings and thus undermine the translation of intervention from a specialized setting to a child's daily life. As indicated above, a growing body of research has demonstrated the use of functional analysis procedures in a variety of treatment settings, such as outpatient clinics, schools, and homes (Cooper & Harding, 1993; Cooper et al., 1990; Doggett, Edwards, Moore, Tingstrom, & Wilczynski, 2001; Lohrmann-O'Rourke & Yurman, 2001; Umbreit, 1995). This line of research often includes training procedures that facilitate the use of teachers as therapists in functional analysis conditions. These studies typically stress the importance of capitalizing on classroom resources through the use of indirect data collection procedures, as well as descriptive analyses and observations, to aid in the interpretation of functional analysis data.

In a study by Doggett et al. (2001), behavioral consultants assisted general education classroom teachers in conducting an entire functional assessment. The functional analysis component of the assessment was implemented during periods of general classroom instruction. Behavioral consultants trained the teachers and supervised the entire assessment procedure, ensuring that the teachers played a primary role in hypothesis development and data analysis. Similarly, in Umbreit's (1995) research, a teacher was supported in the implementation of a functional analysis that proved successful in identifying a function of a student's challenging classroom behavior. Lohrmann-O'Rourke and Yurman (2001) embedded the functional analysis conditions naturalistically into the general classroom routine. Erbas, Tekin-Iftar, and Yucesoy (2006) evaluated a structured protocol for training teachers in functional analysis procedures. This research indicated that teachers could successfully acquire the target skills necessary for developing and implementing functional analyses. The study also found that teachers' impressions of the social validity of functional analysis procedures were largely positive after formalized training.

We have been extending this line of research at the Douglass Developmental Disabilities Center (DDDC; Palmieri, 2007). Analogue functional analysis procedures are extremely useful for assessing forms of challenging behavior. However, they are generally too time-consuming and resource-intensive to be readily integrated into school settings. As a result, these procedures are largely inaccessible to many professionals who are attempting to assess and treat maladaptive behavior. In addition, these procedures have rarely been used with teachers; for example, Hanley et al. (2003) note that only 3% of 575 studies used teachers as therapists. A brief assessment can be considered valid when it closely replicates the findings of extended assessment procedures (Derby et al., 1992). The study by Palmieri (2007) assessed a classroom functional analysis procedure that was based upon the initial conditions described by Iwata et al. (1982/1994).

Five students enrolled at the DDDC participated in this study. They were identified for functional analyses through referrals to the DDDC's behavioral consultation unit. Analogue functional analyses were run in a private assessment room equipped with a work table and four chairs. The classroom functional analyses were implemented in each student's natural classroom environment. The order of the two functional analysis procedures was alternated for each participant.

In each case, a teacher interview, a descriptive assessment, preference assessments, an analogue functional analysis, and a classroom functional analysis were conducted. The student-specific information needed for the development of the descriptive data collection sheets and each functional analysis was obtained through semistructured interviews with each participant's teachers, using the Teacher Interview/Condition Development Form (TI/CDF). The descriptive assessment consisted of antecedent–behavior–consequence (ABC) data collection. Case-specific ABC data sheets were developed. Data were analyzed for function (attention, escape, tangible, automatic reinforcement), based upon the recorded antecedents and consequences. Immediately preceding each set of functional analysis sessions, a multiple-stimulus-without-replacement (MSWO) preference assessment was conducted to identity currently preferred tangible items. The format for the preference assessment followed that outlined by DeLeon and Iwata (1996). The analogue functional analysis was based upon the conditions (toy play, alone, social attention, and demand) described by Iwata et al. (1982/1994). Conditions lasted 10 minutes, with behavior analysts serving as therapists.

Each classroom analysis was conducted with the teacher serving as therapist. The model used 5-minute sessions and implemented the following conditions: toy play (control), social attention, demand, and tangible. Condition parameters were modified from those used in Iwata et al. (1982/1994) for use within the natural classroom environment.

Prior to the analysis, the teacher received brief training from a graduate-level behavior analyst. In addition to verbal information, the teacher was given a brief written description of the condition protocols and was provided with visual prompts that outlined crucial condition components. All information presented in the classroom functional analysis condition descriptions was specifically reviewed with the teacher, allowing him or her time to ask questions and receive clarifications using case examples. Each teacher was equipped with an earpiece that enabled the behavior analyst to communicate from outside the classroom throughout the assessment. Through the earpiece, the teacher was given prompts for establishing the contingencies for each session and for providing reinforcement when necessary.

After all analyses were completed, the functional analyses for each case were evaluated by two highly experienced raters for agreement on indicated function. Similarly, the functional analyses were also compared for function correspondence with the ABC data.

Case Example: Gary

Gary was referred for assessment due to screaming and hand pressing (forcefully pressing one hand to his face in the region just below the nose). He was a 13-year-old boy diagnosed with autistic disorder who had been a student at the DDDC for several years. Gary used a digital augmented communication system and was able to participate in most classroom and community activities. The teacher interview revealed that Gary's screaming and hand pressing had been present to varying degrees over several years. Recently, however, these behaviors had begun to substantially impair his ability to participate successfully in instruction or social activities. The TI/CDF indicated that the target topographies of the behaviors often occurred together, across a variety of times and locations, and were most common during nonpreferred work periods and when Gary was restricted from watching or fast-forwarding and rewinding highly preferred videos. His teacher reported that the challenging behaviors were least likely when he was allowed free access to highly preferred foods, videos, and the VCR control.

ABC data were collected on Gary during four sessions distributed across a variety of times, days, and DDDC settings. Descriptive data analysis indicated work demands and restricted access to preferred items as the stimuli most likely to precede Gary's target behaviors. Analysis of consequence events identified increased access to preferred items and extinction as the most likely environmental responses. The ABC data also suggested a variable schedule of escape from demands following screaming or hand-pressing. Evaluations of the data by raters unaware of the hypotheses being examined indicated escape and restricted access as potential maintaining variables for Gary's screaming and hand pressing.

MSWO preference assessments conducted before each functional analysis session consistently indicated items such as *Thomas the Tank Engine* and *Barney* videos, popcorn, and chips as Gary's most highly preferred tangibles. Treatment fidelity checks verified implementation integrity at 100% for all components of the analysis. Interrater reliability averaged 92% on screaming and 96% on handpressing. Gary's analogue functional analysis consisted of 20 conditions of a standard functional analysis, followed by 10 conditions of pairwise comparisons between the tangible and toy play and demand and toy play conditions. In total, the analysis required 250 minutes of testing. Evaluation by unaware raters indicated that Gary's screaming and hand pressing were maintained by negative reinforcement in the form of escape from demands and positive reinforcement in the form of access to preferred items.

During the standard analysis, average responses per minute across conditions were as follows: toy play (0.20), attention (0.39), demand (1.16), tangible (1.45), and ignore (3.08). One outlier point during the first ignore session accounted for the elevated rate during that condition. The pairwise comparisons of the tangible and toy play conditions rendered rates of 1.06 and 0.20, respectively, and comparisons between demand and toy play conditions yielded rates of 1.79 and 0.87.

Gary's classroom functional analysis consisted of 24 standard conditions and required 120 minutes of testing. During the classroom analysis, the average responses per minute across conditions were as follows: toy play (0.77), attention (0.56), demand (0.67), and tangible (1.46). Evaluations of the data by unaware raters again indicated that Gary's screaming and hand pressing were maintained by negative reinforcement in the form of escape from demands and positive reinforcement in the form of access to preferred items.

Function correspondence analyses evaluated Rater 1's and Rater 2's scorings to assess agreement among the ABC assessment, classroom analysis, and analogue analysis. In combined format, full agreement was scored among all three assessment procedures, with positive reinforcement in the form of access to preferred items and negative reinforcement in the form of escape from demands identified as the likely maintaining variables for Gary's screaming and hand pressing. Gary's performance across all conditions is summarized in Figures 12.1 and 12.2.

The data collected from Palmieri's (2007) study provide information on a series of components relevant to supporting the use of classroom-based functional analysis. The correspondence among the raters' evaluations of

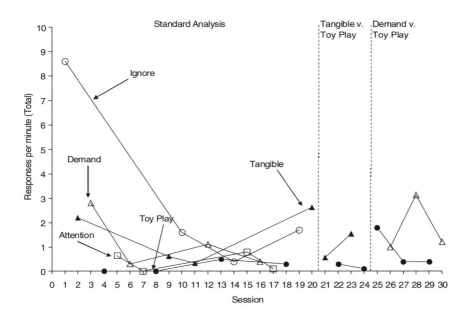

FIGURE 12.1. Gary's analogue functional assessment. From Palmieri (2007). Copyright 2007 by Mark J. Palmieri. Reprinted by permission.

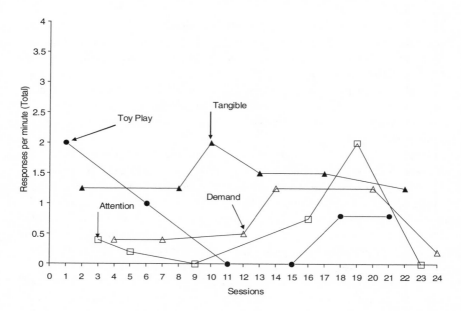

FIGURE 12.2. Gary's classroom functional assessment. From Palmieri (2007). Copyright 2007 by Mark J. Palmieri. Reprinted by permission.

the functional analysis data indicated that across all the cases in this study, 93% yielded full or partial agreement scores between the classroom and analogue functional analyses. This correspondence level strongly supports classroom analysis as a viable behavior assessment strategy. Table 12.1 summarizes the interrater agreement for each participant across each condition.

In addition, the classroom model typically required far less time than the analogue model. On average, the classroom analyses took 135 minutes of testing time, whereas the analogue analyses required 314 minutes. This difference resulted in an average time saving of 54% (range = 40–74%) when the classroom analysis was used. The ability of trained teachers and school-based behavior support staff to serve as therapists during a classroom functional analysis is critical to this procedure's feasibility for being incorporated in school settings (Doggett et al., 2001; Lohrmann-O'Rourke & Yurman, 2001; Umbreit, 1995). Training in Palmieri's (2007) study required less than 15 minutes and was done immediately before the start of the functional analysis sessions. The training components were efficient; they provided a general outline and goals of the functional analysis, and then gave specific instructions for implementing each session. Brief role plays with the teacher and consultant gave a sample of how the conditions

TABLE 12.1. Agreement on Function between Raters

Student	Analysis comparison					
	CFA	AFA	ABC	CFA	ABC	AFA
Gary	*Full agreement* • Escape • Access to preferred items	• Escape • Access to preferred items	*Full agreement* • Escape • Access to preferred items	• Escape • Access to preferred items	*Full agreement* • Escape • Access to preferred items	• Escape • Access to preferred items
Stephon	*Partial agreement* • Escape • Access to preferred items	• Escape	*Full agreement* • Escape • Access to preferred items	• Escape • Access to preferred items	*Partial agreement* • Escape • Access to preferred items	• Escape
Andre	*Partial agreement* • Attention • Access to preferred items • Automatic reinforcement	• Automatic reinforcement • Attention	*Partial agreement* • Escape • Access to preferred items, Attention	• Attention • Access to preferred items • Automatic reinforcement	*Partial agreement* • Escape • Access to preferred items • Attention	• Automatic reinforcement • Attention
Benjamin	*Partial agreement* • Automatic reinforcement • Attention • Access to preferred items	• Automatic reinforcement	*Partial agreement* • Attention • Escape	• Automatic reinforcement • Attention • Access to preferred items	*No agreement* • Attention • Escape	• Automatic reinforcement
Matthew	*Full agreement* • Access to preferred items • Escape	• Access to preferred items • Escape	*No agreement* • Automatic reinforcement • Attention	• Access to preferred items • Escape	*No agreement* • Automatic reinforcement • Attention	• Access to preferred items • Escape

Note. CFA, classroom functional analysis; AFA, analogue functional analysis; ABC, antecedent–behavior–consequence analysis.

349

would run. The two-way communication system allowed the teacher and trainer to communicate discreetly during the analysis while the consultant stayed in a separate room behind a one-way mirror. The treatment fidelity checks indicated that after training, every teacher was able to implement the critical condition components with 100% integrity. This training procedure was consistent across staff members and was applied to teachers and teaching assistants with varying level of experience. In addition, the teachers indicated that they felt engaged, highly interested in the process, and very motivated to participate in the development and implementation of the behavior support plans.

Both the interview and descriptive assessment procedures provided meaningful support for conducting comprehensive, individualized functional analyses. The importance of incorporating descriptive assessment procedures into functional analyses has been stressed repeatedly (Aikman, Garbutt, & Furniss, 2003; Cooper & Harding, 1993; Cooper et al., 1992; Doggett et al., 2001; Steege et al., 2007; Tiger, Hanley & Bessette, 2006; Umbreit, 1995). Data from the indirect and descriptive assessments facilitated developing clear definitions for the topographies of challenging behavior, as well as identifying likely antecedent and consequence events, relevant individual-specific environmental manipulations, important natural environmental relationships (e.g., divided adult attention with a particular peer), and behavior topographies that tended to covary.

School settings are often the first locations where assessments of aberrant behavior are conducted. Brief, naturalistic, and accessible functional analysis procedures may encourage function-driven analyses and treatments to be incorporated more successfully into clients' natural environments. Analysis methods that can be completed quickly, while maintaining procedural integrity and validity, are the most likely to be adopted into educational settings (Derby et al., 1992). The Palmieri (2007) study identified components of a successful classroom analysis model. Research in this area will continue to support the development of sound, efficient, and naturalistic assessments necessary for equalizing the integrity of service delivery between highly controlled clinical settings and the natural environments where most clients receive support.

CURRENT DIAGNOSTIC ASSESSMENT PRACTICES IN MODEL SCHOOLS

In addition to adopting empirically supported behavioral assessment methods in the classroom, schools need to be able to use state-of-the-art tools for doing traditional psychological assessments. Doing assessments of children who are being considered for classification for special services is an important role for many school psychologists. There are a number of diagnostic tools available for this purpose when one wishes to determine whether a child has an ASD. Recently we asked the senior administrators of 11 educational programs for young children with ASD to describe the assessment tools they used in making a decision about admitting a child to their program (Handleman & Harris, 2008). These public, private, and university-based programs included the Alpine Learning Center in Paramus, New Jersey; the Autism Center at the University of Washington in Seattle (formerly the University of Colorado Affiliated Program for Developmental Disabilities); Ascent in Deer Park, New York; Comprehensive Application of Behavior Analysis for Schooling (CABAS) at Columbia University, New York, New York; the Children's Units at the State University of New York at Binghamton; the DDDC at Rutgers, The State University of New Jersey, New Brunswick, New Jersey; Groden Center in Providence, Rhode Island; Learning Experiences: An Alternative Program for Preschoolers and Parents (LEAP) at the University of Colorado in Denver; Summit Academy in Getzville, New York; the Pyramid Model at the Cape Henlopen School District in Sussex County, Delaware; and the Valley Program in Bergen County, New Jersey.

Most of the programs rely on the school district sending each child to provide diagnostic information, and two of them did no additional psychological assessment beyond those data. The other nine programs reaffirmed the diagnostic status of each child prior to admission. Among the most frequently used diagnostic tools were the Autism Diagnostic Observation Schedule (Lord, Rutter, DiLavore, & Risi, 1999), which was employed in five programs, and the *Autism Diagnostic Interview—Revised* (Lord, Rutter, & LeCouteur, 1994), used by four programs. Five of the programs used the Childhood Autism Rating Scale (CARS; Schopler, Reichler, & Renner, 1988) as part of their admissions process, and six programs reported that they relied on Diagnostic and Statistical Manual of Mental Disorders, fourth edition, text revision (DSM-IV-TR) criteria (American Psychiatric Association, 2000). Most of the programs used more than one of these diagnostic tools.

For cognitive assessment, two programs used a version of the Stanford–Binet (Roid, 2003; Thorndike, Hagen, & Sattler, 1986); two used a Wechsler test (Wechsler, 1991); and the Mullen Scales of Early Learning (Mullen, 1995) and McCarthy Scales of Children's Abilities (McCarthy, 1972) were each reported by one program. In looking at developmental skills, four of the model programs used the original Vineland Adaptive Behavior Scales (Sparrow, Balla, & Cicchetti, 1984), and one used the Learning Accomplishment Profile (LeMay, Griffen, & Sanford, 1977). Two programs said they used the Preschool Language Scale, Fourth Edition (Zimmerman, Steiner, & Pond, 2002) to assess speech and language.

Case Example: Isaac

Isaac was a 5-year-old boy suspected of having an ASD diagnosis, whose parents were moving into Pennsylvania from another state. The Commonwealth of Pennsylvania uses a system in which geographically defined, government-funded special education agencies (called "intermediate units" or "IUs") provide special education support to school districts if the districts determine that they do not have the resources to provide education for a given student. In Isaac's case, he was moving into a district that did not have its own autistic support classes, and therefore there was a strong possibility that the district would contract with the IU to provide his educational programming within an IU-run autistic support class. Therefore, as part of his transition process, the school district requested that the IU conduct an evaluation of Isaac's current educational needs.

As a first step, the IU school psychologist did a comprehensive review of Isaac's past records (e.g., previous evaluation reports, individualized education program [IEP] assessments by outside professionals, etc.). The IU school psychologist then interviewed Isaac's former out-of-state preschool teacher over the phone. Usually, once information of this kind has been gathered, the IU school psychologist observes the new student in the family's home to gain an initial impression of the student's potential to respond to a testing situation; the psychologist also interviews the parents, to fill in the gaps in the information already gathered from the youngster's formal records, and to learn about the parents' own expectations for their child. However, because Isaac's parents were moving to the area during the summer and the school psychologist would be on vacation, this information was gathered over the phone near the end of the school year. Although this was not an optimal format, the information obtained via phone was useful in deciding which evaluative tools and strategies would be most successful in obtaining a valid assessment of Isaac's abilities.

The record review and phone interviews revealed that Isaac had been attending a special education preschool class for children with "developmental delays"; however, much of the information suggested that he might have an ASD. Since the question of diagnosis was unclear, it was decided that the IU's evaluation should include a diagnostic component. The records also described Isaac as a child with some speech, although he tended to speak in abbreviated sentences that were often laced with jargon. Furthermore, he was described as an easily distracted child who found it difficult to stay on task for longer than a few minutes. He would, however, spend long periods of time playing with toy trains, and he could name all of the *Thomas the Tank Engine* characters. Isaac generally did not respond to social interactions or praise, but he did enjoy gross motor play and tickling. He was reported to have age-appropriate fine and gross motor skills, so there was no need for a physical therapist or occupational therapist to be part of the evaluative team. Because of his speech and language delays, it was decided that the IU's speech–language therapist would conduct her own assessment, which would be incorporated into the subsequent evaluation report.

When Isaac's case was examined systemically, various issues become apparent. On an individual level, Isaac's skills and behavioral presentation would have a significant influence on his ability to respond to testing, as well as on decisions about eventual classroom placement. Another aspect to consider was that he was moving into a school district with a special education administrator who was very open to the IU's input (unfortunately, this is not always the case). This positive relationship would help make the evaluative process run smoothly. It was also noted that Isaac's parents were highly educated and knowledgeable regarding his needs, as well as about special education law—factors that needed to be respected in working with them. Of special significance was the fact that his parents were adamant that Isaac had the right to attend a classroom in his own neighborhood.

On an organizational level, the IU psychologist had to remember that the school district was ultimately in charge of Isaac's educational programming, even though the IU staff would be conducting the actual assessment. This relationship was not immediately obvious and needed to be clarified for his parents. Another organizational issue to consider was that there was only one IU primary elementary classroom for students with ASD in Isaac's school district, and there were insufficient students on the autism spectrum to warrant funding another. The IU's autistic support classrooms are stratified according to functioning level, and because his parents were adamant that Isaac attend a class in his home district, there was a potential issue if his skills did not match those of the students in the one available classroom.

On a federal/state level, it was important to help Isaac's parents understand the difference between services provided to preschoolers and those available for school-age students, because Isaac was leaving the preschool system and entering school-age education. For example, although social service agencies are responsible for providing therapies and educational support for preschoolers with developmental delays, once a child reaches school age, the home school district is responsible for his or her educational needs. Also, although the emphasis for preschool support services is on addressing the entire family's needs, the focus narrows to the child's educational needs once the child is in public school. This loss of family support can be disheartening to parents, so it was important for the social worker to provide Isaac's parents with the names of local social service agencies that could continue to address their needs outside the realm of education.

Isaac was assessed in mid-August, after the IU staff members returned from their summer vacations. The school psychologist and speech–language therapist each completed an independent evaluation. The school psychologist used various tools during her assessment, including the fourth edition of the Stanford–Binet (Thorndike et al., 1986) and the second edition of the AAMR Adaptive Behavior Scales—School (Lambert, Nihiri, & Leland, 1993). She had extensive experience in using the DSM-IV-TR diagnostic criteria (American Psychiatric Association, 2000), and used these criteria along with the CARS (Schopler et al., 1988) to make a diagnostic assessment. Achievement tests were not used, because the preschool staff members had done this assessment just before Isaac left their system.

During testing, the school psychologist made numerous adaptations to the prescribed protocol in order to obtain a meaningful understanding of Isaac's abilities. For example, because Isaac was able to stay on task for a maximum of 30 minutes, the assessment involved four shorter testing sessions rather than an attempt to complete the testing in one sitting. Also, edible reinforcers, tickles, and access to train toys were provided contingent upon Isaac's staying on task, but not upon the accuracy of his responding. Testing took place in the speech room, where there were minimal distractions. To decrease Isaac's frustration, visual cues were provided regarding how much time was left for each task before he received a break. The test's prescribed wording for giving instructions was simplified occasionally, in order to assure comprehension. Time limits were extended as needed, to guarantee that Isaac's true skills were reflected. All testing took place in the morning, since it was reported that Isaac was best able to stay on task during this time period. Each of these modifications to standardized testing protocol was noted in Isaac's evaluation report.

Once the school psychologist's evaluation was completed, the results were combined with the speech–language pathologist's test data and incorporated into Isaac's evaluation report. A meeting was held including the parents, school district staff, and the IU evaluators to review the testing results and discuss Isaac's educational needs. The team agreed that Isaac's behavioral profile, developmental history and diagnostic assessment by the school psychologist warranted a DSM-IV-TR diagnosis of autistic disorder (American Psychiatric Association, 2000). Subsequently, a new IEP was developed with everyone's input. It became apparent that Isaac was notably less adept at many activities than were the students in the only IU autistic support elementary classroom in his home school district, and therefore the district and IU staff agreed that placement in a more intensive IU autistic support classroom located in a neighboring school district would be the best setting for him. Because of their belief that Isaac had the right to be educated in his home district, the parents were initially hesitant. However, after they observed the proposed class, they recognized that the benefits of the specialized autistic support classroom outweighed the advantages of his attending a class in his home school district. Isaac began attending his new classroom the following week.

CHAPTER SUMMARY

In many school settings, there is a troubling disconnection between effective research on demonstrated methods for the assessment and treatment of students with ASD and actual school-based practice. The responsibility for solving the problem of information transfer resides both with the investigators who develop and attempt to disseminate these innovative tools, and with the educational personnel whose students could benefit from their application. These are problems best solved by improved two-way communication that begins early in the process of developing the new methods and continues through the successful introduction of the methods in the schools. Accomplishing that goal requires not only good-faith effort on the part of the key players—including researchers, teachers, school psychologists, and principals—but support from school board members, government officials, and others who are in a position to set meaningful and realistic goals for the schools.

REFERENCES

American Psychiatric Association. (2000). *Diagnostic and statistical manual of mental disorders* (4th ed., text rev.). Washington, DC: Author.

Aikman, G., Garbutt, V., & Furniss, F. (2003). Brief probes: A method for analyzing the function of disruptive behaviour in the natural environment. *Behavioural and Cognitive Psychotherapy, 31,* 215–220.

Carr, E. G., & Durand, M. V. (1985). Reducing behavior problems through functional communication training. *Journal of Applied Behavior Analysis, 18,* 111–126.

Cooper, J. O., Heron, T. E., & Heward, W. L. (1987). *Applied behavior analysis.* Columbus, OH: Merrill.

Cooper, L. J., & Harding, J. (1993). Extending functional analysis procedures to outpatient and classroom settings for children with mild disabilities. In J. Reichle & D. P. Wacker (Eds.), *Communicative alternatives to challenging behavior: Integrating functional assessment and intervention strategies* (pp. 41–62). Baltimore: Brookes.

Cooper, L. J., Wacker, D. P., Sasso, G., M., Reimers, T. M., & Donn, L. K. (1990). Using parents as therapists to evaluate appropriate behavior of their children: Application to a tertiary diagnostic clinic. *Journal of Applied Behavior Analysis, 23,* 285–296.

Cooper, L. J., Wacker, D. P., Thursby, D., Plagmann, L. A., Harding, J., Millard, T., et al. (1992). Analysis of the effects of task preferences, task demands, and adult attention on child behavior in outpatient and classroom settings. *Journal of Applied Behavior Analysis, 25,* 823–840.

Derby, K. M., Wacker, D. P., Peck, S., Sasso, G., DeRaad, A., Berg, W., et al. (1994). Functional analysis of separate topographies of aberrant behavior. *Journal of Applied Behavior Analysis, 27,* 267–278.

Derby, K. M., Wacker, D. P., Sasso, G., Steege, M., Northup, J., Cigrand, K., et al. (1992). Brief functional assessment techniques to evaluate aberrant behavior in an outpatient setting: A summary of 79 cases. *Journal of Applied Behavior Analysis, 25,* 713–721.

DeLeon, I. G., & Iwata, B. A. (1996). Evaluation of a multiple-stimulus presentation format for assessing reinforcer preferences. *Journal of Applied Behavior Analysis, 29,* 519–533.

Doggett, R. A., Edwards, R. P., Moore, J. W., Tingstrom, D. H., & Wilczynski, S. M. (2001). An approach to functional assessment in general education classroom settings. *School Psychology Review, 30,* 313–328.

Erbas, D., Tekin-Iftar, E., & Yucesoy, S. (2006). Teaching special education teachers how to conduct functional analysis in natural settings. *Education and Training in Developmental Disabilities, 41,* 28–36.

Glisson, C., & Hemmelgarn, A. (1998). The effects of organizational climate and interorganizational coordination on the quality and outcome of children's service systems. *Child Abuse and Neglect, 22,* 401–442.

Handleman, J. S., & Harris, S. (Eds.). (2008). *Preschool education programs for children with autism* (3rd ed.). Austin, TX: PRO-ED.

Hanley, G. P., Iwata, B. A., & McCord, B. E. (2003). Functional analysis of problem behavior: A review. *Journal of Applied Behavior Analysis, 36,* 147–185.

Harding, J., Wacker, D. P., Cooper, L. J., Millard, T., & Jensen-Kovalan, P. (1994). Brief hierarchical assessment of potential treatment components with children in an outpatient clinic. *Journal of Applied Behavior Analysis, 27,* 291–300.

Iwata, B. A., Dorsey, M. F., Slifer, K. J., Bauman, K. E., & Richman, G. S. (1994). Toward a functional analysis of self-injury. *Journal of Applied Behavior Analysis, 27,* 197–209. (Original work published 1982)

Iwata, B. A., Pace, G. M., Kalsher, M. J., Cowdery, G. E., & Cataldo, M. F. (1990). Experimental analysis and extinction of self-injurious escape behavior. *Journal of Applied Behavior Analysis, 23,* 11–27.

Kratochwill, T. R., & Shernoff, E. S. (2003). Evidence-based practice: Promoting evidence-based interventions in school psychology. *School Psychology Quarterly, 18,* 389–408.

Lambert, N., Nihiri, K., & Leland, H. (1993). *AAMR Adaptive Behavior Scales— School: Second Edition.* Austin, TX: PRO-ED.

LeMay, D., Griffen, P., & Sanford, A. (1977). *Learning Accomplishment Profile.* Chapel Hill, NC: Chapel Hill Training–Outreach Project.

Lohrmann-O'Rourke, S., & Yurman, B. (2001). Naturalistic assessment of and intervention for mouthing behaviors influenced by establishing operations. *Journal of Positive Behavior Interventions, 3,* 19–27.

Lonigan, C. J., Elbert, J. C., & Johnson, S. B. (1998). Empirically supported psychosocial interventions for children: An overview. *Journal of Clinical Child Psychology, 27,* 138–145.

Lord, C., Rutter, M., DiLavore, P. C., & Risi, S. (1999). *Autism Diagnostic Observation Schedule—WPS edition (ADOS-WPS).* Los Angeles: Western Psychological Services.

Lord, C., Rutter, M., & LeCouteur, A. (1994). Autism Diagnostic Interview— Revised: A revised version of a diagnostic interview for caregivers of individuals with possible developmental disorders. *Journal of Autism and Developmental Disorders, 24,* 659–685.

McCarthy, D. (1972). *Manual for the McCarthy Scales of Children's Abilities.* New York: Psychological Corporation.

Mullen, E. M. (1995). *Mullen Scales of Early Learning.* Minneapolis, MN: NCS Pearson.

National Research Council. (2001). *Educating children with autism.* Washington, DC: National Academy Press.

Northup, J., Wacker, D., Sasso, G., Steege, M., Cigrand, K., Cook, J., et al. (1991). A brief functional analysis of aggressive and alternative behavior in an outpatient clinic setting. *Journal of Applied Behavior Analysis, 24,* 509–522.

Palmieri, M. J. (2007) *Classroom based functional analysis: A model for assessing challenging behavior within the classroom environment.* Unpublished doctoral dissertation, Rutgers, The State University of New Jersey.

Ringeisen, H., Henderson, K., & Hoagwood, K. (2003). Context matters: Schools and the "research to practice gap" on children's mental health. *School Psychology Review, 32,* 153–168.

Roid, G. (2003). *The Stanford–Binet Intelligence Scales, Fifth Edition.* Itasca, IL: Riverside.

Schopler, E., Reichler, R. J., & Renner, B.R. (1988). *The Childhood Autism Rating Scale.* Los Angeles: Western Psychological Services.

Sparrow, S. S., Balla, D. A., & Cicchetti, D. V. (1984). *Vineland Adaptive Behavior Scales: Interview Edition Survey Form manual.* Circle Pines, MN: American Guidance Service.

Thorndike, R. L., Hagen, E. R., & Sattler, J. M. (1986). *The Stanford-Binet Intelligence Scale: Fourth Edition.* Chicago: Riverside.

Tiger, J, H., Hanley, G. P., & Bessette, K. K. (2006). Incorporating descriptive assessment results into the design of a functional analysis: A case example involving a preschooler's hand mouthing. *Education and Treatment of Children, 29,* 107–124.

Umbreit, J. (1995). Functional assessment and intervention in a regular classroom setting for the disruptive behavior of a student with attention deficit hyperactivity disorder. *Behavioral Disorders, 20,* 267–278.

U.S. Public Health Service. (2000). *Report of the Surgeon General's Conference on Children's Mental Health: A national action agenda.* Washington, DC: U.S. Department of Health and Human Services.

Wechsler, D. (1991). *Wechsler Intelligence Scales for Children—Third Edition.* San Antonio, TX: Psychological Corporation.

Zimmerman, I. L., Steiner, V. G., & Pond, R. E. (2002). *Preschool Language Scale, Fourth Edition.* San Antonio, TX: Psychological Corporation.

CHAPTER THIRTEEN

Alternative Methods, Challenging Issues, and Best Practices in the Assessment of Autism Spectrum Disorders

Sam Goldstein
Sally Ozonoff
Anne Cook
Elaine Clark

The assessment of any complex human condition affected by biopsychosocial factors is challenging even in the best of circumstances. In this chapter, we first briefly review alternative methods for the assessment of autism spectrum disorders (ASD). It is our intent to leave the reader with a broad appreciation of promising assessment approaches in the field of ASD. We then address a number of overarching issues that time and time again confront clinicians in their efforts to assess and diagnose ASD validly and reliably. We begin with a discussion of the risks for under- and overdiagnosis. We then consider the range of assessment options, from a minimal acceptable evaluation to comprehensive batteries and the evaluation of comorbid developmental, behavioral, and medical conditions. Other issues related to assessment—including child compliance, integration of data from different sources, discussing assessment results with caregivers, and emerging ideas about the relationship between symptom severity and daily functional impairment—are also discussed.

ALTERNATIVE METHODS FOR ASSESSING IMPAIRMENTS ASSOCIATED WITH ASD

Many of the methods described in this text have received a lot of attention in the literature. A number of other approaches, however, are promising but have not received as much empirical support with individuals who have ASD. Briefly, some of these approaches include virtual environments, eye-tracking technology, and imaging. What these methods have in common is that they focus not just on individual performance, but on the processes that underlie performance; they represent a shift from explicit assessments to more implicit measurements designed to assess processing differences (Klin, Jones, Schultz, Volkmar, & Cohen, 2002a). Many of these methods require less interaction between the examinee and examiner, and also make use of computer technology, with which many individuals with ASD seem more comfortable than human interaction. This is not to negate the importance of commonly used clinical tools. In fact, the ideal situation would be to use both explicit (e.g., checklists and direct testing and observation) and implicit measures to understand not only differences in performances, but the processes that underlie any differences. Using both types of methods should enable practitioners and researchers alike to develop more effective interventions that address critical social, behavioral, cognitive, and language problems found among individuals with ASD.

Social and Behavioral Assessments

Most methods of assessing social and behavioral functioning involve interviews or observations of individuals as they participate in tasks set up by an examiner. Many of these tasks require some degree of social interaction with the examiner in a laboratory or clinical environment that may (or, more likely, may not) be familiar to the individuals being tested. An unfamiliar assessment setting may exacerbate already existing anxiety and social impairment among individuals with ASD, to the point that it makes them appear even more impaired than they are. Virtual reality displays, however, can immerse an individual in realistic and even familiar assessment environments that are representative of real-world demands, and that may also elicit functional responses, while controlling for variables (e.g., auditory, visual, olfactory, and tactile factors) that could be distracting in clinical testing situations (Trepagnier, 1999). This is thought to result in a more typical behavior display, and thus more valid clinical assessment data (Klin et al., 2002a; Rizzo et al., 2000).

Within the last decade, researchers have attempted to examine individuals' difficulties in social interactions by using assessments that involve processing of facial stimuli. Eye-tracking studies have demonstrated that individuals with ASD process faces differently from typically developing individuals, and that this is correlated with clinical measures of social impairment (e.g., Klin, Jones, Schultz, Volkmar, & Cohen, 2002b; Speer, Cook, Clark, & McMahon, 2007). Improvement of remote eye-tracking technology also allows for the extension of this methodology to very young children and lower-functioning individuals with ASD. An important issue to note, however, is that most studies of face processing have used artificial stimuli, such as "head shots" or movie clips. In these studies, participants are required to give little or no response. Making the assumption that "people with autism interact very 'naturally' with computer technology" (Werry, Dautenhaun, Ogden, & Harwin, 2001, p. 58), several researchers have investigated how socially intelligent agents, such as robots or avatars embedded in virtual environments, can act to diminish and/or mediate the negative impacts of having human examiners conduct testing (Parsons et al., 2000). For example, in virtual environments, individuals can interact with one or more virtual characters in social situations that may feel more realistic and comfortable to these individuals than typical testing scenarios may. Eye movements can be recorded during these interactions. Thus virtual environments may provide more realistic contexts for assessing how individuals with ASD view information in social situations.

Recent technological advances have allowed eye-tracking technology to be combined with neuroimaging methods (e.g., functional magnetic resonance imaging, magnetoencephalography, event-related potentials, etc.), as well as with psychophysiological measures such as heart rate, electrodermal activity, and pupillometry. These implicit measurement techniques can be mapped onto individuals' explicit responses to stimuli in virtual environments. This combination of measures may provide more reliable and more ecologically valid assessments of how individuals with ASD respond in social interactions (see, e.g., Mendozzi, Motta, Barbieri, Alpini, & Pugnetti, 1998; Schilbach et al., 2005). Mapping individuals' explicit responses onto implicit responses may also provide insights into the specific structural or neural differences that underlie ASD-related impairments. Trepagnier (1999) has argued that understanding the variables that underlie differences in how individuals explicitly respond to social stimuli may enable researchers and clinicians to target their interventions more effectively, because they can focus on specific underlying processes, not just overt behaviors.

Language and Cognitive Assessments

Recently researchers have emphasized the importance of assessing both receptive and expressive language abilities, since the language impairments associated with ASD tend to be heterogeneous (e.g., Tager-Flusberg,

2004). Research paradigms used in cognitive psychology provide one possible "implicit" method (Klin et al., 2002a) of assessing receptive language abilities, at least in high-functioning individuals with basic reading skills. Researchers can develop short texts that focus on common areas of language impairment (e.g., pronoun usage, pragmatics, and use of contextual information), and can track individuals' eye movements as they read those texts (cf. Karatekin, 2007). By examining individuals' reading times and patterns of eye fixations for regions of text that reflect problematic aspects of language, evaluators can assess the degree of receptive language processing difficulty these individuals experience, without ever requiring an explicit response (for a review of the use of eye-tracking technology in reading, see Rayner, 1998).

In order to gain a better understanding of the development of language and cognitive impairments in individuals with ASD, Gernsbacher, Geye, and Weismer (2005) have called for more prospective, large-sample, longitudinal studies of children with ASD (see also Nordin & Gillberg, 1998; Tager-Flusberg, 2004). It is often difficult to determine which comes first in ASD, the language impairment or the social impairment. Tracking children longitudinally, in large samples, should make it easier to understand whether or not ASD-related language deficits are related to social impairments and/or to cognitive impairments (Gernsbacher et al., 2005; Joseph & Tager-Flusberg, 2004).

In conclusion, while alternative methods such as these need to be investigated further, there does appear to be a strong need for more approaches that are less explicit and require less social interaction—that is, approaches that are more implicit in nature. We hope that such methods will provide more ecologically valid assessments, and offer greater promise for gaining insights into the underlying processing differences in individuals with and without ASD. Of course, several important questions still need to be addressed before these methods are applied in clinical assessments of individuals suspected of having, or already known to have, ASD. This includes questions about how well these implicit assessment methods generalize to typical "real-world" problems of ASD—in particular, those associated with social relating (Rizzo, Wiederhold, & Buckwalter, 1998; Rizzo et al., 2000).

OVER- AND UNDERDIAGNOSIS

Both over- and underdiagnosis of ASD are significant problems and create assessment challenges. The incidence of ASD in children, based on age of diagnosis, has risen annually. As discussed in Chapter 2 by Lorna Wing and David Potter, there are many possible reasons for these increases.

Changes in diagnostic criteria and in the general public's awareness of ASD are likely to be powerful forces in explaining the increased incidence. As with other developmental conditions that have become increasingly discussed in the popular media, such as attention-deficit/hyperactivity disorder (ADHD), the risk for overdiagnosis of autism and other ASD is very real. Results of the field trials for the *Diagnostic and Statistical Manual of Mental Disorders,* third edition, revised (DSM-III-R) indicated that the definition of autism was too broad and tended to overdiagnose it, particularly in individuals with mental retardation (Croen & Grether, 2003). The DSM-IV-TR definition of autistic disorder (American Psychiatric Association, 2000)—consisting of 12 criteria equally divided among three clusters of symptoms (social interaction, communication/play/imagination, and limited patterns of interest in behavior) and an age-of-onset criterion—appears to have reduced but not eliminated the risk of overdiagnosis of children, particularly those with developmental delays and pragmatic language disorders.

One possible scenario begins with parents observing a behavior such as toe walking or delayed language in their child—behaviors that they have learned through the mass media are associated with ASD. They bring their child to the pediatrician. The physician's knowledge of the condition probably varies greatly, depending on his or her personal interest and experience. A referral may then be made to a community professional, perhaps someone who in his or her daily work doesn't regularly evaluate autism or other ASD. A checklist or screening tool completed by parents and scored by the evaluator may then be used as the sole basis for identifying the child's condition. However, as Jack Naglieri comments in Chapter 3, many of these instruments are poorly developed, with limited validity and reliability. Even with newer, better-developed instruments, it is important for clinicians always to recognize that questionnaires provide statistically based descriptions of behavior, but in and of themselves should not be used to diagnose a disorder. Diagnosis requires not only input from parents regarding the child's everyday functioning and symptoms, but also observation of the child's functioning under the standardized conditions of a structured assessment. Some symptoms are low-base-rate behaviors that may not be apparent during a structured assessment, so parent report is essential. However, parents do not possess the training in typical development, the ability to see subtle signs of dysfunction, and the knowledge of how to diagnose ASD that professionals have. Therefore, both are critical to the diagnostic process, and reliance only on parent-completed checklists may contribute to overdiagnosis.

On the other hand, underdiagnosis is also a significant issue. In essence, any child diagnosed after the age of 3 or 4 represents an initially missed case and is the visible tip of the underdiagnosis iceberg. Studies demonstrate that many children with ASD show signs of their condition by their first birthdays, and almost all by their second birthdays (Wetherby et al., 2004; Yirmiya & Ozonoff, 2007). Early diagnosis is necessary for early intervention, which can have a profound impact on a child's development and outcome, so the field must also work hard to eliminate the problem of underdiagnosis or late diagnosis.

CORE AND COMPREHENSIVE ASSESSMENT BATTERIES

The impairments resulting from ASD are best observed in the natural setting. Ideally, the opportunity to follow a child for days or weeks would be the best way of evaluating and appreciating autistic symptoms and behaviors. However, in clinical practice this is not possible. Instead, a clinician must rely on a combination of structured interactions with the child and reports from parents and other caregivers, who in fact follow the child around. History is one of the clinician's most valuable allies. It is often the case that after completing a careful history, the clinician is well on the way to identifying whether the child may or may not have an ASD. However, it is also critical to include standardized observations of the child by the examiner, as the clinician's trained eye often observes behaviors that parents and other caregivers may not be sensitive to identifying.

In many situations, multiple evaluators (physicians, psychologists, speech pathologists, educators, etc.) will provide input in the assessment process. However, it is important for one individual to act as case coordinator, collecting and organizing the data obtained from different evaluators. This individual then not only integrates the information and explains the implications of the data to parents, but assists in formulating a broad-based treatment plan. This process is particularly important for parents, allowing them the opportunity to ask questions and obtain a complete picture of their child's presentation and needs.

Over the past 100 years, the psychiatric model of assessment formed the framework for the majority of mental health evaluations. Traditionally, psychiatrists do not perform naturalistic observations, nor do they administer standardized tests. Their diagnostic process consists primarily of the collection of data through a careful history. With the development of valid and reliable instruments for the assessment of ASD, and broadening of the types of mental health professionals who see children with ASD, it is now best practice both to collect a detailed history and also to administer standardized direct assessments. Clinicians should set aside sufficient time (typically 90 minutes or more) to obtain a thorough history. As described by Shea and Mesibov in Chapter 5, age-related issues are critical to review. Time should also be directed to obtaining a profile of the child's social behavior, as noted by Gamliel and Yirmiya in Chapter 6; language development, as noted by Paul and Wilson in Chapter 7; intellectual and neuropsychological functioning, as noted by Klinger and colleagues in Chapter 8 and by Corbett and colleagues in Chapter 9; and comorbid medical, developmental, and psychological conditions, as discussed by Deprey and Ozonoff in Chapter 10 and briefly reviewed below.

As discussed in a number of chapters in this volume, children with ASD experience a high rate of comorbid developmental, medical, and psychiatric conditions. The heterogeneity of problems related to ASD necessitates a broad developmental, behavioral, and medical assessment when time allows. A number of instruments are specifically designed to evaluate autistic symptoms and impairments in the clinical setting (e.g., the Autism Rating Scale, Autism Diagnostic Observation Schedule [ADOS], the Childhood Autism Rating Scale, etc.), and these instruments are a critical supplement to a careful history. A comprehensive battery should also include a traditional measure of intelligence when time allows, as well as a measure of neuropsychological processes such as the Cognitive Assessment System (Naglieri & Das, 1997), which uses a Lurian model of brain functions. This model incorporates the assessment of attention, simultaneous, successive, and planning processes, all four of which have been implicated in basic development. Comprehensive batteries should also include measures of motor and perceptual skills, attention, memory, language, and academic achievement; however, these are not always possible, given the time and reimbursement constraints of many assessments. For a more detailed discussion of best practices in constructing assessment batteries for children with ASD, see Ozonoff, Goodlin-Jones, & Solomon (2005).

A number of identifiable medical conditions co-occur with autism at greater than chance levels (for a recent review, see Zafeiriou, Ververi, & Vargiami, 2007). Most commonly, these include fragile X syndrome and tuberous sclerosis. Autistic features are found in many children with fragile X syndrome; one study reported that 47% of participants with this syndrome met autism criteria (Denmark, Feldman, & Holden, 2003). Conversely, however, the fragile X mutation is found at much lower rates in the general population of children with autism, recently estimated at 2% (Zafeiriou et al., 2007). Tuberous sclerosis is found in 1–4% of children with autism (Zafeiriou et al., 2007). Neurological and central nervous system problems are also commonly reported. Up to a third of children with autism develop seizures, although rates tend to be higher in clinic-based studies (Rossi, Posar, & Parmeggiani, 2000) and may be closer to 10–15% in larger community-based samples (Tharp, 2004). Abnormal brain functioning as measured by electroencephalography, neuroimaging, or evoked potentials has consistently been found in a significant percentage of children and adults with autism (for a review, see Pardo & Eberhart, 2007). At a neurostructural level, macrocephaly consistent with brain enlargement is consistently found in 15–20% of children with autism, as well as abnormalities in the cerebellum, amygdala, and several cortical regions (for reviews, see Minshew & Williams, 2007; Pardo & Eberhart, 2007). However, clear patterns of neurological abnormality in autism and other ASD have yet to be identified. Clinicians should be aware of the symptoms and presentation of these associated genetic and medical conditions, and should provide basic screening for these in the course of a thorough evaluation. For in-depth discussions of these conditions, see Goldstein and Reynolds (1999, 2005).

OTHER ISSUES RELATED TO ASSESSMENT

Child Compliance

Although it is traditional to separate children from caregivers for many types of mental health evaluations, this is not recommended for children under the age of 8 being evaluated for ASD. At least one parent should participate as an observer in the evaluation. With young children this participation is invaluable, as children below the age of 5 are typically more comfortable in the presence of their parents, particularly in a novel situation. By involving a parent in the assessment process, the examiner then has a rich resource of parental observations to call upon in understanding the child's behavior within the context of the assessment versus everyday life. Parents should be advised, however, that in general their role in the evaluation room is as observers and secure bases for their children. In most situations, parents want to encourage their children to perform or interact, and may be very uncomfortable watching their children fail items they believe the youngsters are capable of passing. They should be encouraged to observe, but to interact only when asked.

It is not uncommon with young children or those demonstrating resistance to the assessment process to use primary reinforcers. Food reinforcers can be effective in enlisting child compliance. However, it is important for a clinician to recognize that a significant component of assessment is the measurement of a child's intrinsic motivation to meet a new adult and participate spontaneously and actively in the assessment process. Reinforcers can be used as an external means to motivate and shape behavior during the course of the assessment. However, enlisting the child's interest in the assessment process, combined with secondary verbal reinforcement in the form of positive feedback, is a more desirable approach to the assessment process when it is possible.

By its very nature, autism or any other ASD is a condition that impedes and impairs social interaction. A reliable assessment requires the child to participate actively and comply with examiner directions and requests. Many children with ASD struggle against these—not so much because they are oppositional or resistant, but because they lack the bonds of social engagement easily formed between most children and adults. Therefore, it is critical for clinicians to be fully familiar with the procedures they use and prepared with test protocols, materials, and toys at hand at the start of the assessment. Testing sessions must be conducted efficiently and time managed well, so that the child is not left idle and is constantly and meaningfully engaged.

Integration of Data from Different Sources

The risk of overdiagnosing autism or other ASD is minimized when information is collected from multiple sources and a systematic approach to integrating it is utilized. The two biggest challenges facing the clinician in making an ASD diagnosis occur when it is difficult to clearly rule out alternative conditions, and when the data from different sources (e.g., clinician observation vs. parent report) are inconsistent. In such situations, it is often helpful to collect additional information from other informants, such as teachers, or to employ additional high-sensitivity instruments. For example, it has been suggested that using the Socialization domain score from the Vineland Adaptive Behavior Scales, Second Edition, may be helpful when information from different sources is not congruent; the clinician should look for patterns indicative of autism, such as a Socialization standard score far below IQ (Tomanik, Pearson, Loveland, Lane, & Bryant Shaw, 2007). It is critical for clinicians to recognize that neither checklists, symptom counts, nor tests make diagnoses; rather, clinicians make diagnoses. In 1993, John Werry suggested that the term "diagnosis" may be used in different ways by different individuals, but typically implies a process of defining what problems are present so as to allow the application of professional knowledge. Although there are critics of the accuracy of the diagnostic process for autism, it has the highest reliability among the child diagnoses in DSM-IV-TR. Clinicians should keep in mind that the diagnosis of autism or any other ASD, based on the premises and model for the diagnostic nomenclature, must be made first and foremost on clinical symptomatology and historical grounds. As Werry (1993) noted, "it is up to the diagnostician to decide which data are relevant, how to weight them and how to aggregate them into a final judgement" (p. 143).

Several authors have suggested a sequence of questions clinicians must ask themselves as the data are evaluated in the diagnostic process. Schaughency and Rothlind (1991) have suggested four key questions that must be answered, regardless of the diagnosis in question:

1. Does the child meet criteria for one or more DSM conditions?
2. Are there alternative explanations for the symptoms?
3. Are the symptoms developmentally inappropriate?
4. Do the symptoms impair the child's functioning?

Adapting these questions to the differential diagnostic process for ASD, we propose the following steps:

1. Collect information from parents, using a valid and reliable measure, about current concerns and functioning.
2. Use a structured direct assessment measure such as the ADOS to provide opportunities for the display of specific autistic behaviors and to organize observations of the child's strengths and weaknesses.
3. Integrate and apply this information to the DSM criteria.
4. Rule out alternative explanations for the symptoms.

In addition, a clinician should examine whether a child has difficulties or developmentally inappropriate behaviors in any other areas that might indicate a comorbid diagnosis.

It is essential for the clinician to organize, present, and summarize all of the data collected in the process of evaluation. The depth and format of a written report are matters of individual preference. The report should include a summary of the developmental history, analysis of parent and teacher data, presentation and interpretation of available objective data (including an interaction with or observation of the child), a synthesis of the accumulated data in the diagnostic impression, and recommendations. For some clinicians, this results in a report of 2–3 pages; for others, the report can be 10 pages or more. Although longer reports may not be read carefully by other clinicians, for those who do read them the data presented often provide insights into the child's history, his or her functioning, and the process by which the diagnosis was made. Regardless of the length of the report, this document represents the clinician's work product. It is the product used to explain and transmit the clinician's impressions to others. It is this product that will remain as a record of the evaluation and a standard against which to compare the child's future functioning. Increasingly, such reports are used by schools, institutions of higher education, and even federal agencies to make critical decisions in children's lives.

Some clinicians provide lengthy treatment recommendations. These recommendations, due to their specificity, may be unwanted by other professionals or teachers. For example, classroom recommendations that do not fit within a particular teacher's style and classroom structure stand little chance of being implemented. On the other hand, recommendations that are too general will be difficult to implement, particularly if the service providers are not ASD specialists (e.g., classroom recommendations for teachers). A clinician should strive to achieve a balance between generality and specificity, and to make recommendations that are feasible and reasonable to implement and will improve a child's development and behavior. The clinician should communicate to parents and other professionals a willingness to provide more specific assistance if this is requested and if the clinician is given an understanding of the environment in which recommendations will be implemented.

Discussing Assessment Results with Caregivers

It is essential that parents or other caregivers be provided with a copy of the evaluation report. Clinicians must be willing to share with parents the majority of information and impressions they relay to other professionals. In some situations, parents may wish to have certain sensitive information deleted from the evaluation report before granting permission for it to be released to schools or other community agencies. Particularly for lifelong conditions such as ASD, the parents are the only individuals who will be a consistent presence in their children's lives and can maintain continuity in services. Therefore, they often serve as "case managers," and so it is critical to involve them at every step in the diagnostic and treatment planning process.

Latham and Latham (1995) suggest that when evaluations are used for legal purposes, such as to advocate for services under the Individuals with Disabilities Education Act or the Americans with Disabilities Act, written reports should clearly state that diagnoses are based on history, interview, testing, and clinical observations. A written report should also state whether an impairment substantially limits one or more of an individual's major life activities. Documentation should be supported by citations to an authoritative source (either the DSM-IV-TR or the *International Classification of Diseases*, 10th revision). It is important for clinicians to recognize that a document designed to provide legal support for a diagnosis differs from a document designed to provide structure for an intervention program.

Making the diagnosis of autism or another ASD, when appropriate, is a crucial part of the evaluation. However, helping parents understand the specific problems their child is experiencing and the implications of the diagnosis is even more important. This provides a critical link between diagnosis and intervention. As discussed by Hogan and Marcus in Chapter 11, helping parents view the world through the eyes of their child and understand the reasons for and causes of the child's difficulties facilitates the process of starting treatment. An appreciation of the child's problems allows parents to play an active role and helps them make appropriate decisions for their child. Unless parents are helped to be active participants, even the best diagnoses may not yield compliance with recommendations for treatment.

Because an ASD is a lifelong disorder and must be managed throughout the child's life, it is important to reiterate that parents must first understand the disorder. A clinician must spend sufficient time with a child's parents summarizing and explaining the data, highlighting consistencies and inconsistencies within the data, defining the means by which the diagnosis was made, identifying the behavioral characteristics of the diagnosis, and explaining the rationale for treatment. We also recommend that the clinician focus on what is *right* with the child. That is, he or she should spend a reasonable amount of time discussing the child's assets. Parents must be helped to recognize that they can be the most powerful protectors for their child when they are knowledgeable about the child's disorder, develop a warm relationship with their child, are available, take an interest in the child's education and development, make efforts to bolster the child's self-worth, and meet the child's physical needs. A parent's ability to view the world through the eyes of a child exerts a significant impact on their daily interactions.

We find it helpful to explain test data to parents by placing the child in specific situations and explaining how the child's weaknesses compromise his or her ability to function in and meet the demands of that setting. "A day in the life of your child" is often a helpful way of explaining this to parents. For illustrative purposes, a hypothetical description of 8-year-old Allen is presented below, as it might be given in a report and shared with parents:

> The assessment data have revealed that since early childhood Allen has consistently demonstrated problems with social interaction, communication, and atypical patterns of behavior. Allen was difficult to comfort as an infant. He did not appear to enjoy being held. He struggled to make eye contact and appeared uncomfortable in the hands of caregivers. At 2 years of age, he was still not speaking, nor did he appear very interested in social interaction. He would play with toys in a repetitive manner, more as objects with no particular purpose. He did not appear to enjoy playing peek-a-boo or bouncing on caretakers' knees. He did not point to have his needs met and wouldn't point on direction. By 3 years of age he began speaking; however, his speech was somewhat atypical in pitch, tone, and rhythm. He also began exhibiting an atypical pattern of behavior, including a variety of self-stimulatory activities. An evaluation at 4 years of age indicated normal nonverbal intelligence, but delays in language and social interaction. Nonetheless, at age 5, it was thought that Allen's problems might be the result of mental retardation and/or ADHD. Trials of a number of medications met with limited success.
>
> The assessment data collected indicate that Allen continues to demonstrate problems with social interaction. He does not have a best friend. He still plays with other children in parallel. He does not appear to understand social behavior. Testing reveals normal intelligence, but problems with selective and sustained attention as well as with motor and perceptual skills. Basic academic abilities appear near grade level, despite Allen's inconsistent school performance. Allen also continues to demonstrate a number of idiosyncratic behaviors, including repetitively twirling a piece of rope at times for up to an hour. He is isolated at recess, often walking along the fence at school. Though Allen is very pleasant and can be engaged, his behavior is extremely limited and socially isolated when he is left to his own devices.

Such a description not only helps parents understand the extent and nature of their child's problems, but ties these problems to specific situations, which then allows the clinician to describe a model for intervention and specific strategies that may lead to improvements.

Symptoms versus Daily Functional Impairment

Finally, it is important for clinicians to recognize the increasing focus upon impairment in making psychiatric diagnoses. Symptom presentation and severity, though generally predictive of impairment, are not specifically predictive of type or level of impairment. Children with ASD demonstrate a very wide range of impairments in social, academic, and behavioral areas. Despite the fact that all of these children meet DSM-IV-TR criteria for these diagnoses, the range of impairments can vary so much as to lead clinicians to question specific diagnoses. Preliminary work on the DSM-V, scheduled for publication in 2011, is focusing on impairment as a critical component in making these diagnoses. It is likely that the future diagnosis of autism and other ASD will also include very specific impairment criteria.

CONCLUSION

A recent online Google search for "autism" revealed 2.5 million pages devoted to this topic. A further search for "assessment of autism" yielded over 600,000 pages. From online blogs to scientific meetings, the definition, causes, diagnosis, and treatments of ASD have become front-page, often controversial news. Within the hailstorm of media coverage, pseudoscientific theory, and practices based on belief rather than science, clinicians have been left to negotiate and interpret the maze of knowledge related to ASD. It is our intent that this volume provide a reasoned and reasonable guide for the assessment of ASD. A diverse, current literature of many promising practices may change the manner in which ASD are identified, evaluated, and ultimately diagnosed. In the immediate future, however, the diagnostic criteria for and the assessment of ASD are dependent on measurable, observable patterns of behavior within defined contexts.

REFERENCES

American Psychiatric Association. (2000). *Diagnostic and statistical manual of mental disorders* (4th ed., text rev.). Washington, DC: Author.

Croen, L., & Grether, K. G. (2003). Response: A response to Blixill, Baskin, and Spitzer on Croen et al. (2002). The changing prevalence of autism in California. *Journal of Autism and Developmental Disorders, 32,* 227–230.

Denmark, J. L., Feldman, M. A., & Holden, J. J. A. (2003). Behavioral relationship between autism and fragile X syndrome. *American Journal on Mental Retardation, 108*(5), 314–326.

Gernsbacher, M. A., Geye, H. M., & Weismer, S. E. (2005). The role of language and communication impairments within autism. In P. Fletcher & J. F. Miller (Eds.), *Language disorders and developmental theory* (pp. 73–93). Philadelphia: John Benjamins.

Goldstein, S., & Reynolds, C. R. (Eds.). (1999). *Handbook of neurodevelopmental and genetic disorders in children.* New York: Guilford Press.

Goldstein, S., & Reynolds, C. R. (Eds.). (2005). *Handbook of neurodevelopmental and genetic disorders in adults.* New York: Guilford Press.

Joseph, R. M., & Tager-Flusberg, H. (2004). The relationship of theory of mind and executive functions to symptom type and severity in children with autism. *Development and Psychopathology, 16,* 137–155.

Karatekin, C. (2007). Eye tracking studies of normative and atypical development. *Developmental Review, 27,* 283–348.

Klin, A., Jones, W., Schultz, R., Volkmar, F., & Cohen, D. (2002a). Defining and quantifying the social phenotype in autism. *American Journal of Psychiatry, 159,* 895–908.

Klin, A., Jones, W., Schultz, R., Volkmar, F., & Cohen, D. (2002b). Visual fixation patterns during viewing of naturalistic social situations as predictors of social competence in individuals with autism. *Archives of General Psychiatry, 59,* 809–816.

Latham, P. H., & Latham, P. S. (1995). *Documentation disclosure and the law for individuals with learning disabilities and attention deficit disorder.* Cabin John, MD: National Center for Law and Learning Disabilities.

Mendozzi, L., Motta, A., Barbieri, E., Alpini, D., & Pugnetti, L. (1998). The application of virtual reality to document coping deficits after a stroke: Report of a case. *Cyberpsychology and Behavior, 1,* 79–91.

Minshew, N. J., & Williams, D. L. (2007). The new neurobiology of autism: Cortex, connectivity, and neuronal organization. *Archives of Neurology, 64,* 945–950.

Naglieri, J. A., & Das, J. P. (1997). *Cognitive Assessment System.* Itasca, IL: Riverside.

Nordin, V., & Gillberg, C. (1998). The long-term course of autistic disorders: Update on follow-up studies. *Acta Psychiatrica Scandinavica, 97,* 99–108.

Ozonoff, S., Goodlin-Jones, B. L., & Solomon, M. (2005). Evidence-based assessment of autism spectrum disorders in children and adolescents. *Journal of Clinical Child and Adolescent Psychology, 34,* 523–540.

Pardo, C. A., & Eberhart, C. G. (2007). The neurobiology of autism. *Brain Pathology, 17,* 434–447.

Parsons, S., Beardon, L., Neale, H. R., Reynard, G., Eastgate, R., Wilson, J. R., et al. (2000). *Development of social skills amongst adults with Asperger's syndrome using virtual environments: The AS Interactive Project.* Paper presented at the 3rd International Conference on Disability, Virtual Reality, and Associated Technologies, Alghero, Italy.

Rayner, K. (1998). Eye movements in reading and information processing: 20 years of research. *Psychological Bulletin, 124,* 372–422.

Rizzo, A., Buckwalter, J. G., van der Zaag, C., Neumann, U., Thiebaux, M., Chua,

C., et al. (2000). *Virtual environment applications in clinical neuropsychology*. Paper presented at the IEEE Virtual Reality Conference, New Brunswick, NJ.

Rizzo, A., Wiederhold, M., & Buckwalter, J. G. (1998). Basic issues in the use of virtual environments for mental health applications. In G. Riva, B. K. Weiderhold, & E. Molinari (Eds.), *Virtual environments in clinical psychology and neuroscience* (pp. 21–42). Amsterdam: Ios Press.

Rossi, P. G., Posar, A., & Parmeggiani, A. (2000). Epilepsy in adolescents and young adults with autistic disorder. *Brain and Development, 22,* 102–106.

Schaughency, E. A., & Rothlind, J. (1991). Assessment and classification of attention deficit hyperactivity disorders. *School Psychology Review, 20,* 187–202.

Schilbach, L., Helmert, J. R., Mojzisch, A., Pannasch, S., Velichkovsky, B. M., & Vogeley, K. (2005, July). *Neural correlates, visual attention, and facial expression during social interaction with others*. Paper presented at the meeting of the Cognitive Science Society, Stresa, Italy.

Speer, L. L., Cook, A. E., Clark, E., & McMahon, W. M. (2007). Face processing in children with autism: Effects of stimulus contents and type. *Autism, 11,* 265–277.

Tager-Flusberg, H. (2004). Strategies for conducting research on language in autism. *Journal of Autism and Developmental Disorders, 34,* 75–80.

Tharp, B. R. (2004). Epileptic encephalopathies and their relationship to developmental disorders: Do spikes cause autism? *Mental Retardation and Developmental Disabilities Research Reviews, 10,* 132–134.

Tomanik, S. S., Pearson, D. A., Loveland, K. A., Lane, D. M., & Bryant Shaw, J. (2007). Improving the reliability of autism diagnoses: Examining the utility of adaptive behavior. *Journal of Autism and Developmental Disorders, 37,* 921–928.

Trepagnier, C. G. (1999). Virtual environments for the investigation and rehabilitation of cognitive and perceptual impairments. *NeuroRehabilitation, 12,* 63–72.

Werry, I., Dautenhahn, K., Ogden, B., & Harwin, W. (2000). Can social interaction skills be taught by a social agent?: The role of a robotic mediator in autism therapy. In M. Beynon, C. L. Nehaniv, & K. Dautenhahn (Eds.), *Cognitive technology: Instruments of mind* (4th International Conference, CT 2001, Coventry, UK, August 6–9, 2001, pp. 57–74). Berlin: Springer-Verlag.

Werry, J. S. (1993). Diagnosis. Chapter 7. In J. L. Matson (Ed.), *Handbook of hyperactivity in children* (pp. 137–149). Needham Heights, MA: Allyn & Bacon.

Wetherby, A. M., Woods, J., Allen, L., Cleary, J., Dickinson, H., & Lord, C. (2004). Early indicators of autism spectrum disorders in the second year of life. *Journal of Autism and Developmental Disorders, 34*(5), 473–493.

Wing, L. (1989). Diagnosis of autism. In C. Gillberg (Ed.), *Diagnosis and treatment of autism*. New York: Plenum Press.

Yirmiya, N., & Ozonoff, S. (2007). The very early phenotype of autism. *Journal of Autism and Developmental Disorders, 37,* 1–11.

Zafeiriou, D. I., Ververi, A., & Vargiami, E. (2007). Childhood autism and associated comorbidities. *Brain and Development, 29,* 257–272.

Index

Page numbers followed by an *f* or a *t* indicate figures or tables.

373